T0358928

Vitamin D

Editors

J. CHRISTOPHER GALLAGHER
DANIEL D. BIKLE

ENDOCRINOLOGY AND METABOLISM CLINICS OF NORTH AMERICA

www.endo.theclinics.com

Consulting Editors
ANAT BEN-SHLOMO
MARIA FLESERIU

December 2017 • Volume 46 • Number 4

ELSEVIER

1600 John F. Kennedy Boulevard • Suite 1800 • Philadelphia, Pennsylvania, 19103-2899

http://www.theclinics.com

ENDOCRINOLOGY AND METABOLISM CLINICS OF NORTH AMERICA Volume 46, Number 4
December 2017 ISSN 0889-8529, ISBN 13: 978-0-323-55274-5

Editor: Stacy Eastman
Developmental Editor: Meredith Madeira

Endocrinology and Metabolism Clinics of North America (ISSN 0889-8529) is published quarterly by Elsevier Inc., 360 Park Avenue South, New York, NY 10010-1710. Months of issue are March, June, September, and December. Periodicals postage paid at New York, NY and additional mailing offices. Subscription prices are USD 337.00 per year for US individuals, USD 674.00 per year for US institutions, USD 100.00 per year for US students and residents, USD 423.00 per year for Canadian individuals, USD 834.00 per year for Canadian institutions, USD 490.00 per year for international individuals, USD 834.00 per year for international institutions, and USD 245.00 per year for international and Canadian and foreign students/residents. To receive student/resident rate, orders must be accompanied by name of affiliated institution, date of term, and the signature of program/ residency coordinator on institution letterhead. Orders will be billed at individual rate until proof of status is received. Foreign air speed delivery is included in all *Clinics* subscription prices. All prices are subject to change without notice. **POSTMASTER:** Send address changes to *Endocrinology and Metabolism Clinics of North America*, Elsevier Health Sciences Division, Subscription Customer Service, 3251 Riverport Lane, Maryland Heights, MO 63043. **Customer Service: Telephone: 1-800-654-2452** (U.S. and Canada); **1-314-447-8871** (outside U.S. and Canada). **Fax: 1-314-447-8029. E-mail: journalscustomerservice-usa@elsevier.com (for print support); journalsonlinesupport-usa@elsevier.com (for online support).**

Reprints. For copies of 100 or more, of articles in this publication, please contact the Commercial Rights Department, Elsevier Inc., 360 Park Avenue South, New York, NY 10010-1710; phone: +1-212-633-3874; fax: +1-212-633-3820; E-mail: reprints@elsevier.com.

Endocrinology and Metabolism Clinics of North America is covered in *MEDLINE/PubMed (Index Medicus), EMBASE/Excerpta Medica, Current Contents/Clinical Medicine, Current Contents/Life Sciences, Science Citation Index, ISI/BIOMED, BIOSIS,* and *Chemical Abstracts.*

Contributors

CONSULTING EDITORS

ANAT BEN-SHLOMO, MD
Pituitary Center, Division of Endocrinology, Diabetes and Metabolism, Cedars-Sinai Medical Center, Los Angeles, California, USA

MARIA FLESERIU, MD, FACE
Northwest Pituitary Center, Departments of Medicine and Neurological Surgery, Oregon Health & Science University, Portland, Oregon, USA

EDITORS

J. CHRISTOPHER GALLAGHER, MD
Professor of Medicine and Endocrinology, Director Bone Metabolism Unit, Creighton University School of Medicine, Omaha, Nebraska, USA

DANIEL D. BIKLE, MD, PhD
Professor of Medicine and Dermatology, Department of Medicine, University of California San Francisco, Co-Director SDTU, San Francisco VA Medical Center, San Francisco, California, USA

AUTHORS

DEVENDRA K. AGRAWAL, PhD (Biochem), PhD (Med Sciences), MBA, MS (ITM), FAAAAI, FAHA, FAPS, FIACS
Professor and Chairman, Department of Clinical and Translational Science, The Peekie Nash Carpenter Endowed Chair in Medicine, Creighton University School of Medicine, Omaha, Nebraska, USA

JOHN F. ALOIA, MD
Professor of Medicine, Chief Academic Officer, Dean Winthrop Clinical Campus, Stony Brook School of Medicine, Bone Mineral Research Center, NYU Winthrop Hospital, Mineola, New York, USA

DANIEL D. BIKLE, MD, PhD
Professor of Medicine and Dermatology, Department of Medicine, University of California San Francisco, Co-Director SDTU, San Francisco VA Medical Center, San Francisco, California, USA

NEIL BINKLEY, MD
University of Wisconsin Osteoporosis Clinical Research Program, University of Wisconsin–Madison, Madison, Wisconsin, USA

ROGER BOUILLON, MD, PhD, FRCP
Clinical and Experimental Endocrinology, KU Leuven, Leuven, Belgium

MORAY J. CAMPBELL, MS, PhD
Division of Pharmaceutics and Pharmaceutical Chemistry, The Ohio State University
College of Pharmacy, Columbus, Ohio, USA

GRAHAM D. CARTER, MSc
Vitamin D External Quality Assessment Scheme (DEQAS), Imperial College Healthcare
NHS Trust, Charing Cross Hospital, London, United Kingdom

MARLENE CHAKHTOURA, MD, MSc
Department of Internal Medicine, Division of Endocrinology, Calcium Metabolism and
Osteoporosis Program, WHO Collaborating Center for Metabolic Bone Disorders,
American University of Beirut Medical Center, Beirut, Lebanon

SYLVIA CHRISTAKOS, PhD
Department of Microbiology, Biochemistry and Molecular Genetics, Rutgers, The State
University of New Jersey, Rutgers New Jersey Medical School, Newark, New Jersey, USA

RUBAN DHALIWAL, MD, MPH
Assistant Professor of Medicine, Endocrinology, Diabetes and Metabolism, Director,
Metabolic Bone Disease Center, State University of New York Upstate Medical University
Syracuse, New York, USA

GHADA EL-HAJJ FULEIHAN, MD, MPH
Department of Internal Medicine, Division of Endocrinology, Calcium Metabolism and
Osteoporosis Program, WHO Collaborating Center for Metabolic Bone Disorders,
American University of Beirut Medical Center, Beirut, Lebanon

J. CHRISTOPHER GALLAGHER, MD
Professor of Medicine and Endocrinology, Director Bone Metabolism Unit, Creighton
University School of Medicine, Omaha, Nebraska, USA

CONNY GYSEMANS, PhD
Senior Post-doc, Laboratory of Clinical and Experimental Endocrinology (CEE), KU
Leuven, Leuven, Belgium

GLENVILLE JONES, PhD
Department of Biomedical and Molecular Sciences, Queen's University, Kingston,
Ontario, Canada

MARIE LAURE KOTTLER, MD, PhD
Department of Genetics, University de Basse-Normandie, National Reference Center for
Rare Diseases of Calcium and Phosphorus Metabolism, Caen University Hospital, Caen,
France

RAJIV KUMAR, MD
Division of Nephrology and Hypertension, Departments of Medicine and Biochemistry
and Molecular Biology, Mayo Clinic, Rochester, Minnesota, USA

PAUL LIPS, MD, PhD
Department of Internal Medicine, Endocrine Section, VU University Medical Center,
Amsterdam, The Netherlands

SOFIE MALMSTROEM, MD
University of California San Francisco, San Francisco, California, USA; Lundbeck
Foundation Clinical Research Fellowship Candidate, Department of Endocrinology and
Internal Medicine, Aarhus University Hospital, Aarhus, Denmark

CHANTAL MATHIEU, MD, PhD
Full Professor of Medicine, Laboratory of Clinical and Experimental Endocrinology (CEE), KU Leuven, Leuven, Belgium

J. WESLEY PIKE, PhD
Department of Biochemistry, University of Wisconsin–Madison, Madison, Wisconsin, USA

MAYA RAHME, MSc
Department of Internal Medicine, Division of Endocrinology, Calcium Metabolism and Osteoporosis Program, WHO Collaborating Center for Metabolic Bone Disorders, American University of Beirut Medical Center, Beirut, Lebanon

VIKRANT RAI, MBBS, MS
Department of Clinical and Translational Science, Creighton University School of Medicine, Omaha, Nebraska, USA

IAN R. REID, MD, FRACP
Distinguished Professor, Department of Medicine, Faculty of Medical and Health Sciences, The University of Auckland, Department of Endocrinology, Auckland District Health Board, Auckland, New Zealand

KARL PETER SCHLINGMANN, MD
Department of General Pediatrics, University Children's Hospital, Muenster, Germany

JANICE SCHWARTZ, MD
Professor of Medicine, University of California San Francisco, San Francisco, California, USA

LYNETTE M. SMITH, PhD
Associate Professor, Department of Biostatistics, University of Nebraska Medical Center, Omaha, Nebraska, USA

DONALD L. TRUMP, MD
CEO and Executive Director, Inova Schar Cancer Institute, Professor, Department of Medicine, Virginia Commonwealth University, Fairfax, Virginia, USA

NATASJA VAN SCHOOR, PhD
Department of Epidemiology and Biostatistics, Amsterdam Public Health Research Institute, VU University Medical Center, Amsterdam, The Netherlands

AN-SOFIE VANHERWEGEN, MSc
PhD Student, Laboratory of Clinical and Experimental Endocrinology (CEE), KU Leuven, Leuven, Belgium

LADAN ZAND, MD
Division of Nephrology and Hypertension, Department of Medicine, Mayo Clinic, Rochester, Minnesota, USA

Contents

The central role of hormonal 1,25-dihydroxyvitamin D_3 [1,25(OH)$_2$D$_3$] is to regulate calcium and phosphorus homeostasis via actions in intestine, kidney, and bone. These and other actions in many cell types not involved in mineral metabolism are mediated by the vitamin D receptor. Recent studies using genome-wide scale techniques have extended fundamental ideas regarding vitamin D–mediated control of gene expression while simultaneously revealing a series of new concepts. This article summarizes the current view of the biological actions of the vitamin D hormone and focuses on new concepts that drive the understanding of the mechanisms through which vitamin D operates.

Vitamin D deficiency occurs all over the world, mainly in the Middle East, China, Mongolia, and India. This article focuses on the vitamin D status in adults. Risk groups include older persons, pregnant women, and non-Western immigrants. Adequate vitamin D status, defined as serum 25-hydroxyvitamin D greater than 50 nmol/L, is present in less than 50% of the world population, at least in winter. Preventative strategies, such as increasing fish consumption, fortification of foods, use of vitamin D supplements, and advice for moderate sunlight exposure, are warranted.

Vitamin D insufficiency and deficiency can be diagnosed with measurements of serum 25-hydroxyvitamin D (25OHD). Most vitamin D is derived from sunlight (80%), so serum 25OHD levels are lowest in late winter and early spring. Dietary vitamin D in North America is small, about 100 to 200 IU daily. A recent review of the literature shows many association studies relating vitamin D deficiency and insufficiency to several diseases. Large randomized trials of vitamin D are underway and soon there may be answers as to whether vitamin D is clinically effective and what level of serum 25OHD is necessary.

Widespread variation in 25-hydroxyvitamin D (25(OH)D) assays continues to compromise efforts to develop clinical and public health guidelines regarding vitamin D status. The Vitamin D Standardization Program helps alleviate this problem. Reference measurement procedures and standard reference materials have been developed to allow current, prospective, and retrospective standardization of 25(OH)D results. Despite advances in 25(OH)D measurement, substantial variability in clinical laboratory 25(OH)D measurement persists. Existing guidelines have not used standardized data and, as a result, it seems unlikely that consensus regarding definitions of vitamin D deficiency, inadequacy, sufficiency, and excess will soon be reached. Until evidence-based consensus is reached, a reasonable clinical approach is advocated.

The free hormone hypothesis postulates that only the nonbound fraction (the free fraction) of hormones that otherwise circulate in blood bound to their carrier proteins is able to enter cells and exert their biologic effects. For the vitamin D metabolites less than 1% (0.4% for 1,25(OH) $_2$D and 0.03% for 25(OH)D) is free, with more than 99% bound to the vitamin D–binding protein (DBP) and albumin (approximately 85% and 15%, respectively). Assays to measure the free vitamin D metabolite levels have been developed, and initial studies indicated their value in subjects with altered DBP levels.

Recent understanding has highlighted the importance of extraskeletal role of vitamin D. Despite numerous observational and interventional studies over the last two decades, the apparent divergent clinical findings have intensified the controversy regarding this role of vitamin D in older adults. This article reviews the existing literature and summarizes the current knowledge of vitamin D status and vitamin D supplementation on falls and physical performance, describes the putative mechanisms underlying this association, and reflects on the controversy surrounding vitamin D recommendations in older adults.

One hundred years ago, vitamin D was identified as the cause and cure of osteomalacia. This role remains firmly established. Vitamin D influences skeletal mineralization principally through the regulation of intestinal calcium absorption. It has been proposed that vitamin D has direct beneficial effects on bone (besides the prevention of osteomalacia), but these have been difficult to establish in clinical trials. Meta-analyses of vitamin D trials show no effects on bone density or fracture risk when the baseline 25-hydroxyvitamin D is greater than 40 nmol/L. A daily dose of 400 to 800 IU vitamin D_3 is usually adequate to correct such deficiency.

ENDOCRINOLOGY AND METABOLISM CLINICS OF NORTH AMERICA

ISSUE OF RELATED INTEREST

Medical Clinics of North America, January 2015 (Vol. 99, Issue 1)
Diabetes Management
Irl B. Hirsch, *Editor*

VISIT THE CLINICS ONLINE!
Access your subscription at:
www.theclinics.com

ENDOCRINOLOGY AND METABOLISM CLINICS OF NORTH AMERICA

Foreword

Vitamin D Hormone: Where Do We Stand, Where Are We Heading?

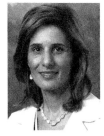 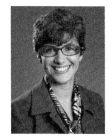

Anat Ben-Shlomo, MD   Maria Fleseriu, MD, FACE
Consulting Editors

J. Christopher Gallagher, MD, a professor of medicine and endocrinology at the Creighton University and Daniel D. Bikle, MD, PhD, a professor of medicine and dermatology at the University of California, San Francisco, both nationally and internationally recognized experts in the vitamin D field, have assembled an excellent team of vitamin D experts around the world to provide our readers with the most updated, state-of-the-art *Endocrinology and Metabolism Clinics of North America* issue on Vitamin D. This issue provides a comprehensive overview on vitamin D physiology and pathophysiology in the skeletal tissue and beyond. It assesses our current knowledge, controversies, and future needs in the global efforts to define low vitamin D levels and determine the best ways to treat it to improve clinical outcomes.

In "Biology and Mechanisms of Action of the Vitamin D Hormone," Drs Pike and Christakos provide a detailed overview on vitamin D synthesis, metabolism, and mechanism of action. They discuss its active metabolites and nuclear vitamin D receptor and consider its activity in regulating calcium and phosphorus homeostasis as well as immune, cardiovascular, skin, and muscle function and cellular growth control.

In "Global Overview of Vitamin D Status," Drs van Schoor and Lips discuss vitamin D levels, deficiency, and treatment requirements in different geographic regions across the globe.

The article, "Dietary Vitamin D Intake for the Elderly Population: Update on the Recommended Dietary Allowance for Vitamin D," by Drs Smith and Gallagher reviews who should be screened for vitamin D deficiency, levels of vitamin D that are considered deficient, insufficient, or sufficient, appropriate dosing to treat the vitamin D– deficient adult and elderly patients, and the metrics used to determine these values.

Endocrinol Metab Clin N Am 46 (2017) xiii–xv
https://doi.org/10.1016/j.ecl.2017.09.002
0889-8529/17/© 2017 Published by Elsevier Inc.

endo.theclinics.com

In their article, "Toward Clarity in Clinical Vitamin D Status Assessment: 25(OH)D Assay Standardization," Drs Binkley and Carter discuss the need for standardization of vitamin D assays and reference ranges in order to properly determine vitamin D status and provide guidelines for treatment. Their discussion summarizes the status of the Vitamin D Standardization Program established in 2010 to develop approaches for standardization of current and prior 25(OH)D data.

In "Current Controversies: Are Free Vitamin Metabolite Levels a More Accurate Assessment of Vitamin D Status than Total Levels?," Drs Bikle, Malmstroem, and Schwartz discuss the rationale for measuring circulating unbound free vitamin D metabolites to more accurately predict vitamin D deficiency status, especially in patients with low vitamin D binding protein and albumin levels.

In their article, "Effect of Vitamin D on Falls and Physical Performance," Drs Dhaliwal and Aloia summarize how vitamin D deficiency and its management affect physical performance, describing potential underlying mechanisms contributing to instability and falls, and discussing the controversy surrounding vitamin D supplement recommendations in the elderly.

Dr Reid discusses the clinical relevance of vitamin D deficiency to bone mineral density and fracture rates in "Vitamin D Effect on Bone Mineral Density and Fractures." The bone effects of vitamin D supplementation with or without calcium are reviewed, and the need for optimizing circulating vitamin D levels is highlighted.

The common occurrence of vitamin D deficiency in obese patients, exacerbated by surgical procedures, including Roux-en-Y gastric bypass and sleeve gastrectomy, is discussed by Drs Chakhtoura, Rahme, and El-Hajj Fuleihan in the article, "Vitamin D Metabolism in Bariatric Surgery." Guidelines for monitoring and replacing vitamin D in these patients are presented.

Pathophysiology and treatment of vitamin D deficiency in patients with chronic kidney disease/end-stage renal failure associated with bone mineral disorders, including secondary hyperparathyroidism and mixed-uremic osteodystrophy, are reviewed by Drs Zand and Kumar in "The Use of Vitamin D Metabolites and Analogues in the Treatment of Chronic Kidney Disease."

In "Vitamin D Receptor Signaling and Cancer," Drs Campbell and Trump review potential mechanisms by which vitamin D and its receptor may regulate cancer growth and treatment resistance as well as the anticancer actions of vitamin D compounds.

In "Role of Vitamin D in Cardiovascular Diseases," Drs Rai and Agrawal explore the association between vitamin D deficiency and cardiovascular disease and consider whether vitamin D supplementation might be beneficial to prevent the disease. As vitamin D deficiency is associated with inflammation and metabolic syndrome, it could represent an important additional risk factor for cardiovascular disease.

Drs Vanherwegen, Gysemans, and Mathieu examine the association between vitamin D deficiency and immune system disorders in "Regulation of Immune Function by Vitamin D and Its Use in Diseases of Immunity." Cellular mechanisms involving vitamin D in immune cells are reviewed, with an emphasis on the effects of vitamin D and its active metabolite on autoimmune diseases, such as diabetes mellitus type 1, systemic lupus erythematosus, and rheumatoid arthritis, as well as chronic bacterial and viral infections.

In "Genetic Diseases of Vitamin D Metabolizing Enzymes," Drs Jones, Kottler, and Schlingmann review key activating and inactivating mutations in cytochrome P450–containing enzymes involved in vitamin D metabolism. They discuss associations between these mutations and vitamin D–dependency rickets and idiopathic infantile hypercalcemia and summarize their symptoms, diagnosis, treatment, and management.

The issue concludes with "Genetic and Racial Differences in the Vitamin D Endocrine System," an article by Dr Bouillon that considers environmental factors, including diet, geographic location, UV-B exposure, and skin color, that determine vitamin D accessibility, as well as genetic factors, such as availability of proteins involved in vitamin D processing and binding, that determine vitamin D metabolism.

We hope you will find this issue on Vitamin D in *Endocrinology and Metabolism Clinics of North America* useful in your daily practice. We thank our guest editors, Dr Gallagher and Dr Bikle, and the authors for this exciting and timely issue and the Elsevier editorial staff for their invaluable help.

Anat Ben-Shlomo, MD
Pituitary Center
Division of Endocrinology Diabetes
& Metabolism
Cedars Sinai Medical Center
8700 Beverly Boulevard
Los Angeles, CA 90048, USA

Maria Fleseriu, MD, FACE
Northwest Pituitary Center
Departments of Medicine and
Neurological Surgery
Oregon Health & Science University
3303 SW Bond Avenue
Portland, OR 97239, USA

E-mail addresses:
benshlomoa@cshs.org (A. Ben-Shlomo)
fleseriu@ohsu.edu (M. Fleseriu)

Preface

Vitamin D: Mechanisms of Action and Clinical Applications

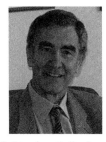 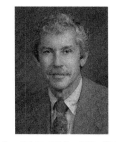

J. Christopher Gallagher, MD   Daniel D. Bikle, MD, PhD
Editors

The vitamin D receptor, through which vitamin D (via its active hormonal form 1,25(OH) 2D) exerts its effects, is found in nearly every tissue in the body. This suggests that vitamin D is likely to play a much greater role in regulating physiologic processes than just that of calcium and phosphate homeostasis. Vitamin D, produced in the skin or absorbed from the diet, must be further metabolized first to its major circulating form, 25(OH)D, and then to its hormonally active form, 1,25(OH)2D. Although the skin is the major source of vitamin D, the liver the major source of 25(OH)D, and the kidney the major source of 1,25(OH)2D, many tissues express the enzymatic machinery (CYP2R1 and CYP27A1 for 25(OH)D production, CYP27B1 for 1,25(OH)2D production) that can metabolize vitamin D to its active forms. Moreover, nearly all tissues also express the enzyme, CYP24A1, that catabolizes both 25(OH)D and 1,25(OH)2D to inactive products. Mutations in these enzymes have profound pathologic effects. These enzymatic mutations are rare, but deficiency of vitamin D is widespread. Given the wide range of tissues and physiologic processes affected by vitamin D, vitamin D deficiency likewise has profound pathologic effects.

Clinical assessment of vitamin D status is generally performed by measurement of serum 25(OH)D. However, this assessment is complicated by the uncertainty about the optimal level of 25(OH)D for vitamin D sufficiency, and whether that level applies to all functions of this hormone. Moreover, vitamin D metabolites are transported in blood bound to the vitamin D binding protein and albumin, which restricts access of the vitamin D metabolites to most cells. The levels of these proteins vary in different pathologic and physiologic conditions, raising the question whether a more accurate assessment of vitamin D nutritional status is the nonbound or free level to which most cells have access.

In this publication, the different articles deal with these aspects of vitamin D, examining its molecular mechanisms of action, metabolism, and impact on various

Endocrinol Metab Clin N Am 46 (2017) xvii–xviii
https://doi.org/10.1016/j.ecl.2017.09.001
0889-8529/17/© 2017 Published by Elsevier Inc.

endo.theclinics.com

physiologic processes with the overall goal of translating what we know into clinical applications.

There is controversy about the clinical effects of vitamin D on various diseases, and the authors have presented a balanced view of the available data. The number of clinical trials where these conditions were primary outcomes is limited by small numbers and relies mainly on meta-analyses. There are several major worldwide trials now underway on different vitamin D doses involving about 100,000 subjects that may produce definitive data on multiple outcomes in the next 5 years and change today's recommendations.

J. Christopher Gallagher, MD
Creighton University Medical Center
2400 Burt Street
Criss 111, Suite 280
Omaha, NE 68131, USA

Daniel D. Bikle, MD, PhD
Department of Medicine
University of California San Francisco
San Francisco VA Medical Center
1700 Clement Street, Room 373
San Francisco, CA 94158, USA

E-mail addresses:
jcg@creighton.edu (J.C. Gallagher)
Daniel.Bikle@ucsf.edu (D.D. Bikle)

Biology and Mechanisms of Action of the Vitamin D Hormone

 CrossMark

J. Wesley Pike, PhD[a],*, Sylvia Christakos, PhD[b]

KEYWORDS

- Mineral homeostasis • Calcemic hormones • Transcription • Target genes • RANKL
- Transient receptor potential vanilloid type-6 (*TRPV6*) • Genome-wide principles
- Genetic linkage

KEY POINTS

- The vitamin D hormone functions to regulate calcium and phosphorus metabolism in higher vertebrates and to control a multitude of additional biological activities linked to the immune and cardiovascular systems, skin and muscle function, cellular growth control, and numerous additional biological processes.
- Virtually all the biological activities of the vitamin D hormone are mediated by the vitamin D receptor, a nuclear receptor protein that functions to control the expression of genes and gene networks in a cell type–selective manner.
- Recent unbiased genome-wide approaches have revealed a series of additional principles through which the vitamin D receptor acts and have provided new insight into vitamin D hormone action.
- Mechanistic studies of specific genes, including vitamin D targets such as *Cyp24a1*, *Spp1*, *IL-17*, *Tnfsf11*, and *Mmp13* have yielded novel genetic and epigenetic templates for understanding the additional complexity associated with vitamin D action.

INTRODUCTION/HISTORICAL PERSPECTIVE

Discovered many decades earlier by Mellanby,[1] McCollum and colleagues,[2] Steenbock,[3] and Windaus and colleagues,[4] vitamin D is now known through ensuing research efforts by many investigators to be converted to 1,25-dihydroxyvitamin D_3 [1,25(OH)$_2$D$_3$], its biologically active form, and to be centrally involved in the regulation of calcium and phosphorus homeostasis in higher vertebrates.[5] The vitamin's

Disclosure: The authors have nothing to disclose.
[a] Department of Biochemistry, University of Wisconsin-Madison, Biochem Addition, Room 543D, 433 Babcock Drive, Madison, WI 53706, USA; [b] Department of Microbiology, Biochemistry and Molecular Genetics, Rutgers, The State University of New Jersey, New Jersey Medical School, 185 South Orange Avenue, Newark, NJ 07103, USA
* Corresponding author.
E-mail address: pike@biochem.wisc.edu

Endocrinol Metab Clin N Am 46 (2017) 815–843
http://dx.doi.org/10.1016/j.ecl.2017.07.001
0889-8529/17/© 2017 Elsevier Inc. All rights reserved.

mode of action involves the regulation of gene expression in specific tissues; this activity is mediated by the nuclear receptor for vitamin D (VDR), a DNA-binding protein that interacts directly with regulatory sequences near target genes and that functions to recruit chromatin-active complexes that participate genetically and epigenetically in modifying transcriptional output.[6–9] Based on these individual features as well as the fact that the VDR is a member of the nuclear receptor family of transcription factor genes, the hormonally active form of vitamin D is the key component of a classic steroid hormone endocrine system.[10–12] However, target genes regulated by vitamin D are not limited to those involved in mineral homeostasis but also include genes that are linked to highly diverse biological processes associated with the cardiovascular and immune systems, the skin, the metabolism of xenobiotics, and numerous additional cellular processes.[13] The vitamin D hormone also controls cellular proliferation and differentiation, implying that, in addition to its broad therapeutic potential in metabolic diseases, it may also be useful in the control of certain cancers.[14] This article provides an overview of the vitamin D system and then focuses on details of the mechanism of action of this hormone in specific cell types, illuminating several of the genes that are involved.

VITAMIN D PRODUCTION AND METABOLISM

It is appropriate in this overview to begin with a brief summary of the gene products that function to synthesize and control the levels of $1,25(OH)_2D_3$ in the blood and that serve to degrade the hormone in target tissues. Importantly and consistent with concepts of endocrinology, at least 2 of these gene products are directly regulated by $1,25(OH)_2D_3$ through important feedback loops. Vitamin D is produced in skin following exposure to sunlight through a process that involves photolysis of cutaneous 7-dehydrocholesterol (provitamin D) to previtamin D followed by isomerization.[15] However, it was soon realized that vitamin D must be metabolically activated further before it can function (**Fig. 1**). Accordingly, the parent vitamin is first hydroxylated in the liver to $25(OH)D_3$ by *CYP2R1*, a 25-hydroxylase (25-OHase).[16,17] This enzyme shows the highest affinity for vitamin D and is likely the most important of the 25-OHases based on genetic evidence that suggests that defects in this gene in humans lead to vitamin D dysfunction.[17,18] However, cytochrome P (CYP) 2R1 knockout mice still produce significant levels of $25(OH)D_3$, suggesting that other hydroxylases may be involved, including mitochondrial *CYP27A1* as well as microsomal *CYP2D11*, *CYP2D25*, *CYP2J2/3*, and *CYP3A4*.[19] Thus, additional work will be required to define all the components of this particular modification to vitamin D in vivo.

The second, and most important, hydroxylation of vitamin D occurs in the kidney through the actions of mitochondrial *CYP27B1*, and results in the synthesis of the active hormone $1,25(OH)_2D_3$[20] (see **Fig. 1**). The validity of this enzyme as the exclusive source of $1,25(OH)_2D_3$ is supported by the subsequent identification of mutations in the *CYP27B1* gene that result in vitamin D–dependency rickets, type 1, which accounts for the $1,25(OH)_2D_3$ deficiency first reported in 1973.[21,22] Importantly, the biochemical and skeletal phenotype of this syndrome has been recapitulated more recently through genetic deletion of the *Cyp27b1* gene in mice using homologous recombination.[23] The activity of renal CYP27B1 is critical to the production and maintenance of physiologic levels of circulating $1,25(OH)_2D_3$.[5] As a consequence, the synthesis and activity of CYP27B1 are tightly regulated by endocrine factors that are elaborated in response to changes in plasma calcium and/or phosphorus levels, most notably parathyroid hormone (PTH)[24] (**Fig. 2**). In addition to PTH, which is

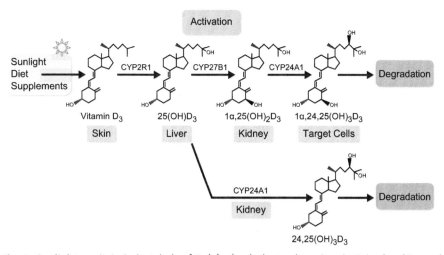

Fig. 1. Sunlight-mediated photolysis of 7-dehydrocholesterol to vitamin D in the skin, and its activation through subsequent sequential hydroxylation in the liver by Cyp2R1 to 25(OH)D$_3$ and by Cyp27b1 to the vitamin D hormone 1,25(OH)$_2$D$_3$ in the kidney. Cyp24a1 initiates the degradation of 25(OH)D$_3$ to 24,25(OH)$_2$D$_3$ in the kidney and the degradation of 1,25(OH)$_2$D$_3$ to 1,24,25(OH)$_3$D$_3$ in all vitamin D target tissues, which results in eventual conversion to calcitroic acid. Alternative degradation pathways in mice also result from Cyp24a1 activity.

induced in response to hypocalcemia and is the major stimulator of 1,25(OH)$_2$D$_3$ production, fibroblast growth factor 23 (FGF23), which requires the transmembrane coreceptor αKlotho, is also an important modulator of vitamin D metabolism[24,25] (see **Fig. 2**). The molecular mechanisms and signaling pathways whereby PTH induces and FGF23 suppresses the expression of renal *CYP27B1* remain undefined at present.[26] Importantly, completion of the vitamin D endocrine circuit involves a potent feedback mechanism through which 1,25(OH)$_2$D$_3$ acts to suppress *CYP27B1* gene

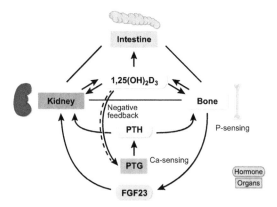

Fig. 2. The regulation of mineral homeostasis in higher vertebrates. The hormones PTH and FGF23 monitor extracellular calcium and phosphate, respectively, and orchestrate the mineral regulating activities of the intestine, kidney and bone through actions on vitamin D metabolism. PTG, parathyroid gland.

expression in the kidney, to downregulate PTH production and secretion by the parathyroid gland, and to upregulate FGF23 expressed in bone.[27,28] A similar negative feedback mechanism seems to exist for FGF23, which acts not only at the kidney to downregulate $CYP27B1$ but may also function in the parathyroid gland to suppress PTH.[29] Several additional factors also regulate $CYP27B1$ expression, including the sex and adrenal hormones, prolactin, and growth hormone.[27] A recent report delineates how prolactin may induce $CYP27B1$ via activation of STAT5.[30] Broad studies also suggest that the expression of $CYP27B1$ may not be restricted to the kidney but that it is synthesized in small amounts in other cell types as well.[31] If correct, this would suggest that circulating levels of $25(OH)D_3$ could control the production of $1,25(OH)_2D_3$ in these cells in either a direct or a paracrine or autocrine manner independently of the kidney. In contrast, the skin may represent a third example in which, in addition to $1,25(OH)_2D_3$, $25(OH)D_3$ is also made internally via expression of CYP2R1.[32,33]

The degradation of $1,25(OH)_2D_3$ is accomplished via the action of CYP24A1, a microsomal enzyme that is expressed basally in the kidney and via $1,25(OH)_2D_3$ induction in this as well as virtually all vitamin D target tissues.[34] This degradation pathway involves a third hydroxylation of $1,25(OH)_2D_3$ at carbon 24 to produce 1,24,25-trihydroxyvitamin D_3 [$1,24,25(OH)_3D_3$] or at carbon 23 to produce 1,25-hydroxyvitamin D_3-26,23-lactone.[27] $25(OH)D_3$, the substrate for $1,25(OH)_2D_3$ production, is also hydroxylated by CYP24A1 in the kidney, leading to the secretion of 24,25-dihydroxyvitamin D_3 ($24,25(OH)_2D_3$) into the blood. Compared with the regulation of CYP27B1, CYP24A1 is reciprocally regulated [stimulated by $1,25(OH)_2D_3$ and suppressed by PTH], an activity that tends to sustain the systemic levels of $1,25(OH)_2D_3$.[35,36] Together, both FGF23 and αKlotho induce CYP24A1 expression, although the mechanisms involved are currently unknown.[26] Because CYP24A1 is present in all vitamin D target cells as well, CYP24A1 can also modulate the intracellular levels, resulting in the control of cellular response to $1,25(OH)_2D_3$. A biological role for the $24,25(OH)_2D_3$ metabolite has been suggested for several decades, although evidence for this hypothesis has yet to emerge in vivo. Although deletion of the $CYP24A1$ gene in the mouse by St-Arnaud[37] resulted in a phenotype of hypercalcemia, hypercalciuria, renal calcification, and skeletal abnormalities, all of these effects were subsequently attributed to the toxicity induced by high circulating levels of $1,25(OH)_2D_3$. Thus, simultaneous excision of the genes for not only $CYP24A1$ but for the VDR as well completely abrogated the toxicity that resulted from these high levels of the hormone.[38] Debilitating mutations within the $CYP24A1$ gene that potentiate response to $1,25(OH)_2D_3$ have been found recently in very young children with idiopathic infantile hypercalcemia and in adults. In adults, patients were characterized by hypercalcemia, hypercalciuria, and recurring kidney stones.[39–42] These findings provide evidence for a critical role of CYP24A1 in humans. As indicated earlier, one of the fundamental actions of $1,25(OH)_2D_3$ in all target cells is to stimulate the expression of $CYP24A1$, thus initiating the means to its own destruction. Surprisingly, although the general mechanism through which $1,25(OH)_2D_3$ induces $CYP24A1$ transcription was thought to be understood at the molecular level, more recent studies have revealed a more complex mode of activation by the vitamin D hormone.[43] This additional complexity represents a paradigm for how most genes are thought to be regulated through distal genomic modulation.[9,44] The molecular mechanisms through which the primary regulators PTH, $1,25(OH)_2D_3$, and FGF23 control the expression of renal $Cyp27b1$ and $Cyp24a1$ remain to be determined, although their actions are likely all transcriptional. These mechanisms are critical to understanding the vitamin D system because these components represent the exclusive enzymatic mediators of the production and degradation of the key metabolite of vitamin D and their levels are frequently aberrant as a consequence of numerous disease processes.

THE ROLES OF VITAMIN D IN CLASSIC AND NONCLASSIC TARGET TISSUES

Calcium and phosphorus homeostasis is orchestrated via the interregulatory actions of PTH and FGF23, respectively[45,46] (see **Fig. 2**). These hormones in turn control the expression of renal *CYP27B1*, which completes the synthesis of 1,25(OH)$_2$D$_3$, acting directly through intestine, kidney, and bone to control mineral balance.[47] Accordingly, these tissues function to acquire calcium and phosphate from the diet, to resorb the ions from glomerular filtrate, and to provide an immediate source of skeletal calcium and phosphate when the diet becomes deficient. Integrating these tissue activities so that plasma calcium and phosphorus concentrations are tightly maintained is central to the function of 1,25(OH)$_2$D$_3$ and to multiple downstream processes linked to normal calcium and phosphate levels such as muscle and nerve function. The intestinal actions of 1,25(OH)$_2$D$_3$ are focused on regulating the production of proteins essential to the processes of dietary calcium and phosphorus absorption, and include such gene products as calbindin D9K (S100g), NCX1, TRPV6, and ATP2B1[48] (**Fig. 3**). The principal action of vitamin D in maintenance of calcium homeostasis is to promote calcium absorption from the intestine. This conclusion is based on the observation that rickets and osteomalacia can be prevented in VDR-null mice fed a prevention diet high in calcium, phosphorus, and lactose.[49,50] In addition, when patients with hereditary 1,25(OH)$_2$D$_3$-resistant rickets are treated with intravenous or high-dose oral calcium, the skeletal phenotypes of these patients are reversed.[51] In the traditional facilitated diffusion model, 1,25(OH)$_2$D$_3$ acts by regulating (1) calcium entry through the apical calcium channel TRPV6, (2) transcellular movement of calcium by binding to the calcium-binding protein calbindin D, and (3) extrusion of calcium from the cell by the plasma membrane Ca-sensitive ATPase PMCA2b (ATP2B1). However, studies in TRPV6-null and calbindin D–null mice have challenged this traditional view. There are no phenotypic differences between calbindin-D$_{9k}$–null or TRPV6-null mice and wild-type mice when dietary calcium level is normal.[52–54] These findings indicate that, under adequate calcium conditions, calbindin-D$_{9k}$ and TRPV6 are redundant for intestinal calcium absorption and suggest compensation by other channels or proteins yet to be identified. In contrast, intestine-specific transgenic expression of TRPV6 has been shown to result in a marked increase in intestinal calcium absorption and bone density in VDR-null mice, indicating a significant role for TRPV6 in the calcium absorptive process.[55] Recent studies suggest the possibility that vitamin D–sensitive calcium uptake is achieved via a complex network of active calcium-regulating components rather than through a single entity.[56] It should also be noted that, although the duodenum has been the focus of research related to 1,25(OH)$_2$D$_3$ regulation of calcium absorption over many years, it is the distal intestine where most ingested calcium is absorbed.[57] Studies in which VDR is expressed or deleted specifically in the distal region of the intestine highlight the importance of the distal as well as proximal segments of the intestine in vitamin D–mediated calcium homeostasis and bone mineralization.[58,59] Studies related to mechanisms involved in 1,25(OH)$_2$D$_3$ regulation of calcium absorption in the distal intestine may suggest new strategies to increase the efficiency of calcium absorption in individuals at risk for bone loss because of aging, bariatric surgery, or inflammatory bowel disease.

1,25(OH)$_2$D$_3$ can also provoke calcium and phosphorus mobilization from the skeleton through a process that involves both the stimulation of bone-resorbing osteoclast activity and the induction of new osteoclast formation from cellular precursors.[60–62]

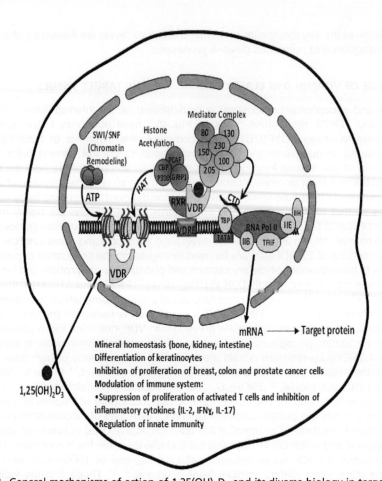

Fig. 3. General mechanisms of action of $1,25(OH)_2D_3$ and its diverse biology in target cells. $1,25(OH)_2D_3$ regulates gene transcription in target cells by binding to VDR. This activated VDR heterodimerizes with RXR and binds to vitamin D response elements (VDREs) in and around target genes. Transcription proceeds through the interaction of the VDR with coactivators and with the transcription machinery. Liganded VDR interacts with steroid receptor coactivator 2 (SRC2; also known as GRIP1), which has histone acetylase (HAT) activity as a primary coactivator. SRC2 can recruit proteins as secondary coactivators, such as CBP/p300, which also have HAT activity. VDR also interacts with mediator complex, which facilitates the activation of the RNA polymerase II holoenzyme through its C-terminal domain, thus promoting formation of the preinitiation complex. The SWI/SNF complex, which remodels chromatin using the energy of ATP hydrolysis, also contributes to activation by VDR. $1,25(OH)_2D_3$ is known to maintain calcium homeostasis and to affect numerous other cell types. Effects on other cell systems include inhibition of proliferation of cancer cells and modulation of the immune system. CBP, CREB binding protein; IFN, interferon; IL, interleukin; mRNA, messenger RNA; TBP, TATA binding protein.

This mechanism takes advantage of the hormone's ability to induce expression of the autocrine tumor necrosis factor (TNF) alpha–like factor RANKL (receptor activator of nuclear factor kappa-B ligand) from chondrocytes, osteoblasts, and osteocytes, as discussed later in this article. Recent studies suggest that $1,25(OH)_2D_3$ may also play an active role in modulating the expression of mineralization regulating factors such as Spp1 (osteopontin), MGP (matrix gla protein), ENPP1 (ectonucleotide pyrophosphatase phosphodiesterase 1) and ENPP2, and ANK (progressive ankylosis protein), and ALPL (intestinal alkaline phosphatase), and perhaps others as well.[63] This overall mechanism of calcium release from bone has a particularly profound consequence when dietary levels of calcium and phosphate are insufficient to maintain extracellular levels, leading to an increase in both PTH and $1,25(OH)_2D_3$ levels. In such cases, maintenance of calcium and phosphorus levels in the blood is prioritized, resulting in bone resorption and a corresponding structural weakening of the skeleton, thereby increasing the risk of bone fracture. Recent studies also suggest that osteocytes, mature osteoblasts that have become fully encased in bone mineral, not only function to control calcium and phosphate release from bone through the production of RANKL and mineralization regulators[64,65] but may also act to remodel bone directly during certain physiologic states such as lactation.[66] This process is prompted by both $1,25(OH)_2D_3$ and PTH-related protein. The actions of these hormones also influence the expression of the *FGF23* gene directly from the osteocyte and perhaps other cell types as well, and its cellular processing and liberation into the circulation, where it controls renal modulation of phosphate levels.[46] It is also important to note that depletion of calcium and phosphorus levels in the blood results in the failure of bone to mineralize via physicochemical principles, resulting in rickets or osteomalacia.[47] Thus, these studies support a direct effect of $1,25(OH)_2D_3$ on bone as well as an indirect role through calcium provision to bone via stimulation of intestinal calcium absorption. If normal serum calcium levels cannot be maintained by intestinal calcium absorption, then $1,25(OH)_2D_3$ acts together with PTH to stimulate osteoclastogenesis and to increase calcium reabsorption from the distal tubules of the kidney.[36] Although the actions of $1,25(OH)_2D_3$ are modest at the kidney, the amount of calcium recovered through reabsorption is highly significant because of the large daily load of calcium that is filtered by this organ.

Central to the orchestration of intestinal, kidney, and bone actions by $1,25(OH)_2D_3$ are the regulatory systems that monitor calcium and phosphorus content in plasma and participate along with the vitamin D hormone in maintaining those levels in the extracellular compartment. In the case of calcium, the level of this ion is continually monitored by the calcium-sensing receptor in the parathyroid gland, which responds by increasing parathyroid gland secretion of PTH when calcium content decreases. Although the consequence of calcium liberation from the skeleton increases phosphate levels as well, both PTH and FGF23 function collectively in the kidney to promote phosphate diuresis through a mechanism involving cellular relocation of multiple sodium-phosphate transporters.[29,67] FGF23 represents the long-sought-after phosphate-regulating hormone or phosphatonin that is induced not only by phosphate when it is in abundance but by $1,25(OH)_2D_3$ as well, although neither of these mechanisms are currently understood.[28,68,69] Linkage of FGF23 to the regulation of phosphate was initially derived from phenotypes associated with tumor-induced osteomalacia, autosomal dominant hypophosphatemic rickets, and X-linked hypophosphatemic syndromes.[70] More recently, studies in which the *Fgf23* gene has been either deleted or overexpressed in the mouse have emerged to strongly support this linkage. With regard to FGF23, a novel mechanism has now been identified whereby FGF23 promotes the redistribution of the phosphate transporters NaPi2a (*Slc34a1*) and NaPi2c (*Slc34a3*) such that proximal tubular reabsorption of phosphate is reduced.[29] FGF23's ability to suppress circulating $1,25(OH)_2D_3$ also results in a reduction in intestinal phosphate uptake. These actions and others in kidney and bone as well as in intestine restore calcium and phosphorus concentrations to their appropriate levels in plasma. Feedback mechanisms via FGF23 (described earlier) then act to prevent phosphorus levels from increasing beyond acceptable limits, thereby maintaining calcium and phosphorus levels within narrow boundaries. The molecular mechanisms whereby $1,25(OH)_2D_3$ orchestrates the expression of several of the genes whose functions are integral to the maintenance of calcium and phosphorus homeostasis are being defined.

$1,25(OH)_2D_3$ is also a regulator of cellular proliferation and differentiation, activities that are similar to those manifested by many of the steroid hormones (see **Fig. 3**). These growth-regulating actions of $1,25(OH)_2D_3$, as well as many additional biological processes that are regulated by $1,25(OH)_2D_3$, highlight not only important physiologic activities of the hormone but potential therapeutic roles for both the hormone and for synthetic vitamin D analogues. These roles include treatments for cancer, control of skin function, regulation of the immune system and autoimmune diseases, and control of cardiovascular disease. For example, studies in VDR-null mice provide direct evidence in vivo that, in the absence of VDR, there is increased sensitivity in response to a chemical carcinogen to the development of a variety of tumors, including skin tumors, tumors of the lymph nodes, and estrogen receptor–negative tumors.[71,72] VDR-null mice also develop hypertension and cardiac hypertrophy.[73] Moreover, VDR-null mice also develop more severe conditions of inflammatory bowel disease that is associated with increased numbers of inflammatory cytokine (interleukin [IL]-17 and interferon gamma)–secreting T cells in experimental models of colitis[74,75] and show alterations in innate and adaptive immunity as well. The biological actions of the vitamin D hormone in several of these nonclassic target tissues are considered elsewhere in this issue. Importantly, the underlying key feature of vitamin D response in all of these nonclassic tissues is expression of the VDR.

THE VITAMIN D RECEPTOR AND GENOMIC MECHANISMS OF ACTION
The Vitamin D Receptor

A binding protein eventually designated the VDR was first discovered in the chicken intestine and then in other tissues, including the parathyroid glands, kidney, and bone.[6,7] This protein's biochemical features, including its retention in chromatin[76] and its ability to bind to DNA[8] identified several years later, suggested that it was similar to other receptors for known steroid hormones and that it likely played a role in transcriptional regulation. Despite much effort that preceded this event, it was the cloning of the chicken *VDR* gene[10] and the human[11] and rat[77] versions of this receptor that followed shortly thereafter that ushered in a new era in vitamin D research. The availability of VDR complementary DNA clones enabled the direct detection of VDR RNA in cells and, following the introduction of reverse transcription polymerase chain reaction (PCR) analysis in the late 1980s, made possible the development of the most sensitive assay for the VDR that is now currently in use. The cloning of the VDR and the domain structure of the receptor that was eventually revealed also confirmed that the VDR was a true steroid receptor and a bona fide member of the steroid receptor gene family.[12,78,79] Equally important, the structural cloning and sequence analysis of the human chromosomal gene[80,81] for the VDR that followed in short order led ultimately to the identification of a series of mutations within the gene that was responsible for the syndrome of hereditary $1,25(OH)_2D_3$-resistant rickets.[82–86] This syndrome had been identified earlier by Bell and colleagues[86] in 1978 and it was thought by several groups of investigators[87–90] to be caused by defects in the VDR gene, a hypothesis that was confirmed during the intervening years.[91] The discovery of mutations in the *VDR* gene, the first for any member of the nuclear receptor family, supported the integral and essential role of the VDR as the sole mediator of the activities of the vitamin D hormone, which was eventually confirmed and extended through recapitulation of the disease phenotype observed in the mouse following deletion of the VDR from this model organism's genome.

General Features of Vitamin D Receptor Action

Sites of DNA binding

Early studies suggested that $1,25(OH)_2D_3$ activated gene expression programs in a wide variety of cells and identified numerous gene candidates for further investigation. Most prominent among these were tissues that expressed the vitamin D–dependent calcium-binding proteins (calbindins),[92,93] and the osteocalcin,[94,95] osteopontin,[96] and CYP24A1[97] proteins, although several others emerged during the following several decades as well. The cloning of many of the genes for these proteins and identification of their structural organization prompted exploration of the mechanisms through which $1,25(OH)_2D_3$ and its receptor could promote their regulation (see **Fig. 3**). These studies, first with human *BGLP* (osteocalcin)[98,99] and subsequently with *Spp1* (osteopontin),[100] *Cyp24a1*,[101–104] and others,[105] suggested that the VDR bound to a 15-bp vitamin D–responsive DNA element (VDRE) composed of 2 directly repeated consensus AGGTCA hexanucleotide half-sites separated by 3 bp that was generally located within a kilobase or so of the promoters for these genes.[99] These features were similar, but not identical, to those for other nuclear receptors. $1,25(OH)_2D_3$ also strongly suppressed the expression of numerous genes, most notably those for *PTH* and *CYP27B1* but also in more recent studies of the *IL-17* gene. Repression of IL-17 transcription by $1,25(OH)_2D_3$ has been reported to involve, in part, dissociation of histone acetylase activity, recruitment of deacetylase, and VDR/retinoid X receptor (RXR) binding to nuclear factor of activated T cell (NFAT) sites[106] (**Fig. 4**). Although some progress has been made, the mechanisms of suppression for these and other downregulated genes have yet to be fully understood but are almost certain to be highly diverse. The presence of unique so-called negative VDREs has been suggested for some negatively regulated genes, although this mechanism has yet to be substantiated.[107]

Heterodimer formation with retinoid X receptors

Accompanying the discovery of the first VDREs was the important finding that VDR binding to these specific DNA sequences depended on an unknown nuclear factor.[108–110] The identity of this protein was subsequently revealed when it was discovered that specific members of the steroid receptor family termed RXRs were capable of forming heterodimeric complexes with the VDR and other members of this class of steroid receptors[111] (see **Fig. 3**). Importantly, $1,25(OH)_2D_3$ promotes heterodimer formation between VDR and RXR, although the cellular location of this interaction currently remains undefined.[110,112] It has been suggested that, in addition to its contribution to DNA binding, RXR may participate in the transcriptional activation process.[113,114] However, recent structural studies suggest that this complex is capable of recruiting only a single coregulatory molecule.[115]

The vitamin D receptor functions to recruit coregulatory complexes that mediate gene regulation

Early studies revealed that transcription factor binding near promoters leads to an interaction with basal transcriptional machinery that enhances gene output. However, it is now known that transcriptional modulation by most DNA-binding transactivators is far more complex and involves the receptor-mediated recruitment of different coregulatory complexes, each with unique functions. Overcoming and/or restoring the inherent repressive state of chromatin requires the presence of regulatory machinery able to shift and/or displace nucleosomes (chromatin remodeling), alter the

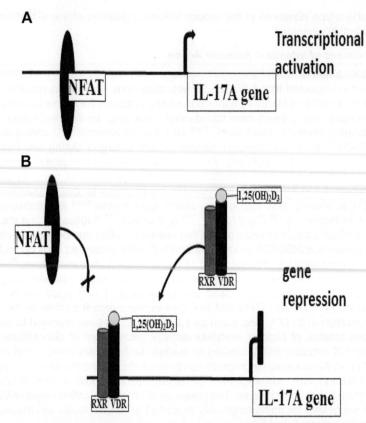

Fig. 4. Mechanism of suppression of the IL-17 gene by 1,25(OH)$_2$D$_3$. Mechanism of repression of IL-17A activated transcription by 1,25(OH)$_2$D$_3$. The negative effect of 1,25(OH)$_2$D$_3$ on IL-17A involves blocking NFAT (an essential regulator of IL-17A gene transcription) from binding to its sites on the IL-17 gene and 1,25(OH)$_2$D$_3$-dependent association of RXR/VDR with the NFAT elements. 1,25(OH)$_2$D$_3$ repression of IL-17A also involves 1,25(OH)$_2$D$_3$-mediated recruitment of histone deacetylase and sequestration of Runx1 (also an important T-cell receptor–mediated transcriptional regulator of IL-17A) by 1,25(OH)$_2$D$_3$/VDR (not shown). (*From* Joshi S, Pantalena LC, Liu XK, et al. 1,25-dihydroxyvitamin D(3) ameliorates Th17 autoimmunity via transcriptional modulation of interleukin-17A. Mol Cell Biol 2011;31(17):3653–69; with permission.)

condensation state and therefore the local architecture of chromatin (histone modifications), create or restrict novel binding sites for additional coregulatory complexes (epigenetic sites), and/or facilitate the entry of RNA polymerase II (RNA pol II) at appropriate times and sites (see **Fig. 3**). Three complexes that participate in these activities that are known to be recruited by the VDR are (1) vertebrate ATPase-containing homologs of the yeast SWI/SNF complex that use the energy of ATP to remodel and reposition nucleosomes[116]; (2) complexes that contain either histone acetyltransferases (HATs) or methyltransferases, deacetyltransferases (HDACs), or histone demethylases, which function to modify the lysine-containing or arginine-containing tails of histone 3 and/or histone 4 at specific locations[117,118]; and (3) mediator complex, thought to facilitate the entry of RNA pol II into the general transcriptional apparatus and perhaps to play a role in transcriptional reinitiation.[119] Other regulatory complexes are also apparent. Several classes of regulatory complexes comprise components of dynamic and highly active mechanisms that are epigenetic and involve the coordinated expression of gene networks across the genome.[120] These programs are widely responsible for development, differentiation, and mature cell function.[121,122] For example, HATs and their reciprocal HDACs regulate the level of epigenetic histone H3 and H4 marks, controlling the degree to which chromatin is condensed and therefore the DNA is accessible for transcription factor binding.[123] The recruitment of these large chromatin regulatory complexes is frequently coordinated by factors such as the p160 family SRC-1, SRC-2, and SRC-3, the HATs CBP and p300, and the corepressors SMRT or NCoR, as well as any of the many HDACs that interact directly with transcription factors such as the VDR.[117] Importantly, activation of the VDR with $1,25(OH)_2D_3$ leads to the creation of a binding site on the VDR protein that mediates the link between the receptor and these coregulatory complexes.[124–126] Recent studies show that the ability of the VDR to recruit several of these coregulatory factors results in striking changes in epigenetic histone marks that facilitate altered gene output.[127–129] Thus, it is clear that, like other DNA-binding proteins, the function of the VDR in a dynamic way is simply to focus the recruitment of transcriptionally active complexes to gene subsets that are integral in a cell-specific manner to vitamin D hormone response. Considerable crystallographic information has now accrued to support not only the structural organization of the VDR/RXR heterodimer but its association with DNA and its recruitment of coregulators.[115] Many of these interactions are prompted by $1,25(OH)_2D_3$ and perhaps differentially affected by analogues of the vitamin D hormone. These differential interactions form the basis for the concept of analogue selectivity in vivo, although this remains controversial for the vitamin D system.

Applying New Methodological Approaches to Study Vitamin D Receptor Action

The recent coupling of chromatin immunoprecipitation initially to tiled microarray analysis (ChIP-chip) and subsequently to next-generation DNA sequencing (ChIP-seq) analysis has revitalized the study of transcription both in vitro and in vivo, providing new methodologies capable of revealing unprecedented detail on a genome-wide scale.[130–132] These techniques permit the site-specific crosslinking of structural chromatin proteins, regulatory transcription factors, and nucleosomes to DNA, and their detection as well as the detection of functional modifications to these components via antibodies at nucleotide level resolution across the genomes of all organisms for which genomic sequence is available. This method and others that focus on direct DNA methylation, detection of presumed structural/functional DNA-bound proteins complexes via DNase1 hypersensitivity analysis, and a multitude of others provide genome-wide annotation not previously attainable, have strikingly advanced factor-based gene regulation, the emerging field of epigenetics, and evaluation of the impact of chromatin epigenetic states on gene regulation as well.[133–137] Although numerous transcriptional principles obtained through earlier studies have been confirmed, others have required extensive revision or radical alteration because of the highly biased and potentially misleading nature of many of the previously used techniques. However, perhaps more important are the many new principles that have emerged as well, particularly when paired with transcriptomic measurements using RNA-seq (sequencing) analysis.[138] Another methodology that deserves mention is one that has enabled the selective editing of the genomes of both cells in culture and model organisms such as mice, rats, and even primates in vivo. This approach, particularly as it relates to the use of the RNA sequence–directed CRISPR/Cas9 method, now permits rapid and inexpensive deletion of not only genes but of the regulatory elements of genes, thereby enabling loss-of-function assessment of their regulatory activities in cells.[139–141] Because of their importance, the results of some of these collective studies that have provided important new insight into the transcriptional mechanism of action of $1,25(OH)_2D_3$ as well as other hormones are discussed later in this article.

Overarching principles of vitamin D receptor interaction at target cell genomes

As indicated earlier, studies using traditional methods coupled in later years to direct ChIP analysis pinpointed the regulatory regions of several vitamin D target genes near their promoters, including *Bglap*, *Spp1*, and *Cyp24a1*.[142] In subsequent studies, the authors used ChIP-chip and then ChIP-seq analyses not only to confirm these findings but to obtain a broader, overarching, genome-wide perspective on binding sites for the VDR in cells (**Box 1**). Focusing on bone osteoblasts, it was discovered using ChIP-chip analysis that we could detect approximately 1000 residual binding sites for the VDR in the absence of $1,25(OH)_2D_3$, which was increased following hormonal treatment to approximately 7000 to 8000.[143] A collection of binding sites such as these has been termed a cellular cistrome. This observation supports the idea that VDR DNA binding is largely hormone dependent.[144] Importantly, a similar analysis of binding sites for RXR revealed a more extensive collection of sites that was only modestly increased through $1,25(OH)_2D_3$ activation, emphasizing our understanding that RXR is a heterodimer partner for not only the VDR but several additional nuclear receptors as well.[111] These findings have been confirmed in similar studies in MSCs (mesenchymal stem cells), osteoblasts, osteocytes, and adipocytes, which also revealed that, although overlap was present, binding sites for the VDR differ significantly across the genome depending on the cell type examined.[144–146] Subsequent studies of VDR-binding sites in Epstein-Barr virus-immortalized human B cells, primary B cells and monocytes,[147] and THP-1 monocytes[148] confirmed each of these findings. Importantly, although genome-wide ChIP-seq analyses have confirmed binding sites for the VDR near the promoters of genes such as *Bglap*, *Spp1*, *Cyp24a1*, and a few others,[144] this technique has been unable to confirm promoter-proximal VDR elements for many genes. These observations highlight the problems inherent to

---

Box 1
Overarching principles of vitamin D action in target cells

VDR binding sites (the cistrome): 2000 to 8000 $1,25(OH)_2D_3$-sensitive binding sites per genome whose number and location are determined as a function of cell type

Active transcription unit for induction: the VDR/RXR heterodimer

Distal binding site locations: dispersed in *cis*-regulatory modules (CRMs, or enhancers) across the genome; located in a cell type–specific manner near promoters but predominantly within introns and distal intergenic regions; frequently located in clusters of elements

VDR/RXR binding site sequence (VDRE): induction mediated by classic hexameric half-sites (AGGTCA) separated by 3 base pairs; repression mediated by divergent sites

Mode of DNA binding: predominantly, but not exclusively, $1,25(OH)_2D_3$ dependent

Modular features: CRMs contain binding sites for multiple transcription factors that facilitate either independent or synergistic interaction

Epigenetic CRM signatures: defined by the dynamically regulated posttranslational histone H3 and H4 modifications

VDR cistromes are highly dynamic: cistromes change during cell differentiation, maturation, and disease activation and thus have consequential effects on gene expression

traditional biased approaches such as plasmid-based transfection methods and the potential for this approach to yield frequent false-positives. Despite this, many of these genes have been shown to retain transcription factors such as C/EBPβ and others through traditional means that have been confirmed via unbiased methods. Thus, the presence of many of these factors at promoter-proximal regions cannot be discounted at present, but must simply be confirmed. In the case of binding sites, de novo motif-finding analyses of the most common DNA sequence elements found in these diverse genome-wide collections of VDR-binding sites has confirmed that a high percentage contain the originally postulated VDRE motif composed of AGGTCA xxg AGGTCA.[144,149] Thus, the consensus VDRE developed initially from that found in the human osteocalcin gene[98,99] is most representative of the sequence with which the VDR can interact at all genomes thus far examined.

The unbiased nature of ChIP-seq analysis has also provided many surprising and perhaps unexpected insights of major significance[150] (see **Box 1**). Perhaps most important, although traditional studies of $1,25(OH)_2D_3$ action identified regions immediately upstream of the transcriptional start sites (TSS) of genes, unbiased ChIP-seq analyses have revealed that regulatory regions for the vitamin D hormone and its receptor are more commonly located in clusters within introns or in intergenic regions tens if not hundreds of kilobases upstream or downstream of regulated genes.[144,145,149] Examples of such distal elements for the VDR abound but can be found in many of the genes whose putative promoter-proximal elements were undetectable by ChIP-seq analysis. They include the mouse *Tnfsf11* (RANKL) gene in bone cells, where at least 5 intergenic regulatory regions for the VDR are located[62]; the *Cyp24a1* gene in numerous cell types in which, in addition to the well-known promoter-proximal element discussed earlier, a complex downstream cluster of regulatory elements exists in both the mouse and the human genes[43]; the *Vdr* gene in bone cells, where both upstream regulatory regions and several intronic elements are present[127,151]; the *TRPV6* gene in intestinal cells, which contains multiple upstream elements[56,152]; the *S100g* gene in the intestine, which also contains multiple upstream elements[56]; and the many target genes, such as *c-FOS* and *c-MYC*, in human colorectal cancer cells as well.[149] Enhancers for other transcription factors have been identified more than a megabase from the genes they are known to regulate, although at present the most distal VDR-binding site is 335 kb upstream of the human *c-MYC* promoter. However, the linear/distal nature of regulatory elements for genes is illusionary, because these distances do not take into account the looping of DNA that brings key regulatory segments into proximity of a gene's promoter region.[153–157] It is also notable that, of the tens of thousands of putative VDREs that naturally occur across the genome based purely on in silico analyses, only a very small proportion of these putative elements are functional because of chromatin restriction.[133,135] In contrast, a peak of activity defined by high-quality ChIP-seq analysis is almost certain to represent a true transcription factor–binding site and provides far more assurance than that developed via direct quantitative PCR–ChIP analysis. An additional observation, as indicated earlier, is the finding through ChIP-seq analysis that most genes are regulated by more than 1 distal regulatory enhancer and, in some cases, by multiple enhancer regions. Recent encyclopedia of DNA elements estimates suggest that genes are regulated by an average of 10 separate enhancers.[135] *Spp1* and *Cyp24a1* represent classic examples, in which additional elements located upstream of the former gene and downstream in the latter mouse and human genes[43,144] have been defined using these unbiased assays. However, the presence of multiple enhancers located at distal sites complicates the studies of gene regulation enormously, as is discussed later.

An additional regulatory feature of genes that has been identified is that of modularity. Thus, individual enhancers generally contain organized arrays of linear DNA sequences capable of assembling distinct, nonrandom transcription factor complexes that can function uniquely to regulate the gene with which they are linked. There are numerous examples, but it is interesting that more than 42% of VDR-binding sites in bone cells are located in enhancers that contain prebound C/EBPβ and the master regulator RUNX2.[144,158] These factors assemble in a highly organized fashion relative to each other, a nucleoprotein structure that the authors have termed an osteoblast enhancer complex. Both RUNX2 and C/EBPβ in this configuration can positively and perhaps negatively influence the overall regulatory activity of $1,25(OH)_2D_3$ and its receptor in unique ways. An alternative arrangement has also been identified in bone cells, as found in the *Mmp13* gene, in which binding sites for the VDR, C/EBPβ, and RUNX2 are dispersed across 3 separate upstream enhancers.[159,160] The activities of these 3 regions are not independent but can influence each other's activity via looping in an overall hierarchical manner to modulate the expression of *Mmp13*. It is likely that many other genes contain this or similar arrangements as well. A collective summary of many of the newly acquired features of vitamin D–mediated gene regulation obtained via genome-wide analyses is provided in **Box 1**.

Genome-wide coregulatory recruitment to target genes via the vitamin D receptor

The function of the VDR is to recruit chromatin-active coregulatory complexes that facilitate modulation of gene output as indicated earlier. Numerous studies at single-gene levels support the capacity of the VDR to recruit these complexes, and recent ChIP-seq analyses support the presence of these complexes on a genome-wide scale as well. Thus, for example, the VDR was found to recruit coactivators such as SRC1, CBP, and MED1, as well as the corepressors NCoR and SMRT in colorectal LS180 cells.[161] This recruitment correlated most profoundly with VDR-binding sites that are linked to genes that are modulated directly by $1,25(OH)_2D_3$. This correlation was not preferentially linked to either upregulated or downregulated genes, as might be expected, suggesting that the roles of these coregulators are not limited specifically to activation or repression and that their activities are likely to be gene-context driven. In contrast, recent studies in liver stellate cells suggested that $1,25(OH)_2D_3$-mediated repression of a profibrotic gene expression program induced by TGFβ does not involve the apparent recruitment of corepressors SMRT and NCoR.[162] In addition to SRC1, CBP, and MED1, Brahma-related gene 1 (BRG1), an ATPase that is a component of the SWI/SNF chromatin remodeling complex, has been reported to play a fundamental role in $1,25(OH)_2D_3$-induced transcription.[163] C/EBP and BRG1 are components of the same complex and are recruited to the C/EBP site of the CYP24A1 gene by $1,25(OH)_2D_3$. PRMT5, a type II protein arginine methyltransferase that interacts with BRG1, represses $1,25(OH)_2D_3$-induced CYP24A1 transcription via its methylation of H3R8 and H4R3. Thus, the SWI/SNF complex can play a role in the silencing as well as in the activation of VDR-mediated transcription.

Identifying underlying early mechanistic outcomes in response to vitamin D receptor /retinoid X receptor binding

The ability of the VDR to recruit epigenetically active coregulatory complexes such as HATs, HDACs, and a variety of histone methyltransferases that regulate chromatin structure, as discussed earlier, suggests that $1,25(OH)_2D_3$ may influence the levels of distinct epigenetic marks imposed by these chromatin modifiers as a means of regulating gene output. Importantly, many such epigenetic marks on histones

H3 and H4 are enriched in regions within gene loci that are uniquely active.[131,132,164,165] Perhaps of most importance are changes in the levels of acetylation at H4K5 (H4K5ac), H3K9 (H3K9ac), and H3K27 (H3K27ac) that reflect alterations in the transcriptional activity of the genes with which they are linked; these modifications generally occur within enhancers that regulate these genes, although they can also occur at locations within genes as well. Regulatory regions that are marked both by genetic and epigenetic information at gene loci are frequently termed variable chromatin modulators.[166] An increase in several of these acetylation marks occurs at specific sites of VDR binding in genes such as *Spp1* and *Cyp24a1*, *Lrp5*, *Tnfsf11*, and the *Vdr* following $1,25(OH)_2D_3$ stimulation[9,165,167] and can be used to define sites of action of $1,25(OH)_2D_3$ even in the absence of evidence for VDR occupancy. These and other findings stimulated a recent assessment of the consequence of VDR binding following $1,25(OH)_2D_3$ treatment on generalized H3 and H4 acetylation at a genome-wide scale in colorectal cells and at more specific histone sites in differentiating bone osteoblasts and osteocytes. All of these studies have revealed a striking increase in the level of H3 and H4 acetylation in response to $1,25(OH)_2D_3$. Although $1,25(OH)_2D_3$ can also provoke enrichment of enhancer methylation marks, these changes are generally gene specific, suggesting that the VDR may retain gene selective functions as well. Overall, histone modification analyses suggest that $1,25(OH)_2D_3$ promotes VDR/RXR binding at sites on cellular genomes that are marked by acetylated H3K9, H3K27, and H4K5, and that these interactions frequently result in an upregulation of acetylation that facilitates enhanced levels of gene expression. These studies provide a global perspective on the actions of vitamin D in several cell types, indicating that the primary role of the VDR is to facilitate the recruitment of chromatin modifiers such as acetyltransferases and deacetyltransferases that function to impose epigenetic histone changes within the enhancers of some, but not all, vitamin D–sensitive target genes.

The dynamic impact of cellular differentiation and disease on vitamin D receptor cistromes and transcriptional outcomes

Perhaps the most important observation made on a genome-wide scale has been the discovery that cellular differentiation exerts a dramatic quantitative and qualitative impact on genomic VDR binding, an effect that correlates directly with the hormone's ability to regulate the differentiating cell's transcriptome in a highly dynamic manner.[144,146] This process is likely responsible for the cell type–specific nature of VDR binding and thus transcriptional outcomes at diverse sets of genes that can be measured in different tissues. A general change in the cellular RNA profile in response to $1,25(OH)_2D_3$ is perhaps not surprising, given that the overall effects of $1,25(OH)_2D_3$ on osteoblast-lineage cells are known to differ significantly depending on the state of bone cell differentiation. This concept of differentiation-induced changes in VDR binding and transcriptional integrity is aptly shown through a detailed examination of the differential expression of several genes, including *Mmp13* in osteoblast precursors and mature mineralizing osteoblasts.[159]

Evans and colleagues[162] recently showed that disease processes can affect VDR cistromes as well. The activation of hepatic stellate cells via the upregulation of TGFβ in the liver induces the expression of a collagen program that causes hepatic fibrosis and can induce cirrhosis of the liver. This disease progression can be ameliorated by simultaneous treatment in vivo with an analogue of vitamin D, and presumably by $1,25(OH)_2D_3$, although this was not tested. The investigators showed that the VDR cistrome that functions normally to suppress the program of collagen expression is altered as a result of TGFβ action, redirecting VDR binding to alternative sites of action away from collagen genes, thereby blunting opposing sites of vitamin D action. Interestingly, although these findings identify an important action of the VDR to prevent liver fibrosis, they also highlight the role of the VDR in the disease-potentiating activation of stellate cells, in a process that could be considered analogous to that of differentiation. Further studies of this system identify the role of the chromatin regulator BRD4 in this activity, and suggest that direct inhibition of this downstream factor by a small molecular regulator can bypass the positive effects of a vitamin D analogue.[168]

Linking Vitamin D Receptor Binding to the Expression of Specific Genes

The problem

ChIP-seq analyses can identify sites of occupancy for transcription factors and confirm that these sites retain epigenetic histone signatures that are consistent with the presence of enhancers. However, they cannot identify the genes to which enhancers are functionally linked, largely because the regulatory regions of genes are frequently located significant distances from gene promoters, and in many cases not contiguous with their target genes.[157,169] These issues are of major concern for studies of mechanisms of gene regulation and of particular relevance to the myriad of genome-wide association studies that have been reported over the past decade. In these studies, single-nucleotide variants can be correlated with a particular biological phenotype or disease risk, but most of the genes whose activities are influenced by these single nucleotide polymorphisms (SNPs) and represent determinants of the phenotype remain to be identified. Much research is currently focused on bioinformatic approaches to establishing linkage between enhancers and the genes they modulate, although this has not yet been accomplished with any certainty.

The solution

The authors and others have taken several approaches in attempts to link distal enhancers to the genes they regulate and to explore the mechanism through which they control the expression of the gene of interest. For example, a preliminary approach is to explore the relationship between the putative target gene's promoter and an identified enhancer using a proximity assay (chromatin conformation capture [3C] or more complex versions thereof), which can provide evidence that the distal element is in physical contact with the candidate gene's promoter, perhaps in a hormone-dependent manner.[156] Importantly, proximity assays have been extended technically to encompass multiple interactions using DNA sequencing and analysis on genome-wide scales as well.[155,170,171] However, this approach with respect to gene-linkage is largely correlative and must generally be confirmed via direct assessment. One approach is to create large minigenes that contain both the potential regulatory regions of genes in the vicinity identified by ChIP-seq analysis and the transcription unit of the putative target.[43] A second and perhaps more robust strategy is to create individual enhancer deletions within the context of the genome, an approach that is most appropriately conducted in the mouse in vivo.[172] An additional approach that has emerged most recently involves direct editing of the genome in either cell lines or in the mouse genome using the RNA-directed CRISPR/Cas9 nuclease method to provoke precise genomic deletions, insertions, and/or mutations at specific gene locations.[159,160] The first 2 of these approaches have been used to examine several genes of relevance to vitamin D biology, including the *Cyp24a1* and *Vdr* genes as well as the more complex *Tnfsf11* gene, and second has been used to explore the *Mmp13* and several other genes. A brief summary of our studies of the *Tnfsf11* and *Mmp13* genes is considered here.

Characterizing the regulatory elements of the *Tnfsf11* (receptor activator of nuclear factor kappa-B ligand) gene

RANKL is a membrane-bound and sometimes soluble TNFα-like factor derived from the *Tnfsf11* gene that strongly induces osteoclast differentiation from hematopoietic precursors.[173,174] The signal transduction pathways that mediate activation of this complex differentiation pathway are now well described.[175] Importantly, the actions of RANKL over the intervening years have been dramatically extended to include immune regulation, mammary gland maturation, thermogenesis, and cardiovascular calcification, to name a few. Despite considerable effort, early attempts using traditional methods to identify regions mediating the regulation of the *Tnfsf11* gene by 1,25(OH)$_2$D$_3$ as well as PTH and cytokines such as IL-6 and oncostatin M in bone cells were largely unsuccessful,[176,177] suggesting that the regulation of this gene might be mediated through more distal sites. Because the mouse and human *TNFSF11* genes are located in gene deserts and bounded on each side by nearly 200 kb of intergenic DNA, the authors explored this gene in osteoblasts for regulation by the vitamin D hormone. Importantly, we used ChIP-chip analysis of both VDR and RXR, and extended our query of mouse *Tnfsf11* to more than 500 kb of DNA surrounding the gene's transcription unit.[62] This initial study, now fully confirmed by ChIP-seq analysis, revealed that although neither VDR nor RXR were present near the *Tnfsf11* promoter region following administration of 1,25(OH)$_2$D$_3$, both were strongly detected at 5 distal regions: −16 (termed D1), −22 kb (D2), −60 kb (D3), −69 kb (D4), and −75/76 kb (D5) upstream of the gene's promoter. Similar follow-on studies revealed that PTH-induced cyclic AMP enhancer binding protein at several of these regulatory regions and cytokine factors such as IL-6 induced transcription factor STAT3 binding at 1 of these enhancers (D5) as well as at a new enhancer at −88 kb (D6). The binding of these and other factors identified across the *Tnfsf11* gene is summarized in **Fig. 5**. These studies suggested that the regulation of *Tnfsf11* expression by 1,25(OH)$_2$D$_3$, PTH, and other hormonal factors is mediated by multiple independent enhancers

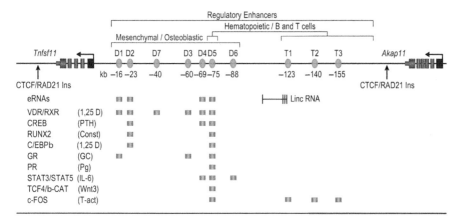

Fig. 5. The *Tnfsf11* gene locus and its osteoblastic and hematopoietic regulatory regions. Arrows indicate the CTCF/RAD21-defined boundaries of the locus, which includes the transcription unit and its upstream noncoding regulatory control regions. Enhancers that mediate osteoblast lineage regulation (D regions) and hematopoietic regulation (T regions) are numbered and indicated in orange ovals. Their distance from the *Tnfsf11* TSS in kilobases is indicated below the ovals. The D5 enhancer is active in both cell lineage types. Factors that have been shown to bind to each enhancer by ChIP-chip and/or ChIP-seq analysis are indicated below the gene locus in orange blocks.

located at significant distances from the gene's TSS. Additional unbiased analysis in T cells revealed a second set of 3 regulatory enhancers located intergenically even further upstream of the *Tnfsf11* TSS between −123 and −155 kb (termed T1–T3)[178,179] (**Fig. 5**). These enhancers, together with the enhancer at D5, mediate the expression of *Tnfsf11* exclusively in hematopoietic B and T cells. Thus, a set of at least 10 independent enhancers has been identified to regulate *Tnfsf11* expression in osteoblast-lineage and hematopoietic-lineage cells when assessed in cultured cell lines.[167] It is these regions that contain single-nucleotide variants (SNPs) of genome-wide significance that seem to influence *TNFSF11* expression and bone mineral density in human populations.

To confirm that these enhancers were responsible for the regulation of *Tnfsf11*, the authors and others individually deleted 3 of the key osteoblast specific enhancers D2, D5, and D6 as well as a single hematopoietic enhancer at −123 kb (T1) from the mouse genome.[180,181] Mice bearing these deletions were then subjected to extensive regulatory and biological phenotyping. The results of these analyses indicate that (1) the D2 enhancer mediates PTH action in osteoblasts,[180] (2) the D5 enhancer reduces basal expression of RANKL in both osteoblasts and hematopoietic cells and mediates both PTH and 1,25(OH)$_2$D$_3$ action in the former tissue,[172,181] (3) the enhancer at D6 limits the regulation of RANKL by inflammatory cytokines, and (4) the enhancer at T1 reduces the basal expression of RANKL exclusively in hematopoietic cells.[181] Biologically, the osteoblast-active enhancers exert profound effects on the skeleton, whereas the hematopoietic cell–active enhancer T1 has no effect. Numerous additional phenotypic responses were identified. The authors conclude from these studies that the *Tnfsf11* gene is regulated congruently both in vitro and in vivo by multiple distal enhancers that retain features that mediate the regulation of *Tnfsf11* expression in unique temporal, hormonal, and tissue-specific fashions.

Studies of the Mmp13 gene

Recent studies have examined the mechanisms through which *Mmp13* expression is regulated in osteoblastic cells in culture by 1,25(OH)$_2$D$_3$ and other hormones.[159] In studies of these cells, 3 regions located upstream of the *Mmp13* gene and bearing epigenetic histone enhancer signatures H3K4me1 and H3K27ac were identified by ChIP-seq analysis. The most proximal of these enhancers, located −10 kb upstream of the *Mmp13* gene bound the VDR, mediating induction by 1,25(OH)$_2$D$_3$, whereas the other two, −20 kb and −30 kb upstream, bound the osteoblast master regulators C/EBPβ and RUNX2, respectively. The authors used CRISPR/Cas9 methods to create a series of homozygous daughter osteoblast cell lines derived from a parental UAMS source that contained deletions of the promoter-proximal region, the −10-kb and −30-kb enhancers, and either VDR or RUNX2, and then examined these lines for basal as well as 1,25(OH)$_2$D$_3$-inducible expression of *Mmp13* transcripts. Loss of the −10-kb enhancer as well as loss of the VDR fully compromised the ability of 1,25(OH)$_2$D$_3$ to promote VDR binding and to induce *Mmp13* expression. Deletion of the promoter-proximal region, the −30-kb enhancer, and RUNX2 expression each dramatically reduced basal expression of *Mmp13*, but surprisingly also reduced the ability of 1,25(OH)$_2$D$_3$ to induce *Mmp13* RNA. Further studies revealed that loss of the −30-kb enhancer or of RUNX2-binding activity affected the actions of the remaining enhancers in a hierarchical manner. These studies using CRISPR/Cas9 methodology disclosed that *Mmp13* enhancers strongly interact with each other as well as with the *Mmp13* gene promoter, and that 1 enhancer mediates a hierarchical, master regulatory action on *Mmp13* expression. Interestingly, PTH response was mediated through RUNX2-binding activity near the *Mmp13* promoter,[160] as suggested by Partridge and colleagues,[182–184] although the enhancer at −30 kb also exerted dominance over this proximal element as well.

CRISPR/Cas9-mediated deletion of the 1,25-dihydroxvyvitamin D₃–inducible Mmp13 enhancer in vivo

To examine the role of the hormone-inducible regulatory enhancer in the *Mmp13* gene in vivo, the authors used the CRISPR/Cas9 approach to delete the −10-kb enhancer region in the *Mmp13* locus in the mouse, obtaining homozygous mice through subsequent cross-breeding.[160] Bone marrow cells from the −10-kb enhancer–deleted mice were then isolated, cultured in osteogenic medium, and examined for response to $1,25(OH)_2D_3$ compared with control mice. Although wild-type cells responded strongly to $1,25(OH)_2D_3$, those derived from the enhancer-deleted mice were resistant. These results confirm the regulatory role of this specific *Mmp13* enhancer in vivo and highlight the utility of the CRISPR/Cas9 approach in defining enhancer activities in vivo.

SUMMARY

This article discusses the metabolic activation of vitamin D to its hormonal form; the mechanism of its action to regulate genes through a specific nuclear receptor; its central homeostatic function to regulate mineral metabolism through genes that include *S100G*, *ATP2B1*, and *TRPV6*; and the regulation of additional genes in the skeleton that include *TNFSF11* (*RANKL*). It also discusses the actions of vitamin D to regulate genes such as *IL-17* in the immune system. New methodologies have emerged in the past few years that now enable detailed studies of these transcriptional mechanisms in unprecedented detail both in cells in culture and in animal models in vivo. These approaches are leading to profound new insights into the mechanisms through which the vitamin D hormone operates not only to control mineral metabolism but to modulate unique cell-specific biology in numerous extraskeletal systems as well. These molecular details have the potential to illuminate novel mechanisms that may be sensitive to newly designed vitamin D therapeutics.

ACKNOWLEDGMENTS

The work cited in this article was supported by numerous grants from the NIH to J.W. Pike and S. Christakos. The authors wish to thank past and current members of their laboratories for their contributions to the individual work described here and the numerous senior collaborators who have also been involved in specific aspects of this research. We also acknowledge Laura Vanderploeg and Puneet Dhawan for artistic contributions to this article.

REFERENCES

1. Mellanby E. An experimental investigation on rickets. Lancet 1919;1:407–12.
2. McCollum E, Simmonds N, Becker J, et al. An experimental demonstration of the existence of a vitamin which promotes calcium deposition. J Biol Chem 1922; 1922:293–8.
3. Steenbock H, Black A. Fat soluble vitamins. XVII. The induction of growth promoting and calcifying properties in a ration by exposure to ultraviolet light. J Biol Chem 1924;61:405–22.

4. Windaus A, Schenck F, von Werden F. Uber das antirachitisch wirksame bestrahlungs-produkt aus 7-dehydrocholesterin. Hoppe-Seyler's Z Physiol Chem 1936;241:100–3.
5. DeLuca HF. Overview of general physiologic features and functions of vitamin D. Am J Clin Nutr 2004;80(6 Suppl):1689S–96S.
6. Brumbaugh P, Haussler M. 1 Alpha,25-dihydroxycholecalciferol receptors in intestine. I. Association of 1 alpha,25-dihydroxycholecalciferol with intestinal mucosa chromatin. J Biol Chem 1974;249(4):1251–7.
7. Brumbaugh PF, Haussler MR. 1a,25-dihydroxycholecalciferol receptors in intestine. II. Temperature-dependent transfer of the hormone to chromatin via a specific cytosol receptor. J Biol Chem 1974;249(4):1258–62.
8. Pike JW, Haussler MR. Purification of chicken intestinal receptor for 1,25-dihydroxyvitamin D. Proc Natl Acad Sci U S A 1979;76(11):5485–9.
9. Pike JW, Meyer MB, Benkusky NA, et al. Genomic determinants of vitamin D-regulated gene expression. Vitam Horm 2016;100:21–44.
10. McDonnell DP, Mangelsdorf DJ, Pike JW, et al. Molecular cloning of complementary DNA encoding the avian receptor for vitamin D. Science 1987;235(4793): 1214–7.
11. Baker AR, McDonnell DP, Hughes M, et al. Cloning and expression of full-length cDNA encoding human vitamin D receptor. Proc Natl Acad Sci U S A 1988; 85(10):3294–8.
12. Evans RM. The steroid and thyroid hormone receptor superfamily. Science 1988;240(4854):889–95.
13. Plum LA, DeLuca HF. Vitamin D, disease and therapeutic opportunities. Nat Rev Drug Discov 2010;9(12):941–55.
14. Feldman D, Krishnan AV, Swami S, et al. The role of vitamin D in reducing cancer risk and progression. Nat Rev Cancer 2014;14(5):342–57.
15. DeLuca HF. The vitamin D story: a collaborative effort of basic science and clinical medicine. FASEB J 1988;2(3):224–36.
16. Cheng JB, Motola DL, Mangelsdorf DJ, et al. De-orphanization of cytochrome P450 2R1: a microsomal vitamin D 25-hydroxilase. J Biol Chem 2003;278(39): 38084–93.
17. Cheng JB, Levine MA, Bell NH, et al. Genetic evidence that the human CYP2R1 enzyme is a key vitamin D 25-hydroxylase. Proc Natl Acad Sci U S A 2004; 101(20):7711–5.
18. Al Mutair AN, Nasrat GH, Russell DW. Mutation of the CYP2R1 vitamin D 25-hydroxylase in a Saudi Arabian family with severe vitamin D deficiency. J Clin Endocrinol Metab 2012;97(10):E2022–5.
19. Zhu JG, Ochalek JT, Kaufmann M, et al. CYP2R1 is a major, but not exclusive, contributor to 25-hydroxyvitamin D production in vivo. Proc Natl Acad Sci U S A 2013;110(39):15650–5.
20. Holick MF, Schnoes HK, DeLuca HF. Identification of 1,25-dihydroxycholecalciferol, a form of vitamin D3 metabolically active in the intestine. Proc Natl Acad Sci U S A 1971;68(4):803–4.
21. Fu GK, Lin D, Zhang MY, et al. Cloning of human 25-hydroxyvitamin D-1 alpha-hydroxylase and mutations causing vitamin D-dependent rickets type 1. Mol Endocrinol 1997;11(13):1961–70.
22. Fraser D, Kooh SW, Kind HP, et al. Pathogenesis of hereditary vitamin-D-dependent rickets. An inborn error of vitamin D metabolism involving defective conversion of 25-hydroxyvitamin D to 1 alpha,25-dihydroxyvitamin D. N Engl J Med 1973;289(16):817–22.

23. Dardenne O, Prud'homme J, Arabian A, et al. Targeted inactivation of the 25-hydroxyvitamin D(3)-1(alpha)-hydroxylase gene (CYP27B1) creates an animal model of pseudovitamin D-deficiency rickets. Endocrinology 2001;142(7): 3135–41.
24. Garabedian M, Holick MF, Deluca HF, et al. Control of 25-hydroxycholecalciferol metabolism by parathyroid glands. Proc Natl Acad Sci U S A 1972;69(7): 1673–6.
25. Quarles LD. Skeletal secretion of FGF-23 regulates phosphate and vitamin D metabolism. Nat Rev Endocrinol 2012;8(5):276–86.
26. Hu MC, Shiizaki K, Kuro-o M, et al. Fibroblast growth factor 23 and Klotho: physiology and pathophysiology of an endocrine network of mineral metabolism. Annu Rev Physiol 2013;75:503–33.
27. Jones G, Prosser DE, Kaufmann M. Cytochrome P450-mediated metabolism of vitamin D. J Lipid Res 2014;55(1):13–31.
28. Shimada T, Hasegawa H, Yamazaki Y, et al. FGF-23 is a potent regulator of vitamin D metabolism and phosphate homeostasis. J Bone Miner Res 2004; 19(3):429–35.
29. Clinkenbeard EL, White KE. Systemic control of bone homeostasis by FGF23 signaling. Curr Mol Biol Rep 2016;2(1):62–71.
30. Ajibade D, Dhawan P, Fechner A, et al. Evidence for a role of prolactin in calcium homeostasis: regulation of intestinal transient receptor potential vanilloid type 6, intestinal calcium absorption, and the 25-hydroxyvitamin D(3) 1alpha hydroxylase gene by prolactin. Endocrinology 2010;151(7):2974–84.
31. Hewison M, Burke F, Evans KN, et al. Extra-renal 25-hydroxyvitamin D3-1alpha-hydroxylase in human health and disease. J Steroid Biochem Mol Biol 2007; 103(3–5):316–21.
32. Bikle DD, Pillai S. Vitamin D, calcium, and epidermal differentiation. Endocr Rev 1993;14(1):3–19.
33. Bikle DD. Vitamin D and the skin. J Bone Miner Metab 2010;28(2):117–30.
34. Omdahl JL, Morris HA, May BK. Hydroxylase enzymes of the vitamin D pathway: expression, function, and regulation. Annu Rev Nutr 2002;22:139–66.
35. Veldurthy V, Wei R, Campbell M, et al. 25-hydroxyvitamin D₃ 24-hydroxylase: a key regulator of 1,25(OH)₂D₃ catabolism and calcium homeostasis. Vitam Horm 2016;100:137–50.
36. Christakos S, Dhawan P, Verstuyf A, et al. Vitamin D: Metabolism, molecular mechanism of action, and pleiotropic effects. Physiol Rev 2016;96(1):365–408.
37. St-Arnaud R. Targeted inactivation of vitamin D hydroxylases in mice. Bone 1999;25(1):127–9.
38. St-Arnaud R, Glorieux FH. 24,25-Dihydroxyvitamin D–active metabolite or inactive catabolite? Endocrinology 1998;139(8):3371–4.
39. Schlingmann KP, Kaufmann M, Weber S, et al. Mutations in CYP24A1 and idiopathic infantile hypercalcemia. N Engl J Med 2011;365(5):410–21.
40. Tebben PJ, Milliner DS, Horst RL, et al. Hypercalcemia, hypercalciuria, and elevated calcitriol concentrations with autosomal dominant transmission due to CYP24A1 mutations: effects of ketoconazole therapy. J Clin Endocrinol Metab 2012;97(3):E423–7.
41. Streeten EA, Zarbalian K, Damcott CM. CYP24A1 mutations in idiopathic infantile hypercalcemia. N Engl J Med 2011;365(18):1741–2 [author reply: 1742–3].
42. Dinour D, Beckerman P, Ganon L, et al. Loss-of-function mutations of CYP24A1, the vitamin D 24-hydroxylase gene, cause long-standing hypercalciuric nephrolithiasis and nephrocalcinosis. J Urol 2013;190(2):552–7.

43. Meyer MB, Goetsch PD, Pike JW. A downstream intergenic cluster of regulatory enhancers contributes to the induction of *CYP24A1* expression by 1alpha,25-dihydroxyvitamin D$_3$. J Biol Chem 2010;285(20):15599–610.

44. Gheldof N, Smith E, Tabuchi T, et al. Cell-type-specific long-range looping interactions identify distant regulatory elements of the CFTR gene. Nucleic Acids Res 2010;38(13):4325–36.

45. Omdahl JL. Interaction of the parathyroid and 1,25-dihydroxyvitamin D3 in the control of renal 25-hydroxyvitamin D3 metabolism. J Biol Chem 1978;253(23): 8474–8.

46. Martin A, David V, Quarles LD. Regulation and function of the FGF23/klotho endocrine pathways. Physiol Rev 2012;92(1):131–55.

47. DeLuca HF, Krisinger J, Darwish H. The vitamin D system: 1990. Kidney Int Suppl 1990;29:S2–8.

48. Hoenderop JGJ, Nilius B, Bindels RJM. Calcium absorption across epithelia. Physiol Rev 2005;85(1):373–422.

49. Amling M, Priemel M, Holzmann T, et al. Rescue of the skeletal phenotype of vitamin D receptor-ablated mice in the setting of normal mineral ion homeostasis: formal histomorphometric and biomechanical analyses. Endocrinology 1999;140(11):4982–7.

50. Masuyama R, Nakaya Y, Katsumata S, et al. Dietary calcium and phosphorus ratio regulates bone mineralization and turnover in vitamin D receptor knockout mice by affecting intestinal calcium and phosphorus absorption. J Bone Miner Res 2003;18(7):1217–26.

51. Hochberg Z, Tiosano D, Even L. Calcium therapy for calcitriol-resistant rickets. J Pediatr 1992;121(5 Pt 1):803–8.

52. Benn BS, Ajibade D, Porta A, et al. Active intestinal calcium transport in the absence of transient receptor potential vanilloid type 6 and calbindin-D9k. Endocrinology 2008;149(6):3196–205.

53. Kutuzova GD, Akhter S, Christakos S, et al. Calbindin D(9k) knockout mice are indistinguishable from wild-type mice in phenotype and serum calcium level. Proc Natl Acad Sci U S A 2006;103(33):12377–81.

54. Kutuzova GD, Sundersingh F, Vaughan J, et al. TRPV6 is not required for 1alpha,25-dihydroxyvitamin D3-induced intestinal calcium absorption in vivo. Proc Natl Acad Sci U S A 2008;105(50):19655–9.

55. Cui M, Li Q, Johnson R, et al. Villin promoter-mediated transgenic expression of transient receptor potential cation channel, subfamily V, member 6 (TRPV6) increases intestinal calcium absorption in wild-type and vitamin D receptor knockout mice. J Bone Miner Res 2012;27(10):2097–107.

56. Lee SM, Riley EM, Meyer MB, et al. 1,25-Dihydroxyvitamin D3 controls a cohort of vitamin D receptor target genes in the proximal intestine that is enriched for calcium-regulating components. J Biol Chem 2015;290(29):18199–215.

57. Wasserman RH. Vitamin D and the dual processes of intestinal calcium absorption. J Nutr 2004;134(11):3137–9.

58. Reyes-Fernandez PC, Fleet JC. Compensatory changes in calcium metabolism accompany the loss of vitamin D receptor (VDR) from the distal intestine and kidney of mice. J Bone Miner Res 2016;31(1):143–51.

59. Christakos S, Seth T, Hirsch J, et al. Vitamin D biology revealed through the study of knockout and transgenic mouse models. Annu Rev Nutr 2013;33: 71–85.

60. Yasuda H, Shima N, Nakagawa N, et al. Identity of osteoclastogenesis inhibitory factor (OCIF) and osteoprotegerin (OPG): a mechanism by which OPG/OCIF inhibits osteoclastogenesis in vitro. Endocrinology 1998;139(3):1329–37.
61. Xiong J, Onal M, Jilka RL, et al. Matrix-embedded cells control osteoclast formation. Nat Med 2011;17(10):1235–41.
62. Kim S, Yamazaki M, Zella L, et al. Activation of receptor activator of NF-kappaB ligand gene expression by 1,25-dihydroxyvitamin D3 is mediated through multiple long-range enhancers. Mol Cell Biol 2006;26(17):6469–86.
63. Lieben L, Masuyama R, Torrekens S, et al. Normocalcemia is maintained in mice under conditions of calcium malabsorption by vitamin D-induced inhibition of bone mineralization. J Clin Invest 2012;122(5):1803–15.
64. Bonewald LF. Osteocytes as dynamic multifunctional cells. Ann N Y Acad Sci 2007;1116:281–90.
65. Bonewald LF, Johnson ML. Osteocytes, mechanosensing and Wnt signaling. Bone 2008;42(4):606–15.
66. Qing H, Ardeshirpour L, Pajevic PD, et al. Demonstration of osteocytic perilacunar/canalicular remodeling in mice during lactation. J Bone Miner Res 2012; 27(5):1018–29.
67. Murali SK, Andrukhova O, Clinkenbeard EL, et al. Excessive osteocytic Fgf23 secretion contributes to pyrophosphate accumulation and mineralization defect in hyp mice. PLoS Biol 2016;14(4):e1002427.
68. Shimada T, Mizutani S, Muto T, et al. Cloning and characterization of FGF23 as a causative factor of tumor-induced osteomalacia. Proc Natl Acad Sci U S A 2001; 98(11):6500–5.
69. Yu X, Sabbagh Y, Davis SI, et al. Genetic dissection of phosphate- and vitamin D-mediated regulation of circulating Fgf23 concentrations. Bone 2005;36(6): 971–7.
70. Yu X, White KE. FGF23 and disorders of phosphate homeostasis. Cytokine Growth Factor Rev 2005;16(2):221–32.
71. Zinser GM, Sundberg JP, Welsh J. Vitamin D(3) receptor ablation sensitizes skin to chemically induced tumorigenesis. Carcinogenesis 2002;23(12):2103–9.
72. Zinser G, Welsh J. Effect of vitamin D3 receptor ablation on murine mammary gland development and tumorigenesis. J Steroid Biochem Mol Biol 2004; 89-90(1–5):433–6.
73. Xiang W, Kong J, Chen S, et al. Cardiac hypertrophy in vitamin D receptor knockout mice: role of the systemic and cardiac renin-angiotensin systems. Am J Physiol Endocrinol Metab 2005;288(1):E125–32.
74. Froicu M, Weaver V, Wynn TA, et al. A crucial role for the vitamin D receptor in experimental inflammatory bowel diseases. Mol Endocrinol 2003;17(12): 2386–92.
75. Cantorna MT. Mechanisms underlying the effect of vitamin D on the immune system. Proc Nutr Soc 2010;69(3):286–9.
76. Haussler MR, Myrtle JF, Norman AW. The association of a metabolite of vitamin D3 with intestinal mucosa chromatin in vivo. J Biol Chem 1968;243(15):4055–64.
77. Burmester JK, Maeda N, DeLuca HF. Isolation and expression of rat 1,25-dihydroxyvitamin D3 receptor cDNA. Proc Natl Acad Sci U S A 1988;85(4):1005–9.
78. Jin CH, Kerner SA, Hong MH, et al. Transcriptional activation and dimerization functions in the human vitamin D receptor. Mol Endocrinol 1996;10(8):945–57.
79. McDonnell D, Scott R, Kerner S, et al. Functional domains of the human vitamin D3 receptor regulate osteocalcin gene expression. Mol Endocrinol 1989;3(4): 635–44.

80. Hughes MR, Malloy PJ, Kieback DG, et al. Point mutations in the human vitamin D receptor gene associated with hypocalcemic rickets. Science 1988; 242(4886):1702–5.

81. Miyamoto K, Kesterson R, Yamamoto H, et al. Structural organization of the human vitamin D receptor chromosomal gene and its promoter. Mol Endocrinol 1997;11(8):1165–79.

82. Hughes M, Malloy P, O'Malley B, et al. Genetic defects of the 1,25-dihydroxyvitamin D3 receptor. J Recept Res 1991;11(1–4):699–716.

83. Malloy P, Hochberg Z, Tiosano D, et al. The molecular basis of hereditary 1,25-dihydroxyvitamin D3 resistant rickets in seven related families. J Clin Invest 1990;86(6):2071–9.

84. Ritchie H, Hughes M, Thompson E, et al. An ochre mutation in the vitamin D receptor gene causes hereditary 1,25-dihydroxyvitamin D3-resistant rickets in three families. Proc Natl Acad Sci U S A 1989;86(24):9783–7.

85. Sone T, Scott R, Hughes M, et al. Mutant vitamin D receptors which confer hereditary resistance to 1,25-dihydroxyvitamin D3 in humans are transcriptionally inactive in vitro. J Biol Chem 1989;264(34):20230–4.

86. Brooks MH, Bell NH, Love L, et al. Vitamin-D-dependent rickets type II. Resistance of target organs to 1,25-dihydroxyvitamin D. N Engl J Med 1978; 298(18):996–9.

87. Eil C, Liberman UA, Rosen JF, et al. A cellular defect in hereditary vitamin-D-dependent rickets type II: defective nuclear uptake of 1,25-dihydroxyvitamin D in cultured skin fibroblasts. N Engl J Med 1981;304(26):1588–91.

88. Pike J, Dokoh S, Haussler M, et al. Vitamin D3–resistant fibroblasts have immunoassayable 1,25-dihydroxyvitamin D3 receptors. Science 1984;224(4651): 879–81.

89. Sone T, Marx S, Liberman U, et al. A unique point mutation in the human vitamin D receptor chromosomal gene confers hereditary resistance to 1,25-dihydroxyvitamin D3. Mol Endocrinol 1990;4(4):623–31.

90. Lin N, Malloy P, Sakati N, et al. A novel mutation in the deoxyribonucleic acid-binding domain of the vitamin D receptor causes hereditary 1,25-dihydroxyvitamin D-resistant rickets. J Clin Endocrinol Metab 1996;81(7):2564–9.

91. Malloy PJ, Tasic V, Taha D, et al. Vitamin D receptor mutations in patients with hereditary 1,25-dihydroxyvitamin D-resistant rickets. Mol Genet Metab 2014; 111(1):33–40.

92. Christakos S, Gabrielides C, Rhoten WB. Vitamin D-dependent calcium binding proteins: chemistry, distribution, functional considerations, and molecular biology. Endocr Rev 1989;10(1):3–26.

93. Gill RK, Christakos S. Identification of sequence elements in mouse calbindin-D28k gene that confer 1,25-dihydroxyvitamin D3- and butyrate-inducible responses. Proc Natl Acad Sci U S A 1993;90(7):2984–8.

94. Price PA, Baukol SA. 1,25-Dihydroxyvitamin D3 increases synthesis of the vitamin K-dependent bone protein by osteosarcoma cells. J Biol Chem 1980; 255(24):11660–3.

95. Lian JB, Stein GS, Stewart C, et al. Osteocalcin: characterization and regulated expression of the rat gene. Connect Tissue Res 1989;21(1–4):61–8 [discussion: 69].

96. Prince CW, Butler WT. 1,25-Dihydroxyvitamin D3 regulates the biosynthesis of osteopontin, a bone-derived cell attachment protein, in clonal osteoblast-like osteosarcoma cells. Coll Relat Res 1987;7(4):305–13.

97. Haussler MR, Chandler JS, Pike JW, et al. Physiological importance of vitamin D metabolism. Prog Biochem Pharmacol 1980;17:134–42.

98. Kerner SA, Scott RA, Pike JW. Sequence elements in the human osteocalcin gene confer basal activation and inducible response to hormonal vitamin D3. Proc Natl Acad Sci U S A 1989;86(12):4455–9.

99. Ozono K, Liao J, Kerner SA, et al. The vitamin D-responsive element in the human osteocalcin gene. Association with a nuclear proto-oncogene enhancer. J Biol Chem 1990;265(35):21881–8.

100. Noda M, Vogel RL, Craig AM, et al. Identification of a DNA sequence responsible for binding of the 1,25-dihydroxyvitamin D3 receptor and 1,25-dihydroxyvitamin D3 enhancement of mouse secreted phosphoprotein 1 (SPP-1 or osteopontin) gene expression. Proc Natl Acad Sci U S A 1990;87(24):9995–9.

101. Ohyama Y, Ozono K, Uchida M, et al. Identification of a vitamin D-responsive element in the 5'-flanking region of the rat 25-hydroxyvitamin D3 24-hydroxylase gene. J Biol Chem 1994;269(14):10545–50.

102. Ohyama Y, Ozono K, Uchida M, et al. Functional assessment of two vitamin D-responsive elements in the rat 25-hydroxyvitamin D3 24-hydroxylase gene. J Biol Chem 1996;271(48):30381–5.

103. Zierold C, Darwish HM, DeLuca HF. Identification of a vitamin D-response clement in the rat calcidiol (25-hydroxyvitamin D3) 24-hydroxylase gene. Proc Natl Acad Sci U S A 1994;91(3):900–2.

104. Zierold C, Darwish H, DeLuca H. Two vitamin D response elements function in the rat 1,25-dihydroxyvitamin D 24-hydroxylase promoter. J Biol Chem 1995; 270(4):1675–8.

105. Carlberg C. Molecular basis of the selective activity of vitamin D analogues. J Cell Biochem 2003;88(2):274–81.

106. Joshi S, Pantalena LC, Liu XK, et al. 1,25-dihydroxyvitamin D(3) ameliorates Th17 autoimmunity via transcriptional modulation of interleukin-17A. Mol Cell Biol 2011;31(17):3653–69.

107. Demay MB, Kiernan MS, DeLuca HF, et al. Sequences in the human parathyroid hormone gene that bind the 1,25-dihydroxyvitamin D3 receptor and mediate transcriptional repression in response to 1,25-dihydroxyvitamin D3. Proc Natl Acad Sci U S A 1992;89(17):8097–101.

108. Liao J, Ozono K, Sone T, et al. Vitamin D receptor interaction with specific DNA requires a nuclear protein and 1,25-dihydroxyvitamin D3. Proc Natl Acad Sci U S A 1990;87(24):9751–5.

109. Sone T, Ozono K, Pike JW. A 55-kilodalton accessory factor facilitates vitamin D receptor DNA binding. Mol Endocrinol 1991;5(11):1578–86.

110. Sone T, Kerner S, Pike JW. Vitamin D receptor interaction with specific DNA. Association as a 1,25-dihydroxyvitamin D3-modulated heterodimer. J Biol Chem 1991;266(34):23296–305.

111. Mangelsdorf DJ, Evans RM. The RXR heterodimers and orphan receptors. Cell 1995;83(6):841–50.

112. Kliewer SA, Umesono K, Mangelsdorf DJ, et al. Retinoid X receptor interacts with nuclear receptors in retinoic acid, thyroid hormone and vitamin D3 signalling. Nature 1992;355(6359):446–9.

113. Thompson PD, Remus LS, Hsieh JC, et al. Distinct retinoid X receptor activation function-2 residues mediate transactivation in homodimeric and vitamin D receptor heterodimeric contexts. J Mol Endocrinol 2001;27(2):211–27.

114. Pathrose P, Barmina O, Chang CY, et al. Inhibition of 1,25-dihydroxyvitamin D3-dependent transcription by synthetic LXXLL peptide antagonists that target the activation domains of the vitamin D and retinoid X receptors. J Bone Miner Res 2002;17(12):2196–205.

115. Orlov I, Rochel N, Moras D, et al. Structure of the full human RXR/VDR nuclear receptor heterodimer complex with its DR3 target DNA. EMBO J 2012;31(2): 291–300.

116. Carlson M, Laurent BC. The SNF/SWI family of global transcriptional activators. Curr Opin Cell Biol 1994;6(3):396–402.

117. Smith CL, O'Malley BW. Coregulator function: a key to understanding tissue specificity of selective receptor modulators. Endocr Rev 2004;25(1):45–71.

118. Rachez C, Freedman LP. Mechanisms of gene regulation by vitamin D(3) receptor: a network of coactivator interactions. Gene 2000;246(1–2):9–21.

119. Lewis BA, Reinberg D. The mediator coactivator complex: functional and physical roles in transcriptional regulation. J Cell Sci 2003;116(Pt 18):3667–75.

120. Arrowsmith CH, Bountra C, Fish PV, et al. Epigenetic protein families: a new frontier for drug discovery. Nat Rev Drug Discov 2012;11(5):384–400.

121. Xie W, Schultz MD, Lister R, et al. Epigenomic analysis of multilineage differentiation of human embryonic stem cells. Cell 2013;153(5):1134–48.

122. Gifford CA, Ziller MJ, Gu H, et al. Transcriptional and epigenetic dynamics during specification of human embryonic stem cells. Cell 2013;153(5):1149–63.

123. Ho L, Crabtree GR. Chromatin remodelling during development. Nature 2010; 463(7280):474–84.

124. McInerney EM, Rose DW, Flynn SE, et al. Determinants of coactivator LXXLL motif specificity in nuclear receptor transcriptional activation. Genes Dev 1998;12(21):3357–68.

125. Perissi V, Staszewski LM, McInerney EM, et al. Molecular determinants of nuclear receptor-corepressor interaction. Genes Dev 1999;13(24):3198–208.

126. Westin S, Kurokawa R, Nolte RT, et al. Interactions controlling the assembly of nuclear-receptor heterodimers and co-activators. Nature 1998;395(6698): 199–202.

127. Zella LA, Meyer MB, Nerenz RD, et al. Multifunctional enhancers regulate mouse and human vitamin D receptor gene transcription. Mol Endocrinol 2010;24(1): 128–47.

128. Meyer MB, Zella LA, Nerenz RD, et al. Characterizing early events associated with the activation of target genes by 1,25-dihydroxyvitamin D_3 in mouse kidney and intestine in vivo. J Biol Chem 2007;282(31):22344–52.

129. Martowicz ML, Meyer MB, Pike JW. The mouse RANKL gene locus is defined by a broad pattern of histone H4 acetylation and regulated through distinct distal enhancers. J Cell Biochem 2011;112(8):2030–45.

130. Hoffman MM, Ernst J, Wilder SP, et al. Integrative annotation of chromatin elements from ENCODE data. Nucleic Acids Res 2013;41(2):827–41.

131. Ernst J, Kellis M. Discovery and characterization of chromatin states for systematic annotation of the human genome. Nat Biotechnol 2010;28(8):817–25.

132. Ernst J, Kheradpour P, Mikkelsen TS, et al. Mapping and analysis of chromatin state dynamics in nine human cell types. Nature 2011;473(7345):43–9.

133. Thurman RE, Rynes E, Humbert R, et al. The accessible chromatin landscape of the human genome. Nature 2012;489(7414):75–82.

134. Bernstein BE, Stamatoyannopoulos JA, Costello JF, et al. The NIH roadmap epigenomics mapping consortium. Nat Biotechnol 2010;28(10):1045–8.

135. Kellis M, Wold B, Snyder MP, et al. Defining functional DNA elements in the human genome. Proc Natl Acad Sci U S A 2014;111(17):6131–8.

136. Stamatoyannopoulos JA. What does our genome encode? Genome Res 2012; 22(9):1602–11.

137. Maurano MT, Wang H, John S, et al. Role of DNA methylation in modulating transcription factor occupancy. Cell Rep 2015;12(7):1184–95.
138. Wang Z, Gerstein M, Snyder M. RNA-Seq: a revolutionary tool for transcriptomics. Nat Rev Genet 2009;10(1):57–63.
139. Cong L, Ran FA, Cox D, et al. Multiplex genome engineering using CRISPR/Cas systems. Science 2013;339(6121):819–23.
140. Hille F, Charpentier E. CRISPR-Cas: biology, mechanisms and relevance. Philos Trans R Soc Lond B Biol Sci 2016;371(1707). pii:20150496.
141. Singh A, Chakraborty D, Maiti S. CRISPR/Cas9: a historical and chemical biology perspective of targeted genome engineering. Chem Soc Rev 2016; 45(24):6666–84.
142. Kim S, Shevde N, Pike J. 1,25-Dihydroxyvitamin D3 stimulates cyclic vitamin D receptor/retinoid X receptor DNA-binding, co-activator recruitment, and histone acetylation in intact osteoblasts. J Bone Miner Res 2005;20(2):305–17.
143. Meyer MB, Goetsch PD, Pike JW. Genome-wide analysis of the VDR/RXR cistrome in osteoblast cells provides new mechanistic insight into the actions of the vitamin D hormone. J Steroid Biochem Mol Biol 2010;121(1–2):136–41.
144. Meyer MB, Benkusky NA, Lee CH, et al. Genomic determinants of gene regulation by 1,25-dihydroxyvitamin D_3 during osteoblast-lineage cell differentiation. J Biol Chem 2014;289(28):19539–54.
145. Meyer MB, Benkusky NA, Sen B, et al. Epigenetic plasticity drives adipogenic and osteogenic differentiation of marrow-derived mesenchymal stem cells. J Biol Chem 2016;291(34):17829–47.
146. St John HC, Bishop KA, Meyer MB, et al. The osteoblast to osteocyte transition: epigenetic changes and response to the vitamin D3 hormone. Mol Endocrinol 2014;28(7):1150–65.
147. Ramagopalan SV, Heger A, Berlanga AJ, et al. A ChIP-seq defined genome-wide map of vitamin D receptor binding: associations with disease and evolution. Genome Res 2010;20(10):1352–60.
148. Heikkinen S, Väisänen S, Pehkonen P, et al. Nuclear hormone 1α,25-dihydroxyvitamin D3 elicits a genome-wide shift in the locations of VDR chromatin occupancy. Nucleic Acids Res 2011;39(21):9181–93.
149. Meyer MB, Goetsch PD, Pike JW. VDR/RXR and TCF4/β-catenin cistromes in colonic cells of colorectal tumor origin: impact on c-FOS and c-MYC gene expression. Mol Endocrinol 2012;26(1):37–51.
150. Ong CT, Corces VG. Enhancer function: new insights into the regulation of tissue-specific gene expression. Nat Rev Genet 2011;12(4):283–93.
151. Lee SM, Meyer MB, Benkusky NA, et al. Mechanisms of enhancer-mediated hormonal control of vitamin D receptor gene expression in target cells. J Biol Chem 2015;290(51):30573–86.
152. Meyer MB, Watanuki M, Kim S, et al. The human transient receptor potential vanilloid type 6 distal promoter contains multiple vitamin D receptor binding sites that mediate activation by 1,25-dihydroxyvitamin D_3 in intestinal cells. Mol Endocrinol 2006;20(6):1447–61.
153. Deng W, Blobel GA. Do chromatin loops provide epigenetic gene expression states? Curr Opin Genet Dev 2010;20(5):548–54.
154. Deng W, Lee J, Wang H, et al. Controlling long-range genomic interactions at a native locus by targeted tethering of a looping factor. Cell 2012;149(6):1233–44.
155. Deng W, Blobel GA. Manipulating nuclear architecture. Curr Opin Genet Dev 2014;25:1–7.

156. Deng W, Blobel GA. Detecting long-range enhancer-promoter interactions by quantitative chromosome conformation capture. Methods Mol Biol 2017;1468: 51–62.
157. Whalen S, Truty RM, Pollard KS. Enhancer-promoter interactions are encoded by complex genomic signatures on looping chromatin. Nat Genet 2016;48(5): 488–96.
158. Meyer MB, Benkusky NA, Pike JW. The RUNX2 cistrome in osteoblasts: characterization, down-regulation following differentiation, and relationship to gene expression. J Biol Chem 2014;289(23):16016–31.
159. Meyer MB, Benkusky NA, Pike JW. Selective distal enhancer control of the Mmp13 gene identified through clustered regularly interspaced short palindromic repeat (CRISPR) genomic deletions. J Biol Chem 2015;290(17): 11093–107.
160. Meyer MB, Benkusky NA, Onal M, et al. Selective regulation of Mmp13 by 1,25(OH)2D3, PTH, and Osterix through distal enhancers. J Steroid Biochem Mol Biol 2015. http://dx.doi.org/10.1016/j.jsbmb.2015.1009.1001.
161. Meyer MB, Pike JW. Corepressors (NCoR and SMRT) as well as coactivators are recruited to positively regulated 1α,25-dihydroxyvitamin D3-responsive genes. J Steroid Biochem Mol Biol 2013;136:120–4.
162. Ding N, Yu RT, Subramaniam N, et al. A vitamin D receptor/SMAD genomic circuit gates hepatic fibrotic response. Cell 2013;153(3):601–13.
163. Seth-Vollenweider T, Joshi S, Dhawan P, et al. Novel mechanism of negative regulation of 1,25-dihydroxyvitamin D3-induced 25-hydroxyvitamin D3 24-hydroxylase (Cyp24a1) Transcription: epigenetic modification involving crosstalk between protein-arginine methyltransferase 5 and the SWI/SNF complex. J Biol Chem 2014;289(49):33958–70.
164. Meyer MB, Benkusky NA, Pike JW. Profiling histone modifications by chromatin immunoprecipitation coupled to deep sequencing in skeletal cells. Methods Mol Biol 2015;1226:61–70.
165. Pike JW, Meyer MB, St John HC, et al. Epigenetic histone modifications and master regulators as determinants of context dependent nuclear receptor activity in bone cells. Bone 2015;81:757–64.
166. Deplancke B, Alpern D, Gardeux V. The genetics of transcription factor DNA binding variation. Cell 2016;166(3):538–54.
167. Pike JW, Lee SM, Meyer MB. Regulation of gene expression by 1,25-dihydroxyvitamin D3 in bone cells: exploiting new approaches and defining new mechanisms. Bonekey Rep 2014;3:482.
168. Ding N, Hah N, Yu RT, et al. BRD4 is a novel therapeutic target for liver fibrosis. Proc Natl Acad Sci U S A 2015;112(51):15713–8.
169. Ong CT, Corces VG. Modulation of CTCF insulator function by transcription of a noncoding RNA. Dev Cell 2008;15(4):489–90.
170. Denker A, de Laat W. A long-distance chromatin affair. Cell 2015;162(5):942–3.
171. Denker A, de Laat W. The second decade of 3C technologies: detailed insights into nuclear organization. Genes Dev 2016;30(12):1357–82.
172. Galli C, Zella LA, Fretz JA, et al. Targeted deletion of a distant transcriptional enhancer of the receptor activator of nuclear factor-kappaB ligand gene reduces bone remodeling and increases bone mass. Endocrinology 2008; 149(1):146–53.
173. Suda T, Takahashi N, Udagawa N, et al. Modulation of osteoclast differentiation and function by the new members of the tumor necrosis factor receptor and ligand families. Endocr Rev 1999;20(3):345–57.

174. Lacey DL, Timms E, Tan HL, et al. Osteoprotegerin ligand is a cytokine that regulates osteoclast differentiation and activation. Cell 1998;93(2):165–76.
175. Boyle WJ, Simonet WS, Lacey DL. Osteoclast differentiation and activation. Nature 2003;423(6937):337–42.
176. Kitazawa R, Kitazawa S. Vitamin D(3) augments osteoclastogenesis via vitamin D-responsive element of mouse RANKL gene promoter. Biochem Biophys Res Commun 2002;290(2):650–5.
177. Kitazawa S, Kajimoto K, Kondo T, et al. Vitamin D3 supports osteoclastogenesis via functional vitamin D response element of human RANKL gene promoter. J Cell Biochem 2003;89(4):771–7.
178. Bishop KA, Coy HM, Nerenz RD, et al. Mouse Rankl expression is regulated in T cells by c-Fos through a cluster of distal regulatory enhancers designated the T cell control region. J Biol Chem 2011;286(23):20880–91.
179. Bishop KA, Wang X, Coy HM, et al. Transcriptional regulation of the human TNFSF11 gene in T cells via a cell type-selective set of distal enhancers. J Cell Biochem 2015;116(2):320–30.
180. Onal M, St John HC, Danielson AL, et al. Deletion of the distal Tnfsf11 RI -D2 enhancer that contributes to PTH-mediated RANKL expression in osteoblast lineage cells results in a high bone mass phenotype in mice. J Bone Miner Res 2016;31(2):416–29.
181. Onal M, St John HC, Danielson AL, et al. Unique distal enhancers linked to the mouse Tnfsf11 gene direct tissue-specific and inflammation-induced expression of RANKL. Endocrinology 2016;157(2):482–96.
182. Selvamurugan N, Jefcoat SC, Kwok S, et al. Overexpression of Runx2 directed by the matrix metalloproteinase-13 promoter containing the AP-1 and Runx/RD/Cbfa sites alters bone remodeling in vivo. J Cell Biochem 2006;99(2):545–57.
183. Shimizu E, Selvamurugan N, Westendorf JJ, et al. Parathyroid hormone regulates histone deacetylases in osteoblasts. Ann N Y Acad Sci 2007;1116:349–53.
184. Shimizu E, Nakatani T, He Z, et al. Parathyroid hormone regulates histone deacetylase (HDAC) 4 through protein kinase A-mediated phosphorylation and dephosphorylation in osteoblastic cells. J Biol Chem 2014;289(31):21340–50.

Global Overview of Vitamin D Status

Natasja van Schoor, PhD[a],*, Paul Lips, MD, PhD[b]

KEYWORDS

- Adults • Global • Vitamin D status

KEY POINTS

- Vitamin D deficiency occurs all over the world, mainly in the Middle East, China, Mongolia, and India.
- Risk groups for vitamin D deficiency include older persons, pregnant women, and non-western immigrants.
- Prevention of vitamin D deficiency is feasible with moderate sunlight exposure, consumption of fatty fish and vitamin D-fortified foods, and the use of vitamin D supplements.
- The required dose in healthy older persons is about 400 to 800 IU per day, the higher dose with low sun exposure or pigmented skin.
- Patients with osteoporosis and older institutionalized persons require 800 IU per day.
- A vitamin D3 supplement of 400 IU per day can be recommended for adults who do not have sun exposure or have a pigmented skin.
- The goal of prevention should be to increase serum 25-hydroxyvitamin D levels to more than 50 nmol/L in all countries all year long.

INTRODUCTION

Many studies have been published describing the vitamin D status in different populations, most of them in individual countries. Vitamin D status is assessed by measuring 25-hydroxyvitamin D, or 25(OH)D. According to the Institute of Medicine, vitamin D deficiency occurs when the serum 25(OH)D concentration is below 30 nmol/L (12 ng/mL).[1] However, opinions differ on whether the optimal serum 25(OH)D for skeletal effects, and possibly muscle strength and nonclassical effects, should be 50 nmol/L as according to the Institute of Medicine[1,2] or 75 nmol/L as according to the Endocrine Society.[3] Despite that there is no complete agreement about the required levels for

Disclosure: P. Lips gave advice to Friesland Campina Nederland BV, Dairy Industry.
[a] Department of Epidemiology and Biostatistics, Amsterdam Public Health Research Institute, VU University Medical Center, Van der Boechorststraat 7, Amsterdam 1081 BT, The Netherlands;
[b] Department of Internal Medicine, Endocrine Section, VU University Medical Center, PO Box 7057, Amsterdam 1007 MB, The Netherlands
* Corresponding author.
E-mail address: nm.vanschoor@vumc.nl

Endocrinol Metab Clin N Am 46 (2017) 845–870
http://dx.doi.org/10.1016/j.ecl.2017.07.002
0889-8529/17/© 2017 Elsevier Inc. All rights reserved.

endo.theclinics.com

optimal health, most clinicians agree that clinical vitamin D deficiency only occurs when serum 25(OH)D is lower than 25 or 30 nmol/L (10 or 12 ng/mL).[2,4,5]

Different studies use different assays. As a consequence, a considerable variation may occur up to 25% in the section of the population needing treatment because of vitamin D deficiency.[6] Currently, liquid chromatography, followed by tandem mass spectrometry (LC-MS/MS) has become the gold standard due to its better precision compared with immunoassays. It also allows separate measurement of $25(OH)D_2$ and $25(OH)D_3$. The Vitamin D External Quality Assessment Scheme (DEQAS) now distributes sera to around 1100 laboratories. Participating laboratories receive the results as the difference between their laboratory and the overall mean value.[7] The Vitamin D Standardization Program (VDSP) uses standards provided by the National Institute of Standardization Technology (NIST) to decrease variation and improve the accuracy of the assays.[8,9] Frozen samples from existing studies can also be used to standardize existing serum 25(OH)D data. In **Fig. 1**, it can be seen how serum 25(OH)D values of the Longitudinal Aging Study Amsterdam (LASA) were standardized using the VDSP protocol as part of the ODIN study.[10] In this way, an unbiased comparison between different studies from different countries becomes feasible.

In recent years, numerous studies describing the vitamin D status have been published and excellent reviews have been performed.[11,12] In this article, we include a selection of the larger studies published in the last decade if available using standardized serum 25(OH)D assessment. It also includes studies presenting the vitamin D status in 1 or more continents performed in a central laboratory. In these studies, interlaboratory variation is not a problem. In the next sections, some important determinants of poor vitamin D status in adults, the vitamin D status in different continents, and implications for the future are described.

DETERMINANTS OF POOR VITAMIN D STATUS IN ADULTS

Vitamin D3 is produced in the skin under the influence of the ultraviolet light of the sun and is for a smaller part available form dietary sources. Although sufficient exposure to sunlight is important for the production of vitamin D3, too much sunlight exposure is not recommended because of the increased risk of skin cancer. Factors influencing the production of vitamin D_3 from sunlight are the duration of sunlight exposure; the

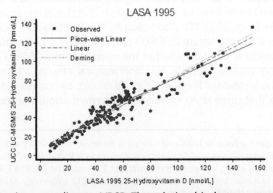

Fig. 1. Standardization according to VDSP. The relationship between serum 25(OH)D in a sample of the LASA (Longitudinal Aging Study Amsterdam) measured by original 25(OH) D assay and standardized LC-MS/MS at UCC (University College Cork). Original Nichols assay: mean 53.2; SD 24.0; median 50.9. VDSP-calibrated: mean 49.1; SD 18.7; median 48.4. Best fit: piecewise linear regression fit (R2 = 0.89). (Figure constructed as part of the ODIN project. Published with permission from Dr Kevin Cashman.)

available ultraviolet light, which varies with latitude, season, and time of the day; skin pigmentation; and the use of sunscreen. Risk groups for poor vitamin D status in adults include older persons, pregnant women, and non-Western immigrants. In older persons, dermal synthesis of vitamin D3 is less efficient. In addition, older persons, especially nursing home residents, may be less mobile and may have less sunlight exposure. In non-Western immigrants migrating to countries with limited sunshine, risk factors such as a pigmented skin, sun-avoiding behavior, a covering clothing style, and a diet low in fish and dairy products may play an important role. The lower the actual sun exposure, the more nutrition becomes important, especially the consumption of fatty fish, vitamin D-fortified foods and vitamin D supplements. Fortification of milk or dairy products is practiced in the United States, Sweden, Finland, and Ireland.

VITAMIN D STATUS IN NORTH AMERICA (INCLUDING CANADA AND MEXICO)

In **Table 1**, a selection of studies examining the vitamin D status in North America is presented. The largest study in North America is the National Health and Nutrition Examination Survey (NHANES). Several NHANES studies on vitamin D status were published. In a recent article, the vitamin D status of a representative sample of the US population (aged $\geq$1 year) in the period 2007 to 2010 was published using LC-MS/MS standardized to international reference materials (n = 15,652).[13] In this publication, data were presented according to age group (from 1–5 to $\geq$60 years), sex, race-ethnicity, and different vitamin D metabolites, that is, 25(OH)D$_3$, 25(OH)D$_2$, and C3-epimer of 25(OH)D$_3$. Prevalence of serum 25(OH)D below 30 and 50 was higher in the age group 20 to 39 years than in the age group 60 years and older. Relatively high serum concentrations of 25(OH)D2 were observed in the age group 60 years or older, probably as a consequence of widespread prescription of vitamin D2 supplements. In the total population (including children and adolescents), mean serum 25(OH)D was lowest in non-Hispanic blacks (46.6 nmol/L) and highest in non-Hispanic whites (75.2 nmol/L). Also, the data of the Canadian Health Measures Survey (CHMS) were standardized using the VDSP reference measurement system.[14] In the total population (including children and adolescents), average 25(OH)D was 58.3 nmol/L and 36.8% had a concentration below 50 nmol/L.[14]

VITAMIN D STATUS IN SOUTH AMERICA

The number of studies published on vitamin D status in South America has been growing (**Table 2**). In several studies, a very high prevalence of persons having serum 25(OH)D below 50 nmol/L was observed. In institutionalized women living in Argentina, 86% of the women had a serum 25(OH)D below 50 nmol/L(86%).[15]

VITAMIN D STATUS IN EUROPE

Many reports describe the vitamin D status in most European countries (**Table 3**). Studies performed in Eastern Europe have been summarized in a recent review.[16] Data from surveys performed in Iceland, Norway, Ireland, the United Kingdom, the Netherlands, Germany, and Greece have recently been standardized by LC-MS/MS and a NIST standard in the framework of the European ODIN (Food-based solutions for optimal vitamin D nutrition and health through the life cycle) study,[10] enabling more reliable comparison between countries. It is apparent that vitamin D status is usually better in Nordic than in Mediterranean countries despite higher latitude and less sunshine. This may be caused by the high intake of cod, cod liver, and cod liver oil in Norway and Sweden; a lighter skin; and more sun bathing.[17] In multicenter

Table 1
Vitamin D status in North America (including Canada and Mexico)

Country Latitude Degree North or South (N/S)	Reference	Study Population	Number	Age (y)	25(OH)D Mean ± SD nmol/l	<25 nmol/L %	<50 nmol/L %	Comments
Canada	Sarafin et al,[14] 2015	Men and women	11,336	3–79	58.3 (SE: 0.9)	7.4 (<30)	36.8 (<50)	Representative sample (CHMS), standardized data
Canada	Green-Finestone et al,[40] 2011	Men and women	1912	35–70+	70.4 (SE: 0.55)	2.3 (<27.5)	20.4	Population-based sample from 7 cities (CaMos)
Canada	Langlois et al,[41] 2010	Community-dwelling	5306	6–79 6–11 12–19 20–39 40–59 60–79	67.7 (65.3–70.1)[a] 75.0 (70.3–79.7)[a] 68.1 (63.8–72.4)[a] 65.0 (61.0–69.0)[a] 66.5 (63.8–69.2)[a] 72.0 (69.4–74.5)[a]	.1 (<27.5) 0.6 (<37.5) — — — —	—	Representative sample of Canada (Atlantic provinces, Quebec, Ontario, the Prairies, British Columbia)
Canada (Newfoundland, Labrador) 47–58 N	Sloka et al,[42] 2009	*Pregnant women* End of winter End of summer	304 289	—	52.1 68.6	6.6 (deficient) 1.7 (deficient)	89 (insufficient) 64 (insufficient)	—
Canada (Northern Alberta) 53 ± 3 N	Chao et al,[43] 2013	Workers	6101	42 ± 14	84 ± 42	3 (<27.5) 8 (<37.5)	40 (37.5–75)	—
Canada (Calgary) 51 N	Aucoin et al,[44] 2013	Refugee women	461	20–45 y	46.2 (44.1–48.3)[a]	21	61	—
Canada (Sherbrooke) 45 N	Lacroix et al,[45] 2014	Pregnant women (6–13 wk)	655	28.4 ± 4.5	63.0 ± 18.8	—	26.7	—
USA	Schleiger et al,[13] 2016	Men and women	3349 3377 3602	20–39 40–59 60+	64.6 (62.2–66.9) 67.9 (66.0–69.9) 71.0 (68.9–73.0)	8.2 (<30) 5.9 (<30) 5.7 (<30)	30 24 22	Representative sample (NHANES), standardized data, race-ethnicity differences observed

Location	Reference	Population	No.	Age	25(OH)D	22.3 (<30)	55.4	Comments
USA	Gernand et al,[46] 2013	Pregnant women (<26 wk)	2048	<20–30+	51.2 ± 27.2	22.3 (<30)	55.4	12 medical centers across USA
USA	Shea et al,[47] 2011	*Older adults*						Random sample of well-functioning older adults (70–81 y) (Health ABC study)
		Black	977	70–81	52.5 ± 26.0	9	54	
		White	1607		73.0 ± 27.3	2	18	
USA	Ginde et al,[48] 2010	Pregnant	928	13–44	65 (61–68)[a]	7	33	Representative sample (NHANES)
		Nonpregnant	5173		59 (57–61)[a]	10	42	
USA (Alabama, Minnesota, California, Pennsylvania, Oregon)	Orwoll et al,[49] 2009	Older men from general community	1606	73.8 ± 5.9	62.8 ± 19.8	2.9	25.7	—
USA (rural Southwest Alaska) 63N	Fohner et al,[50] 2016	Yup'ik Alaska native people	743	14–93	77 ± 31.5	—	—	—
USA (Minnesota)	Campagna et al,[51] 2013	Immigrant & refugee	1378	—	—	15.1	60.0	—
USA (Massachusetts) 41–42 N	Penrose et al,[52] 2012	Refugees	2610	23 median age at arrival	—	—	43	25(OH)D<50 nmol/L most prevalent in refugees from Middle East
USA (Eastern Nebraska) 41 N	Lappe et al,[53] 2006	Rural postmenopausal white women	1179	66.7 ± 7.3	71.8 ± 20.3 April–Oct: 71.1 ± 20.0	4 (<37.5)	14.4	—
Mexico (Toluca) 19 N	Clark et al,[54] 2015	Healthy subjects	585	41.1 ± 15	52.3	2.0	43.6	—

a 95% Confidence interval.
Abbreviations: CaMos, Canadian Multicentre Osteoporosis Study; SE, standard error of the mean.

Table 2
Vitamin D status in South America

City, State Latitude Degree N/S	Reference	Study Population	Number	Age (y)	Mean ± SD nmol/l	25(OH)D		Comments
						<25 nmol/L %	<50 nmol/L %	
Guatemala (Quetzaltenango) 14 N	Sud et al,[55] 2010	Healthy older Mayans	108	69.0 ± 7.2	53.3 ± 15.0	—	46.3	—
Ecuador (Andes mountains and coastal regions)	Orces,[56] 2015	Older adults participating in national health survey	2374	71.0 ± 8.3	60–69 y 69.0 ± 28.8 70–79 y 63.8 ± 24.3 ≥80 y 64.8 ± 33.0	—	21.6	—
Brazil (Joao Pessoa) 7 S	Issa et al,[57] 2016	Random sample of elderly	142	≥60	64.1 ± 8.2	—	40.8 (<75)	—
Brazil (Sao Paulo) 23 S	Lopes et al,[58] 2014	Community-dwelling elderly	908	72.8 ± 4.8	48.5 ± 23.3	14.4	58.0	—
Brazil (Sao Paulo) 23 S	Martini et al,[59] 2013	Population-based sample	636	—	Adult men 48.4 ± 22.9 Elderly men 50.9 ± 2.9 Adult women 51.0 ± 26.1 Elderly women 53.9 ± 18.9	—	—	Differences in season of sampling between life stages
Brazil (Sao Paulo) 23 S	Eloi et al,[60] 2016	Database of laboratory results	39,004	2–95	63.9 ± 28.6	—	—	Greater area of Sao Paulo
Chile (Santiago) 33 S	Gonzalez et al,[61] 2007	*Healthy women* Premenopausal	30	32.6 ± 7.4	61.3 ± 19.5	0 (<22.5)	27	Half: winter (June–Sept)
		Postmenopausal	60	63.7 ± 9.7	48.8 ± 24.8	12 (<22.5)	60	Half: summer (Dec–March)
Argentina (Buenos Aires) 34 S	Portela et al,[15] 2010	Institutionalized women	48	81.3 ± 7.9	34.0 ± 15.3	32	86	End of summer

Table 3
Vitamin D status in Europe

Country Latitude Degree N/S	Reference	Study Population	Number	Age (y)	25(OH)D Mean ± SD nmol/l	<25 nmol/L %	<50 nmol/L %	Comments
Norway (Tromso) 69	Cashman et al,[10] 2016	Regionally representative	12,817	30–87	65.0 ± 17.6	0.3	18.6	ODIN
Norway (Oslo) 60	Cashman et al,[9] 2015	—	866	30–76	71.0 ± 19.5 (white)	0.1 (white)	14.9 (white)	—
Norway 60 N	Snellman et al,[62] 2009	Twins	204	—	84.8 ± 27.4	0	8	—
Finland 60–70	Cashman et al,[9] 2015	Nationally representative	4102	29–77	67.7 ± 13.2	0.2	6.6	—
Finland 60–68	Kauppi et al,[63] 2009	—	2736 men 3299 women	51 (30–97) 53 (30–94)	45.1 (5–132) 45.2 (7–134)	—	—	—
Finland 60–68 N	Viljakainen et al,[64] 2010	Mothers Newborns	98 98	30.5 ± 4	45 ± 12 29.2	—	—	—
Finland 60–68 N	Pekkarinen et al,[65] 2010	Older women	1604	62–79	45 (spring) 53 (autumn)	8.6	60.3	—
Iceland 64	Cashman et al,[10] 2016	Adult men and women	5519	66–96	57.0 ± 17.8	4.2	33.6	ODIN, regionally representative
Sweden 58	Melhus et al,[66] 2010	Older men	1194	71	68.7 ± 19.1	0.8	17	MrOs

(continued on next page)

Table 3
(continued)

Country Latitude Degree N/S	Reference	Study Population	Number	Age (y)	25(OH)D Mean ± SD nmol/l	<25 nmol/l %	<50 nmol/L %	Comments
Sweden 56	Buchebner et al,[67] 2014	OPRA women	995	80 (80–81)	78 ± 30	0	16	—
Denmark (Copenhagen) 56	Cashman et al,[9] 2015	Regionally representative	3409	19–72	65.0 ± 19.2	0	23.6	—
UK 50–59	Cashman et al,[10] 2016	Children, teens and adults Nationally representative	1488	1.5–91	47.4 ± 19.8	15.4	56.4	ODIN
UK 51–58 N	Roddam et al,[68] 2007	Patients with fractures	730	52	82 ± 40	—	21.7	—
		Controls	1445	52	81 ± 38		20.9	
UK 51–58 N	Prentice et al,[20] 2008	Nat Diet Nutr. Survey	—	16–80+	—	5–20	20–60	—
Ireland 51–54	Cashman et al,[69] 2013	Nationally representative	1118	18–84	56.4 ± 22.2	6.0	45.0	—
Germany 47–55	Cashman et al,[10] 2016	Nationally representative	6995	18–79	50.1 ± 18.1	4.2	54.5	ODIN
Netherlands 52	Cashman et al,[10] 2016	LASA 2009 Nationally representative	915	61–99	64.7 ± 22.6	2.4	28.5	ODIN

Country	Reference	Cohort/Study	N	Age				Study
Netherlands 52	Cashman et al,[10] 2016	Regionally representative	2625	40–66	59.5 ± 21.7	4.9	33.6	ODIN
Netherlands 52 N	Van Schoor et al,[34] 2008	LASA	1311	75.5 ± 6.6	53.5 ± 24.2	11.3%	48.4	—
Netherlands 52 N	Van Dam et al,[70] 2007	Hoorn cohort — Men / Women	271 / 267	69.4 ± 6.3 / 69.8 ± 6.7	—	Summer: 1.7 / Winter: 6.6	33.7 / 50.9	—
Netherlands 52 N	Van der Meer et al,[22] 2008	Adult women and men — 613: Dutch / Turkish / Moroccan / Surinam Asian / Surinam Creole / African		18–65	67 / 27 / 30 / 24 / 27 / 33	6 / 41 / 37 / 51 / 45 / 19	—	—
Belgium 51	Hoge et al,[71] 2015	Adults	697	42.7 (32–53)	49.3 (35–65)	7.3	51.1	—
France 43–49	Souberbielle et al,[72] 2016	VARIETE Study	892	18–89	60 ± 20	6.3	34.6	—
Spain	Gonzales-Molero et al,[73] 2011	Adults	1262	20–83	56	—	37% in winter	Asturias and Pizarra studies
Italy	Cadario et al,[74] 2015	Women at delivery — Italian 342 / Migrant 191		33.6 ± 5 / 29.8 ± 5.8	44.9 ± 21.2 / 29.7 ± 16.5	18 / 48.4	61.6 / 89.7	Piemonte
Greece	Vallianou et al,[75] 2012	Adults	472	46	—	—	28.6	Athens

Abbreviations: MrOs, Osteoporotic Fractures in Men Study; VARIETE, Establishment of Reference Values for Insulin-like Growth Factor 1 (IGF1) in the General Population.

studies using a central laboratory, a similar reversed north-south gradient is visible in Europe, with a positive correlation between serum 25(OH)D and latitude.[18] In contrast, the expected gradient with a decreasing serum 25(OH)D from south to north was visible in the French SUVIMAX (Supplementation en Vitamins et Mineraux Antioxydants) study, with a mean serum 25(OH)D of 94 nmol/L in the southwest and around 43 nmol/L in the northern regions of France.[19] The National Dietary and Nutrition Survey in the United Kingdom[20] showed a lower serum 25(OH)D in older persons than in adults. In addition, serum 25(OH)D was remarkably low in adolescents and young adults. Vitamin D status was poor in patients with hip fracture and the institutionalized. Very low serum 25(OH)D levels were observed in noninstitutionalized elderly in Switzerland. Also, in Italy and Greece serum 25(OH)D levels were quite low for the abundant sunshine in these countries. This may be caused by a more pigmented skin and by staying inside the home in summer because of the high temperatures. In general, vitamin D status was very poor in immigrants from non-Western countries,[21,22] compared with native people (see **Fig. 3**). In pregnant non-Western immigrants,[23] serum 25(OH)D often was lower than 25 nmol/L or undetectable.

VITAMIN D STATUS IN THE MIDDLE EAST

Vitamin D status was lower in these countries than expected based on the abundant sunshine (**Table 4**). In Turkey, Jordan, and Saudi Arabia, serum 25(OH)D was lower in women than in men. In women, vitamin D status depended on clothing style, being lower in traditionally clothed women than in women with Western-style clothing.[24] Serum 25(OH)D was very low in Saudi-Arabian women, caused by the completely covering clothing style. Comparable data were published in Egypt and Iran. Another explaining factor is the extreme heat leading to indoor life and low sun exposure.

VITAMIN D STATUS IN ASIA

In the last decade, many studies on vitamin D status in Asian countries have been published (**Table 5**). Vitamin D status was poor in patients with hip fracture in Yekaterinburg, Russia,[25] and in older control subjects. A poor vitamin D status was also observed in women and children in Mongolia, where rickets is very common in children.[20] Adolescent boys and girls in China also had very low serum 25(OH)D concentrations.[26] Vitamin D status was lower than expected in India, situated at a latitude between 13° and 27°. A pigmented skin, skin-covering clothes and sun-avoiding behavior may be the cause. Vitamin D status was better in southeastern Asian countries such as Malaysia and Japan.

VITAMIN D STATUS IN AFRICA

The literature on vitamin D status in Africa was recently reviewed.[27] Studies from African countries are summarized in **Table 6**. The vitamin D status in East and West Africa was adequate. The vitamin D status even was very good in patients with tuberculosis. However, in South Africa and in North Africa, low serum 25(OH)D concentrations were observed.[28]

VITAMIN D STATUS IN OCEANIA

Despite its sunny climate, a vitamin D status below 50 nmol/L is not uncommon in Oceania (**Table 7**). In a study performed in 3 different regions in Australia, higher mean 25(OH)D values were observed at lower latitudes, whereas a high prevalence

Table 4
Vitamin D status in the Middle East

Country Latitude Degree N/S	Reference	Study Population	Number	Age (y)	25(OH)D Mean ± SD nmol/l	<25 nmol/L %	<50 nmol/L %	Comments
Turkey	Hekimsoy et al,[76] 2010	Men	119	45.1 ± 17.5	51.8 ± 38.7	—	66.4	Manisa; low levels related to clothing style
		Women	272	45.1 ± 17.2	38.1 ± 28.7		78.7	
Turkey	Buyukuslu et al,[77] 2014	Female students	100	20.9 ± 2.1	65.7 ± 25	—	34.0	Istanbul; Low levels related to clothing style
Iran	Omrani et al,[78] 2006	Adult women	676	42.3 ± 13.4	28.9 ± 23.0	52.2 (<23)	—	Shiraz
Iran	Hosseinpanah et al,[79] 2011	Healthy adults	251	56.7 ± 11.7	45.2 (27.5–77.5)	19.1	53.8 (<37.5)	Controls of a cardiovascular outcomes study
Israel	Saliba et al,[80] 2012	Men	198,834	0->80	54.8 ± 24.2	10.0	45.0	—
		Women			50.7 ± 24.6	16.2	51.8	
Jordan	Nichols et al,[24] 2012	Women	2032	15-50	27.5 (22.7–33.7)	60.3 (<30)	95.7	Low levels related to clothing style
Saudi Arabia	Hussain et al,[81] 2014	Men	3363	0->60	50.5	23.7	—	Riyadh; Serum 25(OH)D <25 nmol/L in 49% of adolescents
		Women	7346		41.9	35.6		
Saudi Arabia	Alfawaz et al,[82] 2014	Men	756	46.9 ± 16.3	35.5 ± 30.6	36.1	72.4	—
		Women	2719			48.8	78.1	
Egypt	Olama et al,[83] 2013	Healthy women	50	33.1 ± 9.7	47.0 ± 13.5	6 (<20)	30	Controls of a fibromyalgia study

Table 5
Vitamin D status in Asia

Country Latitude Degree N/S	Reference	Study Population	Number	Age (y)	25(OH)D Mean ± SD nmol/L	<25 nmol/L %	<50 nmol/L %	Comments
China 40 N	Zhao et al,[84] 2011	Postmenopausal women	1724	64.1 ± 9.2	33.0 ± 13.5	—	89.7	Beijing
China 43.5 N	Yu et al,[85] 2015	Men	178	40.6 ± 13.6	51 ± 15.5	2.2	53.9	Urumqi
China 39.5			191		44 ± 15.7	11.0	66.5	Beijing
China 39.0			265		58.5 ± 16.0	0.8	32.1	Dalian
China 30.3			220		51.5 ± 14.5	3.6	49.1	Hangzhou
China 23.1			223		55.7 ± 12.5	0.4	32.2	Guangzhou
China 43.5		Women	224		41.5 ± 16.5	11.1	77.2	Urumqi
China 39.5			224		37.5 ± 14.8	20.1	79.5	Beijing
China 39.0			215		49.5 ± 15.5	4.2	54.4	Dalian
China 30.3			217		43.2 ± 13.0	6.0	72.4	Hangzhou
China 23.1			216		51.2 ± 11.5	0	47.2	Guangzhou
China 31	Lu et al,[86] 2012	Men	649	45.5 ± 14.8	57.0 median	2	30	Shanghai
		Women	1939	42.2 ± 15.9	50.2 median	3.6	46	
China 39.5	Song et al,[87] 2013	Pregnant women	125	28.4 ± 2.9	28.4 ± 9.5	44.8	96.8	Beijing
China 31.5	Xiao et al,[88] 2015	Pregnant women	5823	26.4 ± 3.1	34.0 median	40.7 (<30)	78.7	Wuxi
China 22	Ke et al,[89] 2015	—	566	19–84	50.6 ± 17	—	55	Macau
China 36	Zhen et al,[90] 2015	Women 7136	7136	40–75	39.2 ± 17.8	—	75.2	Lanzhou
		Men 2902	2902		45.3 ± 15.7			
China 28	Li et al,[91] 2014	Postmenopausal women	578	62.2 ± 6.1	43.5 ± 14.3	—	72.1	Changsha
China 22	Chan et al,[92] 2011	Men	939	72.8 ± 5.1	77.9 ± 20.5	—	5.9	Hong Kong

China 22	Xu et al,[93] 2015	Adults	933	18–44	42–57	—	—	Hong Kong
		Adults	544	45–64	47–69			
		Adults	51	65+	41–56			
Japan 38 N	Nakamura et al,[94] 2015	Men	9084	60.1 ± 9.3	55.9 ± 18.8	—	53.6	Niigata prefecture
		Women		59.3 ± 9.2	45.2 ± 16.6			
Korea	Choi et al,[95] 2011	Women	3878	45.0 ± 19.3	45.5 ± 17.7	10.4	64.5	4th Korea NHANES
		Men	3047	42.4 ± 19.6	53.0 ± 18.7	4.7	47.3	
Korea	Kim et al,[96] 2012	Adolescents boys	1095	10–18	45.9 ± 15.7	11.7	64.2	4th Korea NHANES
		Adolescent girls	967	10–18	42.4 ± 14.7	15.4	72.6	
Malaysia 3	Chee et al,[97] 2010	Postmenopausal women	178	59.7 ± 5.0	60.4 ± 15.6	—	50.6	Kuala Lumpur
Malaysia 3	Moy,[98] 2011	Adults men	158	48.5 ± 5.2	56.2 ± 18.9	—	67.9	Kuala Lumpur
		Women	222		36.2 ± 13.4			
Vietnam	Laillou et al,[99] 2013	Women	541	32.9	44.5	17 (<30)	57	—
		Children	485	3.7	43.4	21 (<30)	58	
Thailand	Pratumvinit et al,[100] 2015	Pregnant women	147	28.9 ± 6.4	61.6 ± 19.3	0.7	34	Bangkok
Cambodia	Smith et al,[101] 2016	Women	725	15–49	69.7 ± 31.2	4.1	29	—
Singapore	Loy et al,[102] 2015	Pregnant women	940	30.5 ± 5.1	81.0 ± 27.2	—	—	41% <75 nmol/L
India	Marwaha et al,[103] 2011	Pregnant women	541	—	23.2 ± 12.2	—	96.3	—
India	Shivane et al,[104] 2011	Young men	558	25–35	47.2 ± 22.2	12.0	62.0	—
		Young women	579		39.5 ± 22.7	26.4	76.1	
Pakistan	Mehboobali et al,[105] 2015	Women	507	18–60	42.3 ± 17.2	—	76	Karachi Low income
		Men	351		60.1 ± 19.3		33	
Pakistan	Junaid et al,[106] 2015	Women	215	28.4 ± 7.2	40.4 ± 34.4	43	73	Lahore

Table 6
Vitamin D status in Africa

Country Latitude Degree N/S	Reference	Study Population	Number	Age (y)	25(OH)D Mean ± SD nmol/l	25(OH)D <25 nmol/L %	25(OH)D <50 nmol/L %	Comments
Morocco	El Maghraoui et al,[107] 2012	Women >50 y	178	58.8 ± 8.2	39.5 ± 29.0	51.6	65.7	Osteoporosis 25%
Ethiopia	Gebreegziabher & Stoecker,[108] 2013	Women	202	30.8 ± 7.8	—	14.8 (<30)	84.2	—
Nigeria	Olayiwola et al,[109] 2014	Adults	240	>60	—	51.4	—	Older Yoruba in Ibadan
Tanzania 2–10 S	Mehta et al,[110] 2009	HIV-infected women Low D / Adequate D	347 / 537	24.6 ± 5 / 24.6 ± 5	60.5 ± 15 / 107.8 ± 22.5	—	—	—
Tanzania	Friis et al,[111] 2013	Healthy adults / Tuberculosis patients	355 / 1223	<25–>55	84.4 ± 25.6 / 110.9 ± 35.7	—	4.3 / 2.5	Case-control study in Mwanza
Tanzania 2–4	Luxwolda et al,[112] 2013	Nonpregnant adults / Pregnant women	88 / 139	33 ± 10	106.8 ± 28.4 / 138.5 ± 35.0	0	1	Traditional outside lifestyle
Guinea-Bissau 10 S	Wejse et al,[113] 2009	Tuberculosis patients	365	37 ± 14	78.3 ± 22.8	—	—	—
South Africa 22–34 S	Haarburger et al,[28] 2009	Unselected	216	all ages	48.3 (5.5–106)	—	37 (<45)	—
South Africa	George et al,[114] 2013	African / Asian Indian	373 / 344	41.6 ± 13.1 / 43.5 ± 12.9	70.9 (51–95) / 41.8 (29–57)	3 (<30) / 15 (<30)	—	Johannesburg
South Africa	Kruger et al,[115] 2011	Adults	179 / 298 / 129 / 52	<50 / 50–60 / 60–70 / >70	77.3 / 71.2 / 66.2 / 64.7	—	—	—

of serum 25(OH)D less than 50 nmol/L was found in Tasmania (67.3%).[29] Also, in pregnant women, a high prevalence of insufficient vitamin D status was observed.

MULTICENTER STUDIES USING A CENTRAL LABORATORY FACILITY

In multicenter studies using a central laboratory facility, the use of different assays for serum 25(OH)D performed in different laboratories is excluded as a source of variation. The Euronut Seneca study in older persons from Mediterranean countries to Scandinavia[30] showed a positive correlation between serum 25(OH)D and latitude, that is, higher values in northern countries, the inverse of what should be expected from sunlight exposure as main source. Similar results were obtained at baseline in the MORE (multiple outcomes for raloxifene evaluation) study, a study on the effect of raloxifene versus placebo in postmenopausal women with osteoporosis,[18] and the bazedoxifene study.[31] In the bazedoxifene study, the correlation between serum 25(OH)D and latitude in continents outside Europe was negative, especially in winter as should be expected (**Fig. 2**). The baseline data of the bazedoxifene study also showed a relationship between serum 25(OH)D and affluence with lower 25(OH)D levels in Eastern Europe than in Western and Northern Europe. The MORE study, the bazedoxifene study, and another global study[18,31,32] were all done in postmenopausal women with osteoporosis. Because women participating in such clinical trials usually are more concerned about their health, it is likely that their vitamin D status was better than in the population. However, all these studies confirm that the vitamin D status in Middle Eastern countries is very poor.

ETHNIC BACKGROUND AND MIGRATION

Vitamin D status in immigrants from non-Western countries was poor in North America, Norway, the Netherlands, and Australia. In the Netherlands, a very low serum 25(OH)D (<25 nmol/L) was found in 41% of persons from Turkish descent, 36% in persons from Moroccan descent, and in 51% of persons from Surinam South Asian descent[22] (**Fig. 3**). A review on this subject concluded that serum 25(OH)D in non-Western immigrants in the Netherlands was much lower than in native Dutch people and was also lower than in people in their country of origin.[33]

IMPLICATIONS AND CONCLUSIONS

Vitamin D deficiency, when longstanding and severe, results in mineralization defects, rickets, or osteomalacia. When less severe it results in bone loss, osteoporosis, and fractures.[4,31,34] The causal relationship between vitamin D deficiency and fractures has been confirmed by randomized placebo-controlled clinical trials and meta-analyses showing that vitamin D supplementation with or without calcium can decrease the incidence of fractures.[35] In epidemiologic studies, vitamin D deficiency is also associated with muscular weakness, decreased physical performance, and falls.[36–38] In recent years, many association studies have been published on vitamin D with nonclassical outcomes, such as autoimmune disease, including type 1 diabetes and multiple sclerosis; infectious diseases, including tuberculosis and respiratory infections; cardiovascular disease; type 2 diabetes; several types of cancer; and depression.[39] However, regarding these nonclassical outcomes, most clinical trials have been negative, that is, they did not result in a decreased incidence of the disease, implicating that the relationship may not be causal. On the other side, the negative health effects from vitamin D deficiency may be considerable because of the great proportion of the population having a poor vitamin D status. Probably more than 50% of the Western-European population has a serum 25(OH)D level below

Table 7
Vitamin D status in Oceania

City, State Latitude Degree N/S	Reference	Study Population	Number	Age (y)	25(OH)D Mean ± SD nmol/l	<25 nmol/L %	<50 nmol/L %	Comments
Pacific Islands 18 S	Heere et al,[116] 2010	*Fijian women* Indigenous Fijian Indian Fijian	*511* 306 205	15–44	76 (73–78)[a] 80 (76–84)[a] 70 (66–74)[a]	—	11	Mean 25(OH)D higher in rural than urban women
Australia (Kalgoorlie) 31 S	Willix et al,[117] 2015	Pregnant Aboriginal Pregnant non-Aboriginal	100 100	24.8 ± 6.2 29.5 ± 5.1	46.7 ± 21.7 65.4 ± 18.4	18 2	56 20	—
Australia (Sydney) 33 S	Hirani et al,[118] 2013	Community dwelling men	1659	—	55.9 ± 22.2	9.6 (<30)	43	—
Australia (Adelaide) 34 S	Gill et al,[119] 2014	Adults	2413	50.6 ± 16.6	69.2 ± 26.4	0.9	22.7	—
Australia (Sydney) 34 S	Bowyer et al,[120] 2009	Pregnant women	971	29.8	52 (range: 17–174)	15	48	—
Australia 30–35 S	Daly et al,[121] 2012	Adults	11,218	≥25	62.8 ± 25.4	4	31	—
Australia (Victoria) 36 S	Davies-Tuck et al,[122] 2015	Early pregnancy	1550	30.0 ± 5.4	47.0 (12–178)	—	55%	Women with 25(OH)D<75 nmol/L were recommended to take 1000 IU/d and had an additional measurement at 28 wk

Country/region	Reference	Population	n	Age (years)				Season	Comments
New Zealand (Auckland) 36 S	Bolland et al,[123] 2008	Adults	21,987	>18	—	—	48	—	—
New Zealand (Auckland)	Wishart et al,[124] 2007	Refugees	869	17 (9–27)[b]	—	17	54	—	—
New Zealand (Auckland) 37 S	Bolland et al,[125] 2006	Community-dwelling men	378	57 ± 11	85 ± 31	Summer 0 Winter 0–2	Summer 0–17 Winter 0–20	—	—
Australia	van der Mei et al,[29] 2007	**Population based** SQ		75+		Winter/spring SQ: 7.1	Winter/spring SQ: 40.5	Winter/spring	3 different studies performed in 3 regions (Southeast Queensland, SQ 27 S; Geelong region, G 38 S; Tasmania, T 43 S)
		Men	211		72.2				
		Women	167		67.0				
		G				G: 7.9	G: 37.4		
		Women	561		75.5				
		T				T: 13.0	T: 67.3		
		Men	298		55.2				
		Women	432		51.1				
New Zealand	Nessvi et al,[126] 2011	Multiethnic sample of adult volunteers	133	18–34	45.2 (SE 1.8)	—	—		2 regions (Auckland 36 S and Dunedin 45 S)
			121	35–49	44.6 (SE 2.0)				
			130	50–64	52.0 (SE 1.9)				
			119	65–85	51.3 (SE 2.0)				
New Zealand (Invercargill, Dunedin) 45–46 S	Rockell et al,[127] 2008	Volunteers	342	—	Late summer: 79 Early spring: 51	—	—		—

[a] 95% confidence interval.
[b] Median (interquartile range).

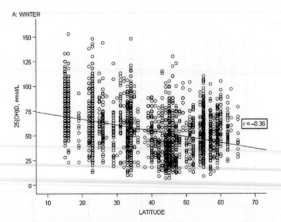

Fig. 2. Serum 25(OH)D according to latitude in winter in 3741 postmenopausal women in 6 continents. Baseline data from the bazedoxifene study, measured in a central laboratory facility. (*Data from* Kuchuk NO, van Schoor NM, Pluijm SM, et al. Vitamin D status, parathyroid function, bone turnover, and BMD in postmenopausal women with osteoporosis: global perspective. J Bone Miner Res 2009;24(4):693–701.)

50 nmol/L in winter.[31] This percentage is lower in North America, and is about similar in South America. The prevalence of vitamin D deficiency was more than 50% in South Africa, and around 20% to 50% in Oceania. The prevalence of severe vitamin D deficiency, serum 25(OH)D<25 nmol/L, was high in the Middle East and several Asian countries, including China, Mongolia, and India. More research on vitamin D deficiency and its prevention in these countries, especially in Asia, is warranted.

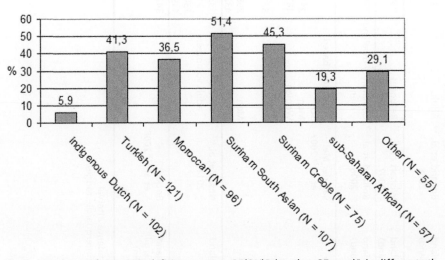

Fig. 3. Prevalence of vitamin D deficiency; serum 25(OH)D less than 25 nmol/L in different ethnicities in the Netherlands. (*Data from* van der Meer IM, Boeke AJ, Lips P, et al. Fatty fish and supplements are the greatest modifiable contributors to the serum 25-hydroxyvitamin D concentration in a multiethnic population. Clin Endocrinol (Oxf) 2008;68(3):466–72.)

In conclusion, to be able to estimate the burden of vitamin D deficiency, more prevalence studies are needed in Eastern Europe, the Middle East, Asia, and Africa. Quality control of the serum 25(OH)D assays should be done at least by participation in a quality-assurance scheme such as DEQAS,[7] and the percent of deviation from the overall mean should be reported. Preferably, results should be standardized by participating in a program such as VDSP.[10]

Prevention of vitamin D deficiency is feasible with moderate sunlight exposure, consumption of fatty fish, vitamin D-fortified foods, and the use of vitamin D supplements. The required dose in healthy older persons is about 400 to 800 IU per day, the higher dose with low sun exposure or pigmented skin. Patients with osteoporosis and older institutionalized persons require 800 IU per day. The required dose in pregnant and lactating women is uncertain but they may need 400 to 800 IU per day. A vitamin D3 supplement of 400 IU/d can be recommended for adults who do not have sun exposure or have a pigmented skin. Adherence to supplements is a problem and requires continuing attention. The goal of prevention should be to increase serum 25(OH)D levels to more than 50 nmol/L in all countries all year long.

REFERENCES

1. Ross AC, Manson JE, Abrams SA, et al. The 2011 report on dietary reference intakes for calcium and vitamin D from the Institute of Medicine: what clinicians need to know. J Clin Endocrinol Metab 2011;96(1):53–8.
2. EFSA (European Food Safety Authority), 2016. Outcome of a public consultation on the Draft Scientific Opinion of the EFSA Panel on Dietetic Products, Nutrition and Allergies (NDA) on Dietary Reference Values for vitamin D. EFSA supporting publication 2016;13(10):EN-1078. 100 pp.
3. Holick MF, Binkley NC, Bischoff-Ferrari HA, et al. Evaluation, treatment, and prevention of vitamin D deficiency: an endocrine society clinical practice guideline. J Clin Endocrinol Metab 2011;96(7):1911–30.
4. Lips P. Vitamin D deficiency and secondary hyperparathyroidism in the elderly: consequences for bone loss and fractures and therapeutic implications. Endocr Rev 2001;22(4):477–501.
5. Need AG, O'Loughlin PD, Morris HA, et al. Vitamin D metabolites and calcium absorption in severe vitamin D deficiency. J Bone Miner Res 2008;23(11):1859–63.
6. Barake M, Daher RT, Salti I, et al. 25-hydroxyvitamin D assay variations and impact on clinical decision making. J Clin Endocrinol Metab 2012;97(3):835–43.
7. Carter GD, Berry JL, Gunter E, et al. Proficiency testing of 25-hydroxyvitamin D (25-OHD) assays. J Steroid Biochem Mol Biol 2010;121(1–2):176–9.
8. Binkley N, Sempos CT. Standardizing vitamin D assays: the way forward. J Bone Miner Res 2014;29(8):1709–14.
9. Cashman KD, Dowling KG, Skrabakova Z, et al. Standardizing serum 25-hydroxyvitamin D data from four Nordic population samples using the Vitamin D Standardization Program protocols: Shedding new light on vitamin D status in Nordic individuals. Scand J Clin Lab Invest 2015;75(7):549–61.
10. Cashman KD, Dowling KG, Skrabakova Z, et al. Vitamin D deficiency in Europe: pandemic? Am J Clin Nutr 2016;103(4):1033–44.
11. Wahl DA, Cooper C, Ebeling PR, et al. A global representation of vitamin D status in healthy populations. Arch Osteoporos 2012;7:155–72.
12. Hilger J, Friedel A, Herr R, et al. A systematic review of vitamin D status in populations worldwide. Br J Nutr 2014;111(1):23–45.

13. Schleicher RL, Sternberg MR, Looker AC, et al. National estimates of serum total 25-hydroxyvitamin D and metabolite concentrations measured by liquid chromatography-tandem mass spectrometry in the US population during 2007-2010. J Nutr 2016;146(5):1051–61.

14. Sarafin K, Durazo-Arvizu R, Tian L, et al. Standardizing 25-hydroxyvitamin D values from the Canadian health measures survey. Am J Clin Nutr 2015; 102(5):1044–50.

15. Portela ML, Monico A, Barahona A, et al. Comparative 25-OH-vitamin D level in institutionalized women older than 65 years from two cities in Spain and Argentina having a similar solar radiation index. Nutrition 2010;26(3):283–9.

16. Pludowski P, Grant WB, Bhattoa HP, et al. Vitamin d status in central europe. Int J Endocrinol 2014;2014:589587.

17. Brustad M, Sandanger T, Aksnes L, et al. Vitamin D status in a rural population of northern Norway with high fish liver consumption. Public Health Nutr 2004;7(6): 783–9.

18. Lips P, Duong T, Oleksik A, et al. A global study of vitamin D status and para-thyroid function in postmenopausal women with osteoporosis: baseline data from the multiple outcomes of raloxifene evaluation clinical trial. J Clin Endocrinol Metab 2001;86(3):1212–21.

19. Chapuy MC, Preziosi P, Maamer M, et al. Prevalence of vitamin D insufficiency in an adult normal population. Osteoporos Int 1997;7(5):439–43.

20. Prentice A. Vitamin D deficiency: a global perspective. Nutr Rev 2008;66(10 Suppl 2):S153–64.

21. Meyer HE, Falch JA, Sogaard AJ, et al. Vitamin D deficiency and secondary hy-perparathyroidism and the association with bone mineral density in persons with Pakistani and Norwegian background living in Oslo, Norway, The Oslo Health Study. Bone 2004;35(2):412–7.

22. van der Meer IM, Boeke AJ, Lips P, et al. Fatty fish and supplements are the greatest modifiable contributors to the serum 25-hydroxyvitamin D concentra-tion in a multiethnic population. Clin Endocrinol (Oxf) 2008;68(3):466–72.

23. van der Meer IM, Karamali NS, Boeke AJ, et al. High prevalence of vitamin D deficiency in pregnant non-Western women in The Hague, Netherlands. Am J Clin Nutr 2006;84(2):350–3 [quiz: 468–9].

24. Nichols EK, Khatib IM, Aburto NJ, et al. Vitamin D status and determinants of deficiency among non-pregnant Jordanian women of reproductive age. Eur J Clin Nutr 2012;66(6):751–6.

25. Bakhtiyarova S, Lesnyak O, Kyznesova N, et al. Vitamin D status among patients with hip fracture and elderly control subjects in Yekaterinburg, Russia. Osteo-poros Int 2006;17(3):441–6.

26. Wu F, Laslett LL, Zhang Q. Threshold effects of vitamin D status on bone health in chinese adolescents with low calcium intake. J Clin Endocrinol Metab 2015; 100(12):4481–9.

27. Prentice A, Schoenmakers I, Jones KS, et al. Vitamin D deficiency and its health consequences in Africa. Clin Rev Bone Miner Metab 2009;7:94–106.

28. Haarburger D, Hoffman M, Erasmus RT, et al. Relationship between vitamin D, calcium and parathyroid hormone in Cape Town. J Clin Pathol 2009;62(6): 567–9.

29. van der Mei IA, Ponsonby AL, Engelsen O, et al. The high prevalence of vitamin D insufficiency across Australian populations is only partly explained by season and latitude. Environ Health Perspect 2007;115(8):1132–9.

30. van der Wielen RP, Lowik MR, van den BH, et al. Serum vitamin D concentrations among elderly people in Europe. Lancet 1995;346(8969):207–10.
31. Kuchuk NO, van Schoor NM, Pluijm SM, et al. Vitamin D status, parathyroid function, bone turnover, and BMD in postmenopausal women with osteoporosis: global perspective. J Bone Miner Res 2009;24(4):693–701.
32. Lips P, Hosking D, Lippuner K, et al. The prevalence of vitamin D inadequacy amongst women with osteoporosis: an international epidemiological investigation. J Intern Med 2006;260(3):245–54.
33. van der Meer IM, Middelkoop BJ, Boeke AJ, et al. Prevalence of vitamin D deficiency among Turkish, Moroccan, Indian and sub-Sahara African populations in Europe and their countries of origin: an overview. Osteoporos Int 2011;22(4): 1009–21.
34. van Schoor NM, Visser M, Pluijm SM, et al. Vitamin D deficiency as a risk factor for osteoporotic fractures. Bone 2008;42(2):260–6.
35. Lips P, Bouillon R, van Schoor NM, et al. Reducing fracture risk with calcium and vitamin D. Clin Endocrinol (Oxf) 2010;73(3):277–85.
36. Wicherts IS, van Schoor NM, Boeke AJ, et al. Vitamin D status predicts physical performance and its decline in older persons. J Clin Endocrinol Metab 2007; 92(6):2058–65.
37. Sohl E, de Jongh RT, Heijboer AC, et al. Vitamin D status is associated with physical performance: the results of three independent cohorts. Osteoporos Int 2013;24(1):187–96.
38. Snijder MB, van Schoor NM, Pluijm SM, et al. Vitamin D status in relation to one-year risk of recurrent falling in older men and women. J Clin Endocrinol Metab 2006;91(8):2980–5.
39. Bouillon R, Carmeliet G, Verlinden L, et al. Vitamin D and human health: lessons from vitamin D receptor null mice. Endocr Rev 2008;29(6):726–76.
40. Greene-Finestone LS, Berger C, de GM, et al. 25-hydroxyvitamin D in Canadian adults: biological, environmental, and behavioral correlates. Osteoporos Int 2011;22(5):1389–99.
41. Langlois K, Greene-Finestone L, Little J, et al. Vitamin D status of Canadians as measured in the 2007 to 2009 Canadian health measures survey. Health Rep 2010;21(1):47–55.
42. Sloka S, Stokes J, Randell E, et al. Seasonal variation of maternal serum vitamin D in Newfoundland and Labrador. J Obstet Gynaecol Can 2009;31(4):313–21.
43. Chao YS, Brunel L, Faris P, et al. Vitamin D status of Canadians employed in northern latitudes. Occup Med (Lond) 2013;63(7):485–93.
44. Aucoin M, Weaver R, Thomas R, et al. Vitamin D status of refugees arriving in Canada: findings from the Calgary refugee health program. Can Fam Physician 2013;59(4):e188–94.
45. Lacroix M, Battista MC, Doyon M, et al. Lower vitamin D levels at first trimester are associated with higher risk of developing gestational diabetes mellitus. Acta Diabetol 2014;51(4):609–16.
46. Gernand AD, Bodnar LM, Klebanoff MA, et al. Maternal serum 25-hydroxyvitamin D and placental vascular pathology in a multicenter US cohort. Am J Clin Nutr 2013;98(2):383–8.
47. Shea MK, Houston DK, Tooze JA, et al. Correlates and prevalence of insufficient 25-hydroxyvitamin D status in black and white older adults: the health, aging and body composition study. J Am Geriatr Soc 2011;59(7):1165–74.

48. Ginde AA, Sullivan AF, Mansbach JM, et al. Vitamin D insufficiency in pregnant and nonpregnant women of childbearing age in the United States. Am J Obstet Gynecol 2010;202(5):436–8.

49. Orwoll E, Nielson CM, Marshall LM, et al. Vitamin D deficiency in older men. J Clin Endocrinol Metab 2009;94(4):1214–22.

50. Fohner AE, Wang Z, Yracheta J, et al. Genetics, Diet, and Season Are Associated with Serum 25-Hydroxycholecalciferol Concentration in a Yup'ik Study Population from Southwestern Alaska. J Nutr 2016;146(2):318–25.

51. Campagna AM, Settgast AM, Walker PF, et al. Effect of country of origin, age, and body mass index on prevalence of vitamin D deficiency in a US immigrant and refugee population. Mayo Clin Proc 2013;88(1):31–7.

52. Penrose K, Hunter AJ, Nguyen T, et al. Vitamin D deficiency among newly resettled refugees in Massachusetts. J Immigr Minor Health 2012;14(6):941–8.

53. Lappe JM, Davies KM, Travers-Gustafson D, et al. Vitamin D status in a rural postmenopausal female population. J Am Coll Nutr 2006;25(5):395–402.

54. Clark P, Vivanco-Munoz N, Pina JT, et al. High prevalence of hypovitaminosis D in Mexicans aged 14 years and older and its correlation with parathyroid hormone. Arch Osteoporos 2015;10:226.

55. Sud SR, Montenegro-Bethancourt G, Bermudez OI, et al. Older Mayan residents of the western highlands of Guatemala lack sufficient levels of vitamin D. Nutr Res 2010;30(11):739–46.

56. Orces CH. Vitamin D status among older adults residing in the littoral and andes mountains in ecuador. ScientificWorldJournal 2015;2015:545297.

57. Issa CT, Silva AS, Toscano LT, et al. Relationship between cardiometabolic profile, vitamin D status and BsmI polymorphism of the VDR gene in non-institutionalized elderly subjects: Cardiometabolic profile, vitamin D status and BsmI polymorphism of the VDR gene in non-institutionalized elderly subjects. Exp Gerontol 2016;81:56–64.

58. Lopes JB, Fernandes GH, Takayama L, et al. A predictive model of vitamin D insufficiency in older community people: from the Sao Paulo aging & health study (SPAH). Maturitas 2014;78(4):335–40.

59. Martini LA Jr, Verly E Jr, Marchioni DM, et al. Prevalence and correlates of calcium and vitamin D status adequacy in adolescents, adults, and elderly from the health survey-Sao Paulo. Nutrition 2013;29(6):845–50.

60. Eloi M, Horvath DV, Szejnfeld VL, et al. Vitamin D deficiency and seasonal variation over the years in Sao Paulo, Brazil. Osteoporos Int 2016;27(12):3449–56.

61. Gonzalez G, Alvarado JN, Rojas A, et al. High prevalence of vitamin D deficiency in Chilean healthy postmenopausal women with normal sun exposure: additional evidence for a worldwide concern. Menopause 2007;14(3 Pt 1):455–61.

62. Snellman G, Melhus H, Gedeborg R, et al. Seasonal genetic influence on serum 25-hydroxyvitamin D levels: a twin study. PLoS One 2009;4(11):e7747.

63. Kauppi M, Impivaara O, Maki J, et al. Vitamin D status and common risk factors for bone fragility as determinants of quantitative ultrasound variables in a nationally representative population sample. Bone 2009;45(1):119–24.

64. Viljakainen HT, Saarnio E, Hytinantti T, et al. Maternal vitamin D status determines bone variables in the newborn. J Clin Endocrinol Metab 2010;95(4):1749–57.

65. Pekkarinen T, Turpeinen U, Hamalainen E, et al. Serum 25(OH)D3 vitamin status of elderly Finnish women is suboptimal even after summer sunshine but is not associated with bone density or turnover. Eur J Endocrinol 2010;162(1):183–9.

66. Melhus H, Snellman G, Gedeborg R, et al. Plasma 25-hydroxyvitamin D levels and fracture risk in a community-based cohort of elderly men in Sweden. J Clin Endocrinol Metab 2010;95(6):2637–45.
67. Buchebner D, McGuigan F, Gerdhem P, et al. Vitamin D insufficiency over 5 years is associated with increased fracture risk-an observational cohort study of elderly women. Osteoporos Int 2014;25(12):2767–75.
68. Roddam AW, Neale R, Appleby P, et al. Association between plasma 25-hydroxyvitamin D levels and fracture risk: the EPIC-Oxford study. Am J Epidemiol 2007; 166(11):1327–36.
69. Cashman KD, Kiely M, Kinsella M, et al. Evaluation of Vitamin D Standardization Program protocols for standardizing serum 25-hydroxyvitamin D data: a case study of the program's potential for national nutrition and health surveys. Am J Clin Nutr 2013;97(6):1235–42.
70. van Dam RM, Snijder MB, Dekker JM, et al. Potentially modifiable determinants of vitamin D status in an older population in the Netherlands: the Hoorn study. Am J Clin Nutr 2007;85(3):755–61.
71. Hoge A, Donneau AF, Streel S, et al. Vitamin D deficiency is common among adults In Wallonia (Belgium, 51 degrees 30' North): findings from the nutrition, environment and cardio-vascular health study. Nutr Res 2015;35(8):716–25.
72. Souberbielle JC, Massart C, Brailly-Tabard S, et al. Prevalence and determinants of vitamin D deficiency in healthy French adults: the VARIETE study. Endocrine 2016;53(2):543–50.
73. Gonzalez-Molero I, Morcillo S, Valdes S, et al. Vitamin D deficiency in Spain: a population-based cohort study. Eur J Clin Nutr 2011;65(3):321–8.
74. Cadario F, Savastio S, Magnani C, et al. High prevalence of vitamin D deficiency in native versus migrant mothers and newborns in the North of Italy: a call to act with a stronger prevention program. PLoS One 2015;10(6):e0129586.
75. Vallianou N, Bountziouka V, Akalestos T, et al. Vitamin D status and health correlates among apparently healthy participants in an urban, sunny region. Cent Eur J Public Health 2012;20(4):262–9.
76. Hekimsoy Z, Dinc G, Kafesciler S, et al. Vitamin D status among adults in the Aegean region of Turkey. BMC Public Health 2010;10:782.
77. Buyukuslu N, Esin K, Hizli H, et al. Clothing preference affects vitamin D status of young women. Nutr Res 2014;34(8):688–93.
78. Omrani GR, Masoompour SM, Sadegholvaad A, et al. Effect of menopause and renal function on vitamin D status in Iranian women. East Mediterr Health J 2006; 12(1–2):188–95.
79. Hosseinpanah F, Yarjanli M, Sheikholeslami F, et al. Associations between vitamin D and cardiovascular outcomes; Tehran lipid and glucose study. Atherosclerosis 2011;218(1):238–42.
80. Saliba W, Rennert HS, Kershenbaum A, et al. Serum 25(OH)D concentrations in sunny Israel. Osteoporos Int 2012;23(2):687–94.
81. Hussain AN, Alkhenizan AH, El SM, et al. Increasing trends and significance of hypovitaminosis D: a population-based study in the Kingdom of Saudi Arabia. Arch Osteoporos 2014;9:190.
82. Alfawaz H, Tamim H, Alharbi S, et al. Vitamin D status among patients visiting a tertiary care center in Riyadh, Saudi Arabia: a retrospective review of 3475 cases. BMC Public Health 2014;14:159.
83. Olama SM, Senna MK, Elarman MM, et al. Serum vitamin D level and bone mineral density in premenopausal Egyptian women with fibromyalgia. Rheumatol Int 2013;33(1):185–92.

84. Zhao J, Xia W, Nie M, et al. The levels of bone turnover markers in Chinese post-menopausal women: Peking Vertebral Fracture study. Menopause 2011;18(11): 1237–43.

85. Yu S, Fang H, Han J, et al. The high prevalence of hypovitaminosis D in China: a multicenter vitamin D status survey. Medicine (Baltimore) 2015;94(8):e585.

86. Lu HK, Zhang Z, Ke YH, et al. High prevalence of vitamin D insufficiency in China: relationship with the levels of parathyroid hormone and markers of bone turnover. PLoS One 2012;7(11):e47264.

87. Song SJ, Zhou L, Si S, et al. The high prevalence of vitamin D deficiency and its related maternal factors in pregnant women in Beijing. PLoS One 2013;8(12): e85081.

88. Xiao JP, Zang J, Pei JJ, et al. Low maternal vitamin D status during the second trimester of pregnancy: a cross-sectional study in Wuxi, China. PLoS One 2015; 10(2):e0117748.

89. Ke L, Mason RS, Mpofu E, et al. Vitamin D and parathyroid hormone status in a representative population living in Macau, China. J Steroid Biochem Mol Biol 2015;148:261–8.

90. Zhen D, Liu L, Quan C, et al. High prevalence of vitamin D deficiency among middle-aged and elderly individuals in northwestern China: its relationship to osteoporosis and lifestyle factors. Bone 2015;71:1–6.

91. Li S, Ou Y, Zhang H, et al. Vitamin D status and its relationship with body composition, bone mineral density and fracture risk in urban central south Chinese postmenopausal women. Ann Nutr Metab 2014;64(1):13–9.

92. Chan R, Chan CC, Woo J, et al. Serum 25-hydroxyvitamin D, bone mineral density, and non-vertebral fracture risk in community-dwelling older men: results from Mr. Os, Hong Kong. Arch Osteoporos 2011;6:21–30.

93. Xu C, Perera RA, Chan YH, et al. Determinants of serum 25-hydroxyvitamin D in Hong Kong. Br J Nutr 2015;114(1):144–51.

94. Nakamura K, Kitamura K, Takachi R, et al. Impact of demographic, environmental, and lifestyle factors on vitamin D sufficiency in 9084 Japanese adults. Bone 2015;74:10–7.

95. Choi HS, Oh HJ, Choi H, et al. Vitamin D insufficiency in Korea–a greater threat to younger generation: the Korea National Health and Nutrition Examination Survey (KNHANES) 2008. J Clin Endocrinol Metab 2011;96(3):643–51.

96. Kim SH, Oh MK, Namgung R, et al. Prevalence of 25-hydroxyvitamin D deficiency in Korean adolescents: association with age, season and parental vitamin D status. Public Health Nutr 2012;17(1):122–30.

97. Chee WS Jr, Chong PN, Chuah KA, et al. Calcium intake, vitamin D and bone health status of post-menopausal Chinese Women in Kuala Lumpur. Malays J Nutr 2010;16(2):233–42.

98. Moy FM. Vitamin D status and its associated factors of free living Malay adults in a tropical country, Malaysia. J Photochem Photobiol B 2011;104(3):444–8.

99. Laillou A, Wieringa F, Tran TN, et al. Hypovitaminosis D and mild hypocalcaemia are highly prevalent among young Vietnamese children and women and related to low dietary intake. PLoS One 2013;8(5):e63979.

100. Pratumvinit B, Wongkrajang P, Wataganara T, et al. Maternal vitamin D status and its related factors in pregnant women in Bangkok, Thailand. PLoS One 2015;10(7):e0131126.

101. Smith G, Wimalawansa SJ, Laillou A, et al. High prevalence of vitamin D deficiency in Cambodian women: a common deficiency in a sunny country. Nutrients 2016;8(5) [pii:E290].

102. Loy SL, Lek N, Yap F, et al. Association of Maternal Vitamin D Status With Glucose Tolerance and Caesarean Section in a Multi-Ethnic Asian Cohort: the Growing Up in Singapore Towards Healthy Outcomes Study. PLoS One 2015; 10(11):e0142239.
103. Marwaha RK, Tandon N, Chopra S, et al. Vitamin D status in pregnant Indian women across trimesters and different seasons and its correlation with neonatal serum 25-hydroxyvitamin D levels. Br J Nutr 2011;106(9):1383–9.
104. Shivane VK, Sarathi V, Bandgar T, et al. High prevalence of hypovitaminosis D in young healthy adults from the western part of India. Postgrad Med J 2011; 87(1030):514–8.
105. Mehboobali N, Iqbal SP, Iqbal MP. High prevalence of vitamin D deficiency and insufficiency in a low income peri-urban community in Karachi. J Pak Med Assoc 2015;65(9):946–9.
106. Junaid K, Rehman A, Jolliffe DA, et al. High prevalence of vitamin D deficiency among women of child-bearing age in Lahore Pakistan, associating with lack of sun exposure and illiteracy. BMC Womens Health 2015;15:83.
107. El Maghraoui A, Ouzzif Z, Mounach A, et al. Hypovitaminosis D and prevalent asymptomatic vertebral fractures in Moroccan postmenopausal women. BMC Womens Health 2012;12:11.
108. Gebreegziabher T, Stoecker BJ. Vitamin D insufficiency in a sunshine-sufficient area: southern Ethiopia. Food Nutr Bull 2013;34(4):429–33.
109. Olayiwola IO, Fadupin GT, Agbato SO, et al. Serum micronutrient status and nutrient intake of elderly Yoruba people in a slum of Ibadan, Nigeria. Public Health Nutr 2014;17(2):455–61.
110. Mehta S, Hunter DJ, Mugusi FM, et al. Perinatal outcomes, including mother-to-child transmission of HIV, and child mortality and their association with maternal vitamin D status in Tanzania. J Infect Dis 2009;200(7):1022–30.
111. Friis H, Range N, Changalucha J, et al. Vitamin D status among pulmonary TB patients and non-TB controls: a cross-sectional study from Mwanza, Tanzania. PLoS One 2013;8(12):e81142.
112. Luxwolda MF, Kuipers RS, Kema IP, et al. Vitamin D status indicators in indigenous populations in East Africa. Eur J Nutr 2013;52(3):1115–25.
113. Wejse C, Gomes VF, Rabna P, et al. Vitamin D as supplementary treatment for tuberculosis: a double-blind, randomized, placebo-controlled trial. Am J Respir Crit Care Med 2009;179(9):843–50.
114. George JA, Norris SA, van Deventer HE, et al. The association of 25 hydroxyvitamin D and parathyroid hormone with metabolic syndrome in two ethnic groups in South Africa. PLoS One 2013;8(4):e61282.
115. Kruger MC, Kruger IM, Wentzel-Viljoen E, et al. Urbanization of black South African women may increase risk of low bone mass due to low vitamin D status, low calcium intake, and high bone turnover. Nutr Res 2011;31(10):748–58.
116. Heere C, Skeaff CM, Waqatakirewa L, et al. Serum 25-hydroxyvitamin D concentration of Indigenous-Fijian and Fijian-Indian women. Asia Pac J Clin Nutr 2010; 19(1):43–8.
117. Willix C, Rasmussen S, Evans S, et al. A comparison of vitamin D levels in two antenatal populations in regional Western Australia–'Tjindoo Ba Thonee Thurra': sunshine for the pregnant belly. Aust Fam Physician 2015;44(3):141–4.
118. Hirani V, Cumming RG, Blyth FM, et al. Vitamin D status among older community dwelling men living in a sunny country and associations with lifestyle factors: the concord health and ageing in men project, Sydney, Australia. J Nutr Health Aging 2013;17(7):587–93.

119. Gill TK, Hill CL, Shanahan EM, et al. Vitamin D levels in an Australian population. BMC Public Health 2014;14:1001.
120. Bowyer L, Catling-Paull C, Diamond T, et al. PTH and calcium levels in pregnant women and their neonates. Clin Endocrinol (Oxf) 2009;70(3):372–7.
121. Daly RM, Gagnon C, Lu ZX, et al. Prevalence of vitamin D deficiency and its determinants in Australian adults aged 25 years and older: a national, population-based study. Clin Endocrinol (Oxf) 2012;77(1):26–35.
122. Davies-Tuck M, Yim C, Knight M, et al. Vitamin D testing in pregnancy: does one size fit all? Aust N Z J Obstet Gynaecol 2015;55(2):149–55.
123. Bolland MJ, Chiu WW, Davidson JS, et al. The effects of seasonal variation of 25-hydroxyvitamin D on diagnosis of vitamin D insufficiency. N Z Med J 2008; 121(1286):63–74.
124. Wishart HD, Reeve AM, Grant CC. Vitamin D deficiency in a multinational refugee population. Intern Med J 2007;37(12):792–7.
125. Bolland MJ, Grey AB, Ames RW, et al. Determinants of vitamin D status in older men living in a subtropical climate. Osteoporos Int 2006;17(12):1742–8.
126. Nessvi S, Johansson L, Jopson J, et al. Association of 25-hydroxyvitamin D3 levels in adult New Zealanders with ethnicity, skin color and self-reported skin sensitivity to sun exposure. Photochem Photobiol 2011;87(5):1173–8.
127. Rockell JE, Skeaff CM, Venn BJ, et al. Vitamin D insufficiency in New Zealanders during the winter is associated with higher parathyroid hormone concentrations: implications for bone health? N Z Med J 2008;121(1286):75–84.

Dietary Vitamin D Intake for the Elderly Population

Update on the Recommended Dietary Allowance for Vitamin D

Lynette M. Smith, PhD[a], J. Christopher Gallagher, MD[b],*

KEYWORDS

- Vitamin D supplementation • IOM • RDA for vitamin D

KEY POINTS

- Incidence of vitamin D deficiency and insufficiency in North America is high.
- Serum 25-hydroxyvitamin D (25OHD) level of 20 ng/mL (50 nmol/L) is clinically important for bone health.
- Clinical studies of vitamin D and vitamin D with calcium show that vitamin D 400 to 800 IU plus calcium 1000 mg daily is a combination that significantly reduces fractures by 10% to 12%. Vitamin D alone is not effective in reducing fractures.
- Ongoing trials with vitamin D are expected to show the risk-benefit of vitamin D on other clinical diseases within 5 years.
- Recommended dietary allowance for vitamin D is as follows: 800 IU needed to reach 25OHD level of 20 ng/mL (50 nmol/L) and vitamin D 1600 IU to reach a serum 25OHD level 30 ng/mL (75 nmol/L). The estimated average requirement is 400 IU for serum 25OHD level 20 ng/mL (50 nmol/L) and 800 IU for serum level of 30 ng/mL (75 nmol/L).

INTRODUCTION: NUTRITIONAL CONSIDERATIONS

Vitamin D deficiency, insufficiency, and sufficiency are 3 categories representing different degrees of the nutritional status of vitamin D, and they are divided according to serum 25-hydroxyvitamin D (25OHD) levels. These categories are not distinct and merge into each other.

Disclosure Statement: The authors have nothing to disclose.

J.C. Gallagher and L.M. Smith were supported by Grant AG28168 from the National Institute on Aging and the Office of Dietary Supplements and by a grant from the Department of Defense (DOD) W81XWH-07-1-201. L.M. Smith is supported also by Great Plains IDEA-CTR Network grant 1U54GM115458-01.

[a] Department Biostatistics, University Nebraska Medical Center, 42nd Street and Emile Street, Omaha, NE 68198, USA; [b] Endocrinology, Creighton University Medical School, 2400 California Plaza, Omaha, NE 68131, USA

* Corresponding author.

E-mail address: jcg@creighton.edu

The Institute of Medicine (IOM) defined vitamin D deficiency as less than 10 ng/mL (25 nmol/L), insufficiency as 10 to 20 ng/mL (25–50 nmol/L), and sufficiency as greater than 20 ng/mL (>50 nmol/L),[1] similar to the definition of the World Health Organization (WHO) in 2003[2] and European Food Safety Association (EFSA) in 2016.[3] An Endocrine Society working group used higher levels, less than 20 ng/mL for deficiency, 20 to 30 ng/mL (75 nmol/L) for insufficiency, and greater than 30 ng/mL (>75 nmol/L) for sufficiency[4] (Table 1). Interest in vitamin D status has led to a 12-fold increase in serum 25OHD tests since 2005.[5]

VITAMIN D DEFICIENCY AND INSUFFICIENCY

A survey from the 3871 adults in the NHANES study carried out on populations in North America shows the relative numbers of the serum 25OHD categories.[6,7] Recent remeasurement of the 25OHD levels as part of a vitamin D standardization program showed the prevalence of insufficiency (12–20 ng/mL) was high at 31%[8] (Table 2).

In most of Northern Europe, the percent of the population with serum 25OHD less than 20 ng/mL (50 nmol/L) is higher because of a combination of social and environmental factors that differ from North America, such as lack of fortification of food and milk, and less exposure to sunlight because of the Northern latitude and cloud cover.[9,10] In certain ethnic groups, such as traditional Arabic women, there is an even higher risk because of cultural habits, such as veiling and purdah, preventing ultraviolet activation of pre-vitamin D in skin.[11]

THE HISTORY OF THE PRESENT RECOMMENDED DIETARY ALLOWANCE FOR VITAMIN D

In determining the recommended dietary allowance (RDA) for vitamin D for the elderly, less than age 50 to 69, and greater than 70 years, the IOM in 2010 performed a comprehensive survey and analysis of literature that linked low levels of vitamin D to the prevalence of several diseases, such as cardiovascular disease, cancer, asthma, bone, and others. The analyses for IOM were conducted by an independent group of epidemiologists and statisticians, Agency for Healthcare Research and Quality (AHRQ)-Tufts, in 2009 and 2011,[12,13] and followed an earlier analysis by another AHRQ-Ottawa group in 2007.[14] Even though there are numerous association studies that linked serum 25OHD levels to various diseases, the epidemiologists found no consistent evidence of a significant effect of vitamin D treatment on any health outcomes other than fractures and bone mineral density (BMD). Thus, the IOM committee decided that only clinical studies related to bone health would be used to derive new dietary reference intakes (DRIs) for vitamin D. To look for a relationship between disorders of calcium metabolism and serum 25OHD levels, the IOM used data on rickets, calcium absorption, fracture risk, and bone health. Clinical studies were reviewed to

Table 1
Categories of low vitamin D (25-hydroxyvitamin D) levels

	IOM, WHO, EFSA		Endocrine Society	
	Serum 25OHD ng/mL	Serum 25OHD nmol/L	Serum 25OHD ng/mL	Serum 25OHD nmol/L
Vitamin D deficiency	<10	25	<20	<50
Insufficiency	10–20	25–50	20–30	50–75
Sufficiency	>20	>50	>30	>75

Table 2
Prevalence of low vitamin D levels

	Serum 25OHD, ng/mL	Original, %	Corrected Values, %
Vitamin D deficiency	<12 (<30 nmol/L)	4	6
Vitamin D insufficiency	12–20 (30–50 nmol/L)	22	31
Vitamin D sufficiency	20–50 (50–125 nmol/L)	55	71

find a dose of vitamin D that would meet the target level of a specified level of serum 25OHD.

Calcium Absorption

A cross-sectional study of calcium absorption and serum 25OHD in 319 patients with a mean age of 67 years shows reduced calcium absorption at mean serum 25OHD levels of 4 ng/mL (9 nmol/L) together with a decrease in serum 1,25-dihydroxyvitamin D.[15] As mean serum 25OHD increased from 4 ng/mL (9 nmol/L) to 7 ng/mL (17 nmol/L), there was an increase in serum 1,25-dihydroxyvitamin D and an increase in calcium absorption from 36% to 56%. The results show that calcium absorption was almost maximal at very low levels of 25OHD, 4 to 7 ng/mL (10–17 nmol/L), and although mean 25OHD increased to 14 ng/mL (35 nmol/L), there was no further increase in calcium absorption. In prospective studies, calcium absorption was reduced at low levels of serum 25OHD ~10 ng/mL (25 nmol/L). After vitamin D treatment, there was an increase in serum 25OHD from 10 ng/mL to 60 ng/mL (150 nmol/L); however, the increase in calcium absorption from 55% to 61% was relatively small, ~6%.[16,17] It is not surprising because calcium absorption is controlled by 1,25-dihydroxyvitamin D and not 25OHD.[18,19]

SERUM PARATHYROID HORMONE AND ITS RELATION TO A SERUM 25-HYDROXYVITAMIN D

Because serum parathyroid hormone (PTH) often increases with vitamin D deficiency and insufficiency in some but not all people, the level at which it normalizes or plateaus has often been used as a marker of vitamin D insufficiency. In the Endocrine Society paper, only 3 studies from the literature were quoted, and they showed a "PTH plateau" at a serum 25OHD level of 30 ng/mL (75 nmol/L).[4] However, there were in fact about 70 studies on serum PTH and 25OHD in the literature at that time, and they showed considerable variation in a "plateau" value for serum 25OHD ranging from 12 ng/mL (30nmol/L) to 40 ng/mL (100 nmol/L); in 7 studies there was no plateau.[19] In a recent analysis of 347,000 laboratory samples, no plateau could be easily identified; thus, a serum PTH plateau is not a reliable marker of vitamin D sufficiency.[20]

BONE

Increased serum PTH is inversely correlated with hip BMD.[21] In an analysis of bone remodeling markers and serum 25OHD in 489 women, a plateau in serum osteocalcin was seen at a serum 25OHD of 17 ng/mL (42 nmol/L), and a plateau in urine N-telopeptides was seen at a plateau at 18 ng/mL (37 nmol/L).[19] Interestingly, other bone data support the importance of the effect of low serum 25OHD less than 20 ng/mL (50 nmol/L) on bone. In a study of 1279 men, BMD was measured over 4.4 years, and rate of bone loss was divided into quartiles; rates of bone loss were increased only in those with serum 25OHD less than 20 ng/mL (50 nmol/L) compared with greater than 20 ng/mL.[22] In 5 case cohort studies of hip fracture in 6562 patients, the relative risk of hip fractures was increased significantly from 1.0 only when serum 25OHD was less than 20 ng/mL (50 nmol/L), and these studies are summarized in a review.[23] There are data also on nonvertebral fractures. In men, nonhip fractures are increased only when serum 25OHD is less than 20 ng/mL (50 nmol/L).[24] In a case cohort study of women from the Women's Health Initiative, Caucasian women showed a lower incidence of nonvertebral fractures when serum 25OHD was greater than 30 ng/mL (75 nmol/L), but in African American and Asian women, fractures were increased when serum 25OHD was increased greater than 20 ng/mL compared with less than 20 ng/mL.[25]

In a recent bone biopsy study, postmortem analysis of bone biopsies was performed in 675 people who had sudden death. They examined the occurrence of osteomalacia in the biopsies and related that to serum 25OHD levels drawn early postmortem.[26] At serum 25OHD levels less than 12 ng/mL (30 nmol/L), more than half of the population failed to demonstrate osteomalacia. At 25OHD levels less than 3 ng/mL, there were ~80/687 cases with normal bone, indicating that factors other than low 25OHD prevented osteomalacia, most obvious factors being that subjects had adequate intake of calcium and phosphorus before death. In the biopsy study, osteoid volume was increased in 7 of 685 (1%) cases when serum 25OHD was between 20 and 30 ng/mL; however, because there was no measurement of mineralization defect, the authors cannot be sure that these 7 cases had osteomalacia. Some might have had hyperparathyroidism.

The totality of these observations support the concept that subjects with levels of serum 25OHD less than 10 ng/mL (50 nmol/L) develop rickets, and malabsorption of calcium and at levels less than 20 ng/mL (50 nmol/L), there is decreased risk of bone loss and fractures. For these reasons, the IOM recommended that the target figure for treatment should be a serum 25OHD of 20 ng/mL (50 nmol/L). A more recent analysis by the EFSA in 2016[2] used similar reasoning and similar conclusions to those of the IOM.

CLINICAL STUDIES OF VITAMIN D

There have been 7 studies on vitamin D alone and 13 studies with vitamin D + calcium on bone. A fundamental flaw is that none of the studies had a dose response design. As a result, meta-analyses have been used to examine the data (please see Ian R. Reid's article, "Vitamin D Effect on Bone Mineral Density and Fractures," in this issue). Regarding vitamin D–only studies, there are few trials in the literature where vitamin D only was compared with placebo, and these were reviewed in 2 meta-analyses.[27,28] On low doses of vitamin D 400 to 1000 IU, there was no reduction in fractures (odds ratio 1.05). In 2 studies, one a large trial of 2256 women age 70 years who were given a single oral high dose annually of vitamin D 500,000 IU, there was unexpectedly a significant increase in fractures within 3 months of dosing in 2 separate years (relative risk [RR] 1.26, confidence interval [CI]: 1.00-1.59).[29] Another study of an annual injection of high-dose vitamin D 300,000 IU showed a significant increase in hip fractures (RR 1.82) in women but not in men (RR 1.1).[30] Thus, vitamin D alone in low doses has no effect on fractures, and large bolus doses increase fractures.

In many clinical trials, vitamin D was combined with calcium supplements, and several different dose combinations of vitamin D and calcium have been used in trials. In a meta-analysis by Tang and colleagues[27] of trials with fracture outcomes but without individual data, there were 5 studies in which the active group was compared with placebo control, and in 8 studies, the control group was calcium. Their analysis showed a significant reduction in fractures of 13% (RR 0.87; 0.77–0.97). In another meta-analysis (DiPART), the investigators obtained individual person data in 7 controlled studies, 3 on vitamin D alone and 4 on vitamin D plus calcium.[28] There was no significant effect of vitamin D alone on fractures (RR 1.01; CI: 0.92–1.12), but a significant effect of vitamin D plus calcium on total fractures (RR 0.92, CI: 0.86-0.99). Hip fractures were marginally reduced on vitamin D plus calcium (RR 0.84, CI: 0.70–1.01, $P<.07$) but not on vitamin D alone (RR 1.09; 0.92–1.29).[28]

In summary, vitamin D alone does not reduce fracture, whereas calcium plus vitamin D supplementation reduces fractures by 8% to 13%. The results of the DIPART analysis show that vitamin D 400 to 800 IU plus 1000 mg calcium is a regimen that prevents fractures. It was not possible for the investigators to define a serum 25OHD level associated with efficacy.

DETERMINATION OF THE RECOMMENDED DIETARY ALLOWANCE IN OLDER PERSONS

There are 3 components to DRIs that are used to determine nutrient intakes for calcium and vitamin D in North America. They are reference intakes for the healthy population and are not therapeutic guidelines for people with diseases, for example, malabsorption syndromes.

Recommended Dietary Allowance

RDA is the average daily dietary intake level estimated to meet the nutrient requirements of nearly all healthy persons in a life stage and gender, that is, it meets the needs of 97.5% of individuals.

The RDA for vitamin D3 can be descriptively defined as the dose that achieves a defined end, for example, it could be the new incidence of type 2 diabetes. In this discussion, the endpoint is a serum 25OHD level of 20 ng/mL (50 nmol/L) or higher in 97.5% of the subjects. It means that for a dose of vitamin D, gender and age specific, 97.5% of subjects in that dose group will have serum 25OHD of at least 20 ng/mL (50 nmol/L).

Regression methodology can also be used for calculating the RDA, in that a dose response curve can be fit to the data, using the linear regression model. From the linear regression model, CIs and prediction intervals can be calculated. CIs are calculated for the mean or *average* response (serum 25OHD) at a dose. Rather than the average response of many individuals, prediction intervals apply to the response of a *new individual*. There is more uncertainty in predicting a serum 25OHD level for an individual than for the average of individuals; therefore, prediction intervals are wider than CIs. Prediction intervals must account for 2 levels of uncertainty: uncertainty in estimating the actual dose response curve and random error for the new individual. Without going into additional detail, linear regression models enable the estimation of 95% prediction limits for each dose level. Because the 95% prediction interval is symmetric about the predicted value (what serum 25OHD a new individual is predicted to have at that dose), 97.5% of values would be greater than the lower prediction limit. Therefore, the RDA can be interpreted as the dose at which a serum 25OHD of 20 ng/mL (50 nmol/L) is greater than the lower prediction limit for a new individual. This prediction interval is a function of the standard deviation of the residuals, the sample size, the sample mean of the independent variables, and the standard deviation of the independent variables.

Prediction intervals are standard and can be calculated easily with statistical software for simple linear regression. However, more complex study designs require advanced statistical techniques for calculating prediction intervals.

In a longitudinal study design, linear mixed effects models that consider correlation within a subject over time are most appropriate. This type of model complicates the calculation of prediction intervals for estimation of the RDA. There is no standard formula for calculating prediction intervals for this type of model such as there is for simple linear regression. Widely accepted in the literature for calculating prediction intervals with linear mixed effects models is a bootstrapping technique. Resampling methodology can be used to calculate CIs and prediction intervals when the distribution is unknown. To perform this calculation, many bootstrap samples are taken (such as 1000) at the subject level, preserving all the time points measured within a subject. The linear mixed effects model is fit for each of the bootstrapped samples, and the predicted values of the random effects (called BLUPS) are found. From this, the 2.5 and 97.5 percentiles are found for each dose. Again, the RDA is the dose at which the 2.5 percentile is greater than 20 ng/mL (50 nmol/L) of serum 25OHD.

Estimated Average Requirement

Estimated average requirement (EAR) is the average daily nutrient intake level estimated to meet the requirements of 50% of the healthy persons for each sex and age group.

The EAR is simpler to calculate than the RDA. The EAR for vitamin D3 can be defined as the dose that achieves a serum 25OD level of 20 ng/mL (50 nmol/L) or a target value of interest in 50% of the subjects. It means that at that dose 50% of subjects in that dose group will have serum 25OHD less than 20 ng/mL (50 nmol/L) and 50% greater than 20 ng/mL (50 nmol/L).

It is also a definition of the median. The median is defined as the middle value of a distribution, where 50% of the observations are greater than and 50% are less than that value. EAR can also be defined as the dose where the median of the serum 25OHD values meets the targeted value of 20 ng/mL. If the serum 25OHD values follow a normal distribution, the mean and median should be approximately equal; so, if all the assumptions from a simple linear regression model (or linear mixed effects model) are met, then the fitted line of the dose response curve corresponds to the mean response. The point where the dose response curve intersects the targeted value (20 ng/mL) is the EAR.

Estimation of the recommended dietary allowance by Institute of Medicine

To find a total vitamin D intake derived from diet and supplements that exceeded a serum 25OHD level of 20 ng/mL (50 nmol/L), the IOM committee in 2011 used several studies from the literature; most studies were single dose, and some used 2 doses.[1] They specifically used studies that were performed in the winter months in Northern countries above a latitude of 49° and from Antarctica 78°S to minimize the effect of sun exposure. Their procedure was to use regression analysis, with a random study effect, and log distribution to estimate a dose response curve. From this, they estimated the EAR of 400 IU/d exceeded a serum 25OHD of 16 ng/mL (40 nmol/L). The RDA was estimated with prediction limits from the average study values and showed that an RDA of 600 IU/d exceeded a serum 25OHD of 20 ng/mL (50 nmol/L).

It should be noted that a more precise analysis would be obtained from prediction limits had individual values been available as pointed out by Veugelers and Ekwaru,[31] although their RDA estimate of 8895 IU daily is clearly incorrect when compared with the authors' dose response curves in the prospective ViDOS and VitaDAS trials, which are described in detail in later discussion. In another analysis, the RDA was estimated from uncontrolled vitamin D supplementation studies and arrived at a figure of 9600 IU daily,[32] an estimate that is clearly incorrect when compared with the authors' dose response curves. The ViDOS study in older women and the VitaDAS study in younger women are dose-ranging studies and were not completed at the time of the IOM report. Nevertheless, the RDA values estimated from the individual subject data in the authors' trials are similar to those in the IOM recommendation (see later discussion).

The most recent analysis in 2016 by EFSA used metaregression.[3] It does not use an RDA figure but an "Adequate Intake," although it is based on a 95% prediction limit with the lower limit being 49 nmol/L (19.6 ng/mL). They conclude that vitamin D3 600 IU/d will meet a target serum 25OHD of 20 ng/mL (50 nmol/L) in nearly everyone.[3] Other groups in Europe, such as the Nordic Council, support the use of 400 IU for an RDA-like figure.[33] The Netherlands recommend 600 IU for ages 50 to 70 years and 800 IU for those older than 70 years.[34] For those younger than 70 years, the target serum 25OHD was 12 ng/mL (30 nmol/L). In England, they chose a serum 25OHD of 25 nmol/L (10 ng/mL) for all ages as protection against adverse musculoskeletal health and recommended vitamin D 400 IU to cover 97.5% of the population[35]

ESTIMATED AVERAGE REQUIREMENT OR RECOMMENDED DIETARY ALLOWANCE

A recent argument has been that nutrient deficiency should be defined by the EAR, which is the nutrient intake for the average of the population.[36] The IOM used a serum 25OHD of 16 ng/mL (40 nmol/L) as the target for the EAR and estimated that vitamin D 400 IU will meet that figure. The RDA for a serum 25OHD of 20 ng/mL (50 nmol/L) is based on 97.5% of the population. Another way to look at it is that 97.5% will have a requirement less than that threshold, and that meeting a goal of 20 ng/mL (50 nmol/L) is more than necessary. In addition, the calculation for RDA was based on wintertime studies. At the authors' latitude of 41°, serum 25OHD increases from winter to summer by about 10 ng/mL (25 nmol/L) from 23 to 32 ng/mL (57–80 nmol/L) (**Fig. 1**); thus, having an EAR rather that an RDA is a reasonable suggestion. Another argument that has been made is that increasing the vitamin intake to achieve an RDA target of 20 ng/mL (50 nmol/L) may push some people into higher 25OHD levels associated with the tolerable upper limit, as suggested by Taylor and colleagues[37] in a statistical model.

Tolerable Upper Level

Tolerable upper level (TUL) is the highest average daily intake of a nutrient that does not increase the risk for adverse health effects for nearly all persons in the population. At the last IOM report, the TUL was increased from 2000 to 4000 IU daily, and much of the reasoning was based on lack of hypercalcemia (it is not a *recommended* intake). However, as another example of an unexpected adverse result of vitamin D, the authors found a significant increase in falls in women taking the higher doses of 4000 and 4800 IU daily; these doses were associated with serum 25OHD levels greater than 40 to 45 ng/mL (100–112 nmol/L) but no hypercalcemia.[38] Thus, the argument made by Taylor and colleagues[37] is reasonable. In epidemiology studies, increased mortalities have been associated with higher serum 25OHD levels of 45 to 50 ng/mL (112–125 nmol/L),[39,40] and in the recent 6-year follow-up of NHANES, there was a reverse J-shaped curve with higher mortality with values less than 40 nmol/L (16 ng/mL) and greater than 120 nmol/L (48 ng/mL).[41]

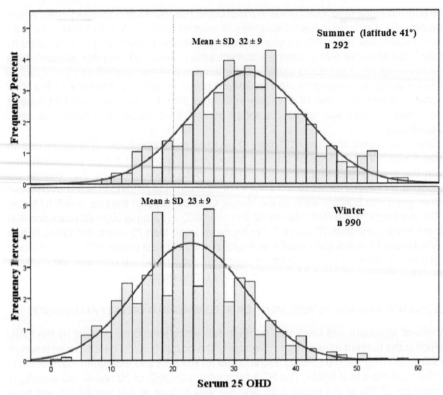

Fig. 1. Seasonal change (cross-sectional) in serum 25OHD in Omaha, latitude 41°. SD, standard deviation.

DOSE RESPONSE IN OLDER CAUCASIAN AND AFRICAN AMERICAN WOMEN

Since the IOM recommendations in 2010, the authors conducted a randomized clinical trial (ViDOS study) to measure the dose response of vitamin D, and through this dose response curve, estimate the RDA and EAR.[42] The study design included randomization of women stratified by race (Caucasian or African American) into 7 dose groups and a placebo group and stratified by body mass index. Doses used were 400, 800, 1600, 2400, 3200, 4000, 4800 IU, and placebo. Inclusion criteria included older women at least 7 years postmenopausal and vitamin D insufficient less than 20 ng/mL (50 nmol/L) at baseline. Exclusion criteria were substantial comorbid conditions or medications that might affect calcium and vitamin D metabolism. A DiaSorin immunoassay was used to measure serum 25OHD in this study. One hundred sixty-three Caucasian women were enrolled as well as 110 African American women. All 163 Caucasian women were enrolled at one site in Omaha, Nebraska, and African American women were enrolled at 2 sites, Nebraska and Indiana. Serum 25OHD was measured at baseline, 6 months, and 12 months.

In the Caucasian women, a quadratic dose response curve was observed. Prediction intervals were calculated with bootstrap methodology for the linear mixed effects model used to fit the data. For the RDA calculation, to reach a serum 25OHD of 30 ng/mL, it was determined that a vitamin D3 dose of 1600 IU/d is required in postmenopausal Caucasian women. To meet a serum level of 20 ng/mL (50 nmol/L) for bone health as recommended by the IOM, an RDA dose for vitamin D_3 of 800 IU/d is required. Although a dose of 600 IU/d was not studied, it can be interpolated from the statistical model that a dose of 600 IU will meet a serum 25OHD level of 20 ng/mL (50 nmol/L). For African American women, a linear dose response curve was the best fit to the data. Prediction limits were calculated the same way as for Caucasian women, and the RDA was found to be 800 IU/d to meet a serum 25OHD level of 20 ng/mL (50 nmol/L), and 1600 IU/d to meet a serum 25OHD of 30 ng/mL (75 nmol/L).[43] To meet an average requirement for serum 25OHD of 30 ng/mL (75 nmol/L), the EAR was calculated as a dose between 800 and 1600 IU/d, and to meet a serum 25OHD level of 20 ng/mL (50 nmol/L), a dose of 400 IU/d for Caucasian women was calculated.[42] In African American women, 400 and 800 IU/d were determined for EAR of serum of 20 ng/mL (50 nmol/L) and 30 ng/mL, respectively.[43]

DOSE RESPONSE IN YOUNGER CAUCASIAN AND AFRICAN AMERICAN WOMEN

The authors conducted a dose response in younger women (VitaDAS study). This study was a randomized placebo controlled clinical trial conducted in both Caucasian and African American women, age range 25 to 45 years, baseline serum 25OHD less than or equal to 20 ng/mL, and similar exclusion criteria to the VidOS study.[44] There were 4 vitamin D dose groups, 400, 800, 1600, 2400 IU/d, or placebo. The DiaSorin assay was used to measure serum 25OHD. There were 119 Caucasian and 79 African American women that completed the study. They were analyzed separately by race, and linear mixed effects models determined a linear dose response curve that best fit the data for both races. The RDA was estimated to be 400 IU in Caucasian and 1200 IU in African American women to reach a serum 25OHD of 20 ng/mL (50 nmol/L). The EAR to meet 20 ng/mL was determined to be 400 IU/d for both races. Because of the smaller number of dose groups and poor compliance compared with older women, it was not possible to use a quadratic curve, and there is more uncertainty about the RDA and EAR.

COMBINING RESULTS FOR ALL AGES

The authors attempted to combine an analysis of ViDOS and VitaDAS studies, young and old, black and white women. In a linear mixed effects model, a dose response curve was fitted, determining if there were interactions between race or study (ViDOS or Vita-DAS) with dose. They determined that there was no interaction between dose and study; however, there was a significant interaction between race and dose. Because of the significant interaction with race, the authors fitted models for each race separately, but combining the studies, so they have a Caucasian dose response curve and an African American dose response curve for young and older women combined.

The best fitting model in Caucasians was a quadratic dose response, shown in **Fig. 2**. One thousand bootstrapped prediction intervals were calculated for each dose, and a dose of 800 IU/d was found to meet a serum 25OHD level of 20 ng/mL (50 nmol/L) because the RDA and 2400 IU would exceed 30 ng/mL (75 nmol/L). The EAR to meet 30 ng/mL was a dose of 800 IU. By 12 months, the estimated combined dose response curve had an average response greater than 20 ng/mL, showing that no supplementation was necessary to meet an EAR of 20 ng/mL. The best fitting model in African Americans was a linear dose response, shown in **Fig. 3**. One thousand bootstrapped prediction intervals were calculated for each dose, and a dose of 800 IU/d was found to meet a serum 25OHD level of 20 ng/mL (50 nmol/L) because the RDA and 2400 IU/ d is required to meet serum 25OHD of 30 ng/mL (75 nmol/L). The lower prediction limit at a dose of 800 IU/d is actually 19 ng/mL. The EAR to meet 30 ng/mL (75 nmol/L) was a dose of 1600 IU. By 12 months, the estimated combined dose response curve had an average response greater than 20 ng/mL (50 nmol/L), showing that no supplementation

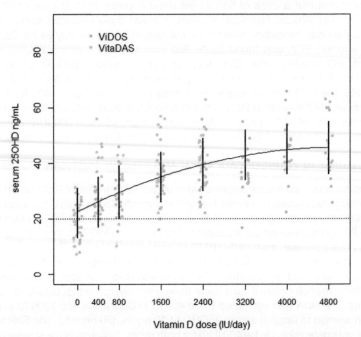

12 mo - ViDOS and VitaDAS Caucasians

Fig. 2. Combined dose response curve in ViDOS and VitaDAS Caucasian subjects. Complete 12-month data are displayed by dose and study with a quadratic dose response curve. Bootstrapped 95% prediction intervals from the linear mixed effects model are shown.

was necessary to meet an EAR of 20 ng/mL (50 nmol/L). A quadratic response may be appropriate for African Americans as well, but with so few individuals at the higher doses, a quadratic curve is difficult to detect. Bootstrapped prediction limits seemed somewhat narrow in this analysis. Further investigation showed that the variability due to the average dose response curve is greater than the variability due to individuals. Therefore, the prediction intervals are being driven by the mean response and not the individual response. When estimating EAR and RDA measurements of serum 25OHD, compliance with the scheduled vitamin D intake is a consideration. Low compliance is defined as less than 80% compliance between the 9- and 12-month visits or an average compliance over the study period of less than 80%. If low compliers are excluded from the model and the bootstrap prediction intervals are recalculated, they are similar to the intervals calculated with the full data. The RDA and EAR do not change if the low compliers are excluded from the estimation. These estimates for the RDA and EAR are summarized in **Table 3**.

Recently, a large study of 328 African Americans aged 40 to 60 years over 3 months compared placebo, vitamin D 1000, 2000, and 4000 IU daily. They estimated that a vitamin D dose of ~1600 IU would exceed serum 25OHD of 20 ng/mL (50 nmol/L).[45] Whether 3 months is long enough to reach a steady state for serum 25OHD on lower doses of vitamin D is a possible limitation of this study.

WHO SHOULD BE SCREENED FOR SERUM 25-HYDROXYVITAMIN D?

This issue was recently addressed by the US Preventive Services Task Force, who examined the evidence on screening for vitamin D deficiency and found insufficient

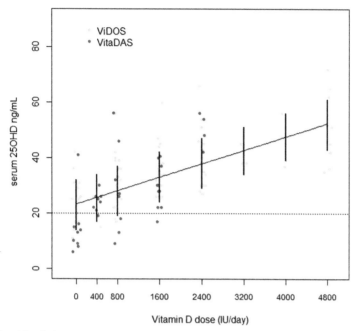

12 mo - ViDOS and VitaDAS African Americans

Fig. 3. Combined dose response curve in ViDOS and VitaDAS African American subjects. Complete 12-month data are displayed by dose and study with a linear dose response curve. Bootstrapped 95% prediction intervals from the linear mixed effects model are shown.

evidence to assess the benefits and harms in asymptomatic people because there was no evidence at the time that treatment of asymptomatic people has benefit on cancer, diabetes, mortality, or risk of fracture.[46] The IOM report recommends an RDA of 600 IU or an EAR of 400 IU to meet the requirements of most people in the

Table 3
Recommended dietary allowance and estimated average requirement estimates based on randomized clinical trials, 1000 bootstrapped samples from linear mixed effects model

Study	Population	EAR 20 ng/mL	EAR 30 ng/mL	RDA 20 ng/mL	RDA 30 ng/mL
ViDOS	Caucasian, age >57	400 IU/d	800–1600 IU/d	800 IU/d (600 IU[a])	1600 IU/d
ViDOS	African American, age >57	0–400 IU/d	800 IU/d	800 IU/d	1600 IU/d
VitaDAS	Caucasian, age 25–45	400 IU/d	800 IU/d	400 IU/d	2400 IU/d
VitaDAS	African American, age 25–45	400 IU/d	1600 IU/d	1200[a] IU/d	2400 IU/d
ViDOS & VitaDAS	Caucasian, young and old combined	0 IU/d	800 IU/d	800 IU/d	2400 IU/d
ViDOS & VitaDAS	African Americans, young and old combined	0 IU/d	1600 IU/d	800 IU/d	2400 IU/d

[a] Based on interpolation.

winter without any risk from taking vitamin D. Therefore, screening healthy individuals for 25OHD levels is not justified. However, screening high-risk patients with fractures, malabsorption syndromes, and other medical conditions related to abnormal calcium and vitamin D metabolism may be clinically beneficial.

SUMMARY

Several groups here and in Europe have arrived at a consensus that an RDA for vitamin D of 400 to 600 IU daily will meet the needs of the population in protecting bone health. The addition of calcium to vitamin D has a protective effect in preventing fractures. Screening for serum 25OHD is unnecessary in normal subjects and not cost-effective; however, patients with clinical problems affecting calcium and vitamin D metabolism may benefit from 25OHD testing. Large ongoing trials involving up to 50,000 subjects will produce results on the effect of vitamin D on several other diseases within 3 to 5 years.

REFERENCES

1. Dietary reference intakes for adequacy: 'calcium and vitamin D', Institute of Medicine. Washington, DC: The National Academies Press; 2011.
2. WHO Scientific Group on the Prevention and Management of Osteoporosis. Prevention and management of osteoporosis: report of a WHO scientific group. Geneva (Switzerland): World Health Organization; 2003.
3. EFSA Technical report. Outcome of a public consultation on the draft scientific opinion of the EFSA panel on dietetic products, nutrition and allergies (NDA) on dietary reference values for vitamin D. Wiley; 2016. 10.1002/(ISSN)1831-4732.
4. Holick MF, Binkley NC, Bischoff-Ferrari HA, et al. Evaluation, treatment, and prevention of vitamin D deficiency: an Endocrine Society clinical practice guideline. J Clin Endocrinol Metab 2011;96:1911-30.
5. Shahangian S, Alspach TD, Astles JR, et al. Trends in laboratory test volumes for Medicare Part B reimbursements, 2000-2010. Arch Pathol Lab Med 2014;138(2): 189-203.
6. Looker AC, Johnson CL, Lacher DA, et al. Vitamin D status: United States (2001-2006). NCHS data brief, no 59. Hyattsville (MD): National Center for Health Statistics; 2011.
7. Bailey RL, Dodd KW, Goldman JA, et al. Estimation of total usual calcium and vitamin D intakes in the United States. J Nutr 2010;140(4):817-22.
8. Binkley N, Dawson-Hughes B, Durazo-Arvizu R, et al. Vitamin D measurement standardization: the way out of the chaos. J Steroid Biochem Mol Biol 2017; 173:117-21.
9. Bruyere O, Decock C, Delhez M, et al. Highest prevalence of vitamin D inadequacy in institutionalized women compared with non-institutionalized women: a case–control study. Womens Health (Lond) 2009;5(1):49-54.
10. Cashman KD, Muldowney S, McNulty B, et al. Vitamin D status of Irish adults: findings from the National Adult Nutrition Survey. Br J Nutr 2012;10:1-9.
11. Holvik K, Meyer HE, Haug E, et al. 2005 Prevalence and predictors of vitamin D deficiency in five immigrant groups living in Oslo, Norway: the Oslo Immigrant study. Eur J Clin Nutr 2005;59(1):57-63.
12. Chung M, Balk EM, Brendel M, et al. Vitamin D and calcium: systematic review of health outcomes. Evidence report/technology assessment no. 183. (Prepared by Tufts Evidence-based Practice Center under Contract No. 290-2007-10055-I).

AHRQ Publication No. 09-E015. Rockville (MD): Agency for Healthcare Research and Quality; 2009.

13. Chung M, Lee J, Terasawa T, et al. Vitamin D with or without calcium supplementation for prevention of cancer and fractures: an updated meta-analysis for the U.S. Preventive Services Task Force. Ann Intern Med 2011;155(12):827–38.

14. Cranney A, Horsley T, O'Donnell S, et al. Effectiveness and safety of vitamin D in relation to bone health. Evidence report/technology assessment no. 158 (Prepared by the University of Ottawa Evidence-based Practice Center (UO-EPC) under Contract No. 290-02-0021). AHRQ Publication No. 07- E013. Rockville (MD): Agency for Healthcare Research and Quality; 2007.

15. Need AG, O'Loughlin PD, Morris HA, et al. Vitamin D metabolites and calcium absorption in severe vitamin D deficiency. J Bone Miner Res 2008;23:1859–63.

16. Gallagher JC, Yalamanchili V, Smith LM. The effect of vitamin D on calcium absorption in older women. J Clin Endocrinol Metab 2012;97(10):3550–6.

17. Gallagher JC, Jindal PS, Smith LM. Vitamin D does not increase calcium absorption in young women: a randomized clinical trial. J Bone Miner Res 2014;29(5): 1081–7.

18. Aloia JF, Dhaliwal R, Shieh A, et al. Vitamin D supplementation increases calcium absorption without a threshold effect. Am J Clin Nutr 2014;99(3):624–31.

19. Sai AJ, Walters RW, Fang X, et al. Relationship between vitamin D, parathyroid hormone and bone health. J Clin Endocrinol Metab 2011;18:1101–12.

20. Valcour A, Blocki F, Hawkins DM, et al. Effects of age and serum 25-OH-vitamin D on serum parathyroid hormone levels. J Clin Endocrinol Metab 2012;97:3989–99.

21. Krall EA, Dawson-Hughes B, Hirst K, et al. Bone mineral density and biochemical markers of bone turnover in healthy elderly men and women. J Gerontol A Biol Sci Med Sci 1997;52(2):M61–7.

22. Ensrud KE, Taylor BC, Paudel ML, et al, Osteoporotic Fractures in Men Study Group. Serum 25-hydroxyvitamin D levels and rate of hip bone loss in older men. J Clin Endocrinol Metab 2009;94:2773–80.

23. Gallagher JC, Sai AJ. Vitamin D insufficiency, deficiency, and bone health. J Clin Endocrinol Metab 2010;95:2630–3.

24. Cauley JA, Parimi N, Ensrud KE, et al, Osteoporotic Fractures in Men (MrOS) Research Group. Serum 25-hydroxyvitamin D and the risk of hip and non-spine fractures in older men. J Bone Miner Res 2012;25:545–53.

25. Cauley JA, Danielson ME, Boudreau R, et al. Serum 25-hydroxyvitamin D and clinical fracture risk in a multiethnic cohort of women: Women's Health Initiative (WHI). J Bone Miner Res 2011;26:2378–88.

26. Priemel M, von Domarus C, Klatte TO, et al. Bone mineralization defects and vitamin D deficiency: histomorphometric analysis of iliac crest bone biopsies and circulating 25-hydroxyvitamin D in 675 patients. J Bone Miner Res 2010; 25(2):305–12.

27. Tang BM, Eslick GD, Nowson C, et al. Use of calcium or calcium in combination with vitamin D supplementation to prevent fractures and bone loss in people aged 50 years and older: a meta-analysis. Lancet 2007;370(9588):657–66.

28. DIPART (Vitamin D Individual Patient Analysis of Randomized Trials) Group. Patient level pooled analysis of 68 500 patients from seven major vitamin D fracture trials in US and Europe. BMJ 2010;340:b5463.

29. Sanders KM, Stuart AL, Williamson EJ, et al. Annual high-dose oral vitamin D and falls and fractures in older women: a randomized controlled trial. JAMA 2010; 303(18):1815–22.

30. Smith H, Anderson F, Raphael H, et al. Effect of annual intramuscular vitamin D on fracture risk in elderly men and women–a population-based, randomized, double-blind placebo-controlled trial. Rheumatology (Oxford) 2007;46(12): 1852–7.

31. Veugelers PJ, Ekwaru JP. A statistical error in the estimation of the recommended dietary allowance for vitamin D. Nutrients 2014;6(10):4472–5.

32. Garland CF, French CB, Baggerly LL, et al. Vitamin D supplement doses and serum 25hydroxyvitamin D in the range associated with cancer prevention. Anticancer Res 2011;31(2):607.

33. Nordic Council of Ministers. Nordic Nutrition Recommendations 2012. Integrating nutrition and physical activity. Copenhagen (Denmark): Nordic Council of Ministers; 2014. p. 627. 10.6027/Nord2014-002.

34. Health Council of the Netherlands. Evaluation of dietary reference values for vitamin D. The Hague: Health Council of the Netherlands; 2012, publication no. 2012/15E. p. 1–138.

35. Scientific Advisory Committee on Nutrition (SACN). Vitamin D and health. 2016. Public Health England. Available at: https://www.gov.uk/government/groups/scientific advisory-committee-on-nutrition.

36. Manson JE, Brannon PM, Rosen CJ, et al. Vitamin D deficiency - is there really a pandemic? N Engl J Med 2016;375(19):1817–20.

37. Taylor CL, Carriquiry AL, Bailey RL, et al. Appropriateness of the probability approach with a nutrient status biomarker to assess population inadequacy: a study using vitamin D. Am J Clin Nutr 2013;97(1):72–8.

38. Smith LM, Gallagher JC, Suiter C. Higher doses of vitamin D increase the incidence of falls. A randomized clinical trial. J Steroid Biochem Mol Biol 2017.

39. Melamed ML, Michos ED, Post W, et al. 25-hydroxyvitamin D levels and the risk of mortality in the general population. Arch Intern Med 2008;168(15):1629–37.

40. Durup D, Jørgensen HL, Christensen J, et al. A reverse J-shaped association of all-cause mortality with serum 25-hydroxyvitamin D in general practice: the CopD study. J Clin Endocrinol Metab 2012;97(8):2644–52.

41. Sempos CT, Durazo-Arvizu RA, Dawson-Hughes B, et al. Is there a reverse J-shaped association between 25-hydroxyvitamin D and all-cause mortality? Results from the U.S. nationally representative NHANES. J Clin Endocrinol Metab 2013;98(7):3001–9.

42. Gallagher JC, Sai AJ, Templin TJ, et al. Dose response to vitamin D supplementation in postmenopausal women: a randomized clinical trial. Ann Intern Med 2012;156:425–37.

43. Gallagher JC, Peacock M, Yalamanchili V, et al. Effects of vitamin D supplementation in older African American women. J Clin Endocrinol Metab 2013;98(3): 1137–46.

44. Gallagher JC, Jindal PS, Smith LM. Vitamin D supplementation in young Caucasian and African American women. J Bone Miner Res 2014;29(1):173–81.

45. Ng K, Scott JB, Drake BF, et al. Dose response to vitamin D supplementation in African Americans: results of a 4-arm, randomized, placebo-controlled trial. Am J Clin Nutr 2014;99(3):587–98.

46. LeFevre ML, U.S. Preventive Services Task Force. Screening for vitamin D deficiency in adults: U.S. Preventive Services Task Force recommendation statement. Ann Intern Med 2015;162(2):133–40.

Toward Clarity in Clinical Vitamin D Status Assessment: 25(OH)D Assay Standardization

Neil Binkley, MD[a],*, Graham D. Carter, MSc[b]

KEYWORDS

- 25-Hydroxyvitamin D • Vitamin D External Quality Assessment Scheme
- National Institute of Standards and Technology • Office of Dietary Supplements
- Standardization/harmonization • Vitamin D Standardization Program • Vitamin D

KEY POINTS

- Substantial variability in 25(OH)D measurement continues to exist between assay methodologies.
- The Vitamin D Standardization Program (VDSP) has developed approaches allowing standardization of current and prior 25(OH)D data.
- It is necessary to use standardized 25(OH)D results in meta-analyses of outcomes potentially related to vitamin D status.
- Based on data from highly sun-exposed individuals, and including consideration of assay variability, it is our opinion that clinicians are well-advised to target 25(OH)D values of ~30 to 40 ng/mL in their patients, although lower levels have been deemed adequate by other panels of experts.

INTRODUCTION

From a clinical perspective, vitamin D status assessment consists of measuring serum total 25-hydroxyvitamin D (25(OH)D), the sum of serum $25(OH)D_2$ and $25(OH)D_3$ concentrations. Although it is possible, perhaps likely, that other vitamin D metabolites (eg, the 3-epimer of 25(OH)D, cholecalciferol, $24,25(OH)_2D$, and $1,25(OH)_2D$) should also be considered in the assessment of vitamin D physiologic status,[1] measurement of these other vitamin D metabolites is currently available only as a research tool.[2] Although other metabolites may be included in the future, it is currently accepted that singular measurement of serum 25(OH)D is the biologic marker of vitamin D status

Disclosure: The authors have nothing to disclose.
[a] University of Wisconsin Osteoporosis Clinical Research Program, University of Wisconsin-Madison, 2870 University Avenue, Madison, WI 53705, USA; [b] Vitamin D External Quality Assessment Scheme (DEQAS), Imperial College Healthcare NHS Trust, Charing Cross Hospital, Fulham Palace Road, London W6 8RF, UK
* Corresponding author.
E-mail address: nbinkley@wisc.edu

Endocrinol Metab Clin N Am 46 (2017) 885–899
http://dx.doi.org/10.1016/j.ecl.2017.07.012
0889-8529/17/© 2017 Elsevier Inc. All rights reserved.

endo.theclinics.com

clinically[3-5] and this is used to define vitamin D deficiency, inadequacy/insufficiency, sufficiency, and excess. However, there is no consensus regarding the 25(OH)D values to define these clinical states; two quite different guidelines exist to define vitamin D status.[3,4] As a result, clinicians and patients may receive different guidance regarding what constitutes "low" vitamin D status.

Despite massive amounts of vitamin D research, existing data do not allow definitive definition of what constitutes vitamin D inadequacy. A primary confounder of efforts to develop consensus clinical and public health guidelines defining vitamin D status is the substantial variability in the multiple 25(OH)D assays used in research studies over the years.[6-9] In our view, prior lack of 25(OH)D assay standardization is the major underlying confounder of attempts to pool research data and thereby develop consensus cut-points.[10]

In the past, there was no internationally recognized reference measurement procedure (RMP) or certified reference materials to allow standardization of total 25(OH)D measurements. This lack of standardization led to substantial variability among the different assay platforms[6-9,11] with resultant chaos in the vitamin D field with varying 25(OH)D values used to define low vitamin D status and thus varying intake recommendations. This is not surprising; different 25(OH)D assays have yielded different results making it difficult, if not impossible, to conduct meaningful meta-analyses, and to pool data from different studies as part of the process of developing consensus on clinical and public health guidelines.[10] Given the use of different primary data, one could expect that vitamin D intake recommendations and definitions of vitamin D inadequacy would differ. Thus, prior lack of 25(OH)D assay standardization is a fundamental source of chaos in the vitamin D field. Standardization of 25(OH)D assays therefore becomes the path toward clinical (and research/public health guideline) clarity. The Vitamin D Standardization Program (VDSP) was developed to address this situation.[12]

Before describing the VDSP and current assay status, a brief history of 25(OH)D measurement seems appropriate.[11] $25(OH)D_3$ was identified and isolated in 1968. Competitive protein binding assays for 25(OH)D were developed in 1971; since then many commercial and "in house" 25(OH)D methodologies have been developed for use in clinical and research settings. Most of the commercially developed methods are immunoassays because this approach is inexpensive, capable of high throughput, and reasonably simple to use and maintain. More recently, there has been a trend toward chromatography-based assays for use in clinical and research laboratories.[6] A summary of current assay performance is noted in the section on performance testing/quality assessment of 25(OH)D assays.

MEASUREMENT OF 25-HYDROXYVITAMIN D

Serum 25(OH)D is notoriously difficult to measure; this is mainly caused by the hydrophobic nature of the molecule, its existence in three structurally different forms ($25(OH)D_3$, $25(OH)D_2$, and 3 epi-25(OH)D), and its tight binding to vitamin D binding protein (DBP). Additionally, the presence of other substances in serum, particularly lipids, can compromise the ability of the binding agent, usually an antibody, to behave identically with the 25(OH)D in samples and standards. These so-called matrix effects can seriously compromise the accuracy of assays, particularly the modern fully automated immunoassays. In the original Haddad and Chyu[13] competitive protein binding assay, matrix effects were overcome by extracting the 25(OH)D with an organic solvent and chromatographing the extract on silicic acid. Early attempts at abandoning the extraction/chromatography step were unsuccessful.[14] The complexities of the Haddad and Chyu method limited its use to specialist laboratories but with an upsurge of interest in vitamin D, commercial manufacturers developed 25(OH)D methods and added them into automated clinical analytical platforms. Indeed, most clinical laboratories now use these automated immunoassays or the more recently introduced liquid chromatography-tandem mass spectrometry (LC-MS/MS) methods.

A fundamental issue with all nonextraction immunoassays is the preparation of suitable standards; in traditional steroid assays this would involve the addition of known amounts of the steroid, usually in ethanol, to analyte-free human serum. Unfortunately, it has proven virtually impossible to remove endogenous 25(OH)D from human serum, probably because of its tight binding to DBP. Some methods have used bovine serum albumin or other matrices, such as horse serum, in which to prepare standards with the result that they may behave differently to the samples. Indeed the use of horse serum by National Institute of Standards and Technology (NIST) in the preparation of an early standard reference material (SRM) rendered it unusable in a popular automated immunoassay. Furthermore, preparing serum standards by adding known amounts of the analyte in ethanol results in underrecovery of vitamin D metabolites; the reason for this is unknown.[15] Given these problems, it is essential that all immunoassay standards are calibrated with a RMP, that is, a rigorous LC-MS/MS method accepted as accurate by the Committee on Traceability in Laboratory Medicine[16] or an assay traceable to an RMP. An alternative approach is to use SRMs, which can be purchased from NIST; these consist of sets of four human sera (SRM972a) with values for $25(OH)D_2$, $25(OH)D_3$, and $3\text{-epi-}25(OH)D_3$ assigned by the NIST RMP. Details are available on the NIST Web site.[17] Additionally, the NIST SRMs now include $24,25(OH)_2D$ concentrations that have been assigned by the NIST RMP for this metabolite.[18] In addition to SRM972a noted previously, NIST also offers calibrating solutions (SRM2972a) suitable for preparing working standards for LC-MS/MS assays.

Although standardization is fundamental, the accuracy of 25(OH)D results can also be compromised by interference from serum proteins in the sample, notably DBP. In the original extraction methods, DBP was excluded by solvent extraction of 25(OH)D, but in the fully automated immunoassays, alternative methods are required to free 25(OH)D from binding proteins and to prevent their interfering in the assay. Manufacturers are understandably reluctant to give details regarding this process, but changing the serum pH seems to be an approach often used to neutralize the potential effects of DBP. Whatever method is used in these automated systems, the assumption is that all 25(OH)D is released from DBP or, at the very least, the same percentage in every standard and sample. However, some evidence suggests that this may not be true; in four of six immunoassay methods examined in a recent study, 25(OH)D results were significantly reduced in samples with higher DBP concentration.[19] That some inaccuracies result from differences in sample DBP concentration would help to explain sample to sample variability within and between the different immunoassay methods (**Figs. 5–7**).

LC-MS/MS methods are not immune from interference, although solvent extraction and chromatography reduces the risk of nonspecific matrix effects. Problems arise when isobars (compounds having the same molecular weight as the analyte being measured) are not resolved by chromatography.[20] Notably, 3-epi-25(OH)D has the same mass as $25(OH)D_3$ and some routine LC-MS/MS methods fail to resolve this metabolites. Although the concentration of the 3-epimer is low in adults (usually <5% of the $25(OH)D_3$ concentration), the 3-epimer is thought to contribute to the consistently positive bias seen in routine LC-MS/MS 25(OH)D assays, especially in those samples with a high 25(OH)D level (because the 3-epimer concentration is highly correlated with the $25(OH)D_3$ concentration). The concentration of the 3-epimer can be high in neonates, and clinicians wishing to assess vitamin D status in this group should check that the method used appropriately identified 3-epi-25(OH)D.

The difficulties in measuring 25(OH)D accurately make participation in an accuracy-based external quality assessment scheme essential. Clinicians and journal editors should be encouraged to require clinical and research laboratories to produce evidence that their 25(OH)D results are accurate.

WHAT IS ASSAY STANDARDIZATION?

It is important to understand the meaning of assay standardization; for 25(OH)D a standardized laboratory measurement is one that is "comparable across measurement system, location and time."[21–23] Every laboratory regardless of the assay used would obtain the same 25(OH)D result (within predetermined statistical limits) on a given sample as would be obtained using one of the internationally recognized gold standard RMPs.[24–27] It is important to recognize that standardization is not the same as "harmonization." Harmonization is a process by which all laboratories report the same value for a given specimen, but that value is not necessarily the true concentration.[23] Standardization takes harmonization a step further such that laboratories using standardized 25(OH)D assays report not only the same value or concentration, but most importantly the true 25(OH)D concentration.

VITAMIN D STANDARDIZATION PROGRAM

The VDSP was organized in 2010 by the National Institutes of Health Office of Dietary Supplements with the goal of promoting standardized total 25(OH)D measurement and thereby improving health around the world.[12] As part of progress to meet this goal, the VDSP developed methods not only to standardize currently available 25(OH)D assays but also to retrospectively calibrate 25(OH)D results from prior studies that have stored serum to current reference measurement procedures. Such retrospective calibration would allow use of these data in meaningful systematic reviews, thereby facilitating use of previously conducted studies in the development of consensus definitions of vitamin D status.

The VDSP is a collaboration among the National Institutes of Health Office of Dietary Supplements, NIST, Centers for Disease Control and Prevention (CDC), Ghent University, College of American Pathologists, Vitamin D External Quality Assessment Scheme (DEQAS), American Association for Clinical Chemistry, International Federation of Clinical Chemistry and Laboratory Medicine, and researchers worldwide including those working directly with national health/nutrition surveys in many countries.

The primary VDSP objective is to promote standardized serum total 25(OH)D measurement by national health/nutrition surveys, assay manufacturers, and research and clinical laboratories. As such, the VDSP developed a reference measurement system necessary to allow standardized 25(OH)D measurement.[28,29] This system includes gold standard RMPs, SRMs with known NIST-determined 25(OH)D values, the VDSP's Standardization Certification Program developed and conducted by CDC,[25] and accuracy-based performance testing or external quality-assessment schemes (proficiency testing/external quality assessment) conducted by the College of American Pathologists or College of American Pathologists Accuracy-Based Vitamin D Performance Testing Scheme and the Vitamin D External Quality Assessment Scheme or DEQAS.[29–31] The VDSP also developed laboratory performance guidelines for gold standard RMPs and for routine laboratories.[32] Those interested in the practical application of the VDSP system to allow traceability of 25(OH)D results to the gold standard RMPs are referred to recent works describing this process.[28,29]

TRACEABILITY

Ensuring that a 25(OH)D assay is traceable to the RMP is initially the responsibility of assay manufacturers and then subsequently of laboratorians directing their clinical laboratories.[21] For health care providers, knowledge that their clinical assay is traceable to the RMP is important, but clinicians are also advised to appreciate that traceability includes guidance for assay bias and variability (% coefficient of variation [CV]). In this regard, the VDSP has adopted 25(OH)D assay performance criteria developed by Stöckl and colleagues.[32] Specifically, for RMPs the limits for total CV and mean bias were less than or equal to 5% and less than or equal to 1.7%, respectively. Less rigorous requirements apply to routine laboratories for which the limits for total CV and mean bias were less than or equal to 10% and less than or equal to 5%, respectively. Thus, for a clinical laboratory 25(OH)D assay to be defined as traceable to the NIST-Ghent-CDC RMPs it must demonstrate a CV less than or equal to 10% and mean bias of less than or equal to 5%.

EFFECT OF USING STANDARDIZED 25-HYDROXYVITAMIN D ASSAYS

It is self-evident to clinicians that use of assays yielding different results on the same serum specimen could confound clinical care, particularly in the case of vitamin D status where fixed cutpoint values are being recommended to define inadequacy, such as 20 ng/mL or 30 ng/mL. As an example, consider the situation noted in **Fig. 1** in which serum aliquots from two individuals were sent to several clinical laboratories. It is apparent that applying a rigid cutpoint to diagnose "low" vitamin D status, without appreciating assay variability, leads a given individual to receiving different diagnoses (low or normal). Widespread use of standardized assays minimizes this situation.

In addition to the effect on individual patient care, assay variability can affect estimates of vitamin D inadequacy on a nation-wide scale. For example, large research

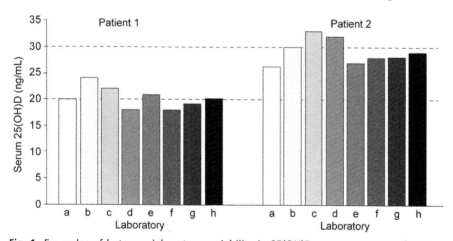

Fig. 1. Examples of between-laboratory variability in 25(OH)D measurement. In these two examples (patient 1 and 2), serum aliquots were sent to eight different clinical laboratories where 25(OH)D was measured in routine clinical manner. It is apparent that applying a simple "cutpoint" approach (depicted here as the *dotted line* at 20 ng/mL for patient 1 and 30 ng/mL for patient 2) would lead the individual patient to being told that their vitamin D status was "normal" or "low" based on the laboratory used. (*Data from* Binkley N, Krueger D, Morgan S, et al. Current status of clinical 25-hydroxyvitamin D measurement: an assessment of between-laboratory agreement. Clin Chim Acta 2010;411:1976–82.)

studies are used not only to define "low" vitamin D status but also to quantify the prevalence of inadequacy. Use of differing assays can yield differing prevalence estimates and retrospective assay standardization can therefore substantially affect the prevalence of vitamin D inadequacy. Importantly, the result of such retrospective standardization can vary from study to study depending on whether the original 25(OH)D assay was positively or negatively biased.[33–37] Two examples from national surveys clearly demonstrate the effect of 25(OH)D assay bias: retrospective standardization of the US NHANES III study increased the prevalence of low vitamin D status (**Fig. 2**A).[37] In contrast, in the German KIGGS study the proportion with low vitamin D status was substantially reduced (see **Fig. 2**B).[35] In summary, it is apparent that 25(OH)D assay standardization can affect clinical care and public health guideline development; without standardization, both of these processes remain suboptimal.

ARE ALL 25-HYDROXYVITAMIN D ASSAY METHODOLOGIES THE SAME?

The VDSP does not require any single analytical approach for 25(OH)D measurement. Indeed, the VDSP methods can be used in the standardization of any currently available 25(OH)D assay. However, it is important that clinicians appreciate differences in assay methodology, because despite following VDSP guidance, there are inherent differences. As a generalization, immunoassays have greater variability than chromatographic ones. This variability becomes clinically important despite following the VDSP guidance to evaluate assay performance using mean bias. For example, two laboratories can have similar mean bias, but substantial variation around the mean. This is illustrated by the results for two laboratories, one using an immunoassay and the other an LC-MS/MS method, respectively (**Fig. 3**). Both laboratories have similar levels of total variance at 6% and 4%. They also have similar values for mean bias (−1% and 2%). These statistics suggest that the two laboratories have similar levels of assay performance. However, as is evident in **Fig. 3**, the variability for the immunoassay is substantially greater.

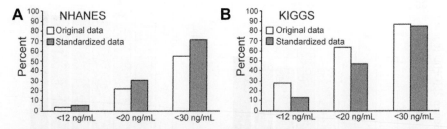

Fig. 2. Impact of assay standardization on the prevalence of persons with serum total 25-hydroxyvitamin D concentrations less than 30, less than 50, and less than 70 nmol/L. Results from the US NHANES III (1988–1994) (*A*) and the German KIGGS study (*B*) Adaptation of the data from two large national surveys reveals the potential effect of retrospective 25(OH)D standardization on vitamin D status prevalence. In the NHANES data (*A*), the prevalence of "low" vitamin D status lower than commonly used cutpoints was increased, whereas in the KIGGS data (*B*), the prevalence was reduced.[35,37] (*Data from* Cashman KD, Dowling KG, Skrabakova Z, et al. Standardizing serum 25-hydroxyvitamin D data from four Nordic population samples using the vitamin D standardization program protocols: shedding new light on vitamin D status in Nordic individuals. Scand J Clin Lab Invest 2015;75(7):549–61; and Schleicher RL, Sternberg MR, Lacher DA, et al. The vitamin D status of the US population from 1988 to 2010 using standardized serum concentrations of 25-hydroxyvitamin D shows recent modest increases. Am J Clin Nutr 2016;104(2):454–461.)

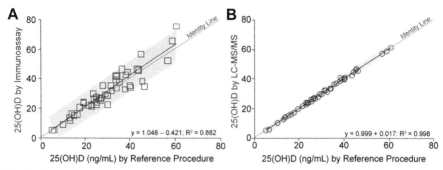

Fig. 3. Illustration of assay variability: immunoassay (*A*) versus LC-MS/MS (*B*). These data, part of a VDSP commutability study, compare reference measurement procedure, that is, "true" 25(OH)D results from two laboratories, one using an immunoassay and the other LC-MS/MS. That substantially less variability is present with the LC-MS/MS method is apparent. The shaded area is the 95% Prediction Interval for the regression line. (*Courtesy of* Christopher Sempos, PhD, National Institutes of Health, Bethesda, MD.)

The clinical "take home message" is that when 25(OH)D results are obtained with an immunoassay, as is often the case in routine clinical care, it should be appreciated that there may be modest variability from the "true" result. Additional considerations surrounding clinical 25(OH)D result variability stem from acceptable assay variation and the use of a fixed cutpoint value to define "low." For example, the VDSP guidance allows up to a 10% CV; in a laboratory with such a CV, a reported 25(OH)D value of 20 ng/mL could be between approximately 16 and 24 ng/mL (**Fig. 4**), that is, either optimal vitamin D status or vitamin D inadequacy if using a 20 ng/mL cutpoint to define low.

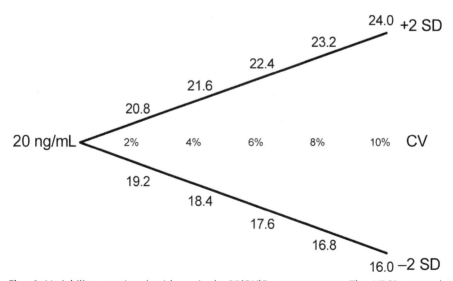

Fig. 4. Variability associated with a single 25(OH)D measurement. The VDSP currently suggests assay performance limits for clinical laboratories that allow a coefficient of variation (%CV) of up to 10%. Assays meeting this criterion are deemed "acceptable." The effect of this variability on a single 25(OH)D value reported as "20 ng/mL" is shown here; the true value lies between 16 and 24 ng/mL. (*Courtesy of* Christopher Sempos, PhD, National Institutes of Health, Bethesda, MD.)

PERFORMANCE TESTING/QUALITY ASSESSMENT OF 25-HYDROXYVITAMIN D ASSAYS

Participation in proficiency testing or external quality assessment schemes has made an important contribution to improving analytical performance in clinical laboratories. The DEQAS is the world's largest specialist external quality assessment for vitamin D metabolites and, since 1989, the quarterly distribution of a large number of samples has facilitated the monitoring of trends in methodology and the performance of individual assays.[8] DEQAS currently has approximately 1000 participating laboratories in 56 countries using about 30 methods or variants of methods (January 2017). Full details of how the scheme operates are found on the DEQAS Web site (www.deqas.org). In brief, five samples of human serum are distributed quarterly. Participating laboratories are given approximately 5 weeks to analyze the samples and return results. The data are used to calculate the All-Laboratory Trimmed Mean and individual Method Means.[38] The DEQAS 25(OH)D scheme became "accuracy based" in 2013 with values assigned by the NIST RMP; this allows participants and manufacturers to check the accuracy of their results against the "true" values. The accuracy of a result is generally expressed as its ×% Bias from the "true" result, the target value provided by NIST; % Bias = {(result−target value)/(target value)*100}.

DEQAS data collected In recent years show an overall improvement in accuracy, that is, bias (**Fig. 5**) and interlaboratory precision (**Fig. 6**); 25(OH)D assay standardization has undoubtedly contributed to this improvement. Unfortunately, there remains considerable sample-to-sample variability in accuracy, particularly in the nonchromatographic immunoassays. This is a problem inherent to this type of assay in which the accuracy of results is affected by the presence (cross-reactivity) of other vitamin D metabolites (eg, $24,25(OH)_2D$, the concentration of which varies from sample to sample). Other constituents of the sample can also give rise to falsely low or falsely high results (matrix effects). Unfortunately this type of interference is inconsistent and contributes to intermethod differences independent of standardization, therefore compromising the approach of using mean bias to compare accuracy of different methods (**Fig. 7**). LC-MS/MS methods are much less prone to intersample variability, although there is a modest overall positive bias, possibly caused by the cross-reactivity of 3-epi-$25(OH)D_3$, which in many assays is not resolved from $25(OH)D_3$.

Most 25(OH)D methods are required to measure "total 25(OH)D," which by definition is the sum of $25(OH)D_3$ and $25(OH)D_2$. Because $25(OH)D_2$ is present in substantial quantity only in individuals supplemented with vitamin D_2, it is important that samples

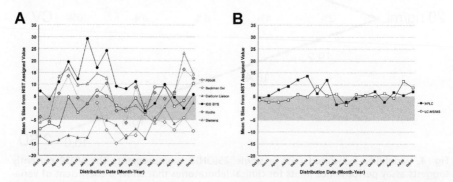

Fig. 5. Mean bias from NIST assigned values in DEQAS. (*A*) Major automated ligand binding assays. (*B*) Chromatographic assays (HPLC [high-performance liquid chromatography] and LC-MS/MS [liquid chromatography tandem mass spectrometry]). Shaded area depicts the limits for routine clinical assays adopted by the VDSP.

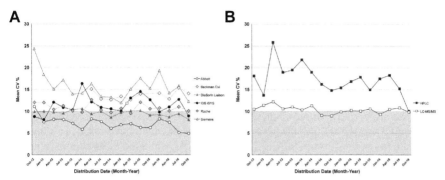

Fig. 6. Mean interlaboratory %CV in DEQAS. (*A*) Major automated ligand binding assays. (*B*) Chromatographic assays (HPLC [high-performance liquid chromatography] and LC-MS/MS [liquid chromatography tandem mass spectrometry]). Shaded area depicts the limits for routine clinical assays adopted by the VDSP.

from these subjects are analyzed by a method that is cospecific for both 25(OH)D$_3$ and 25(OH)D$_2$. At least in the past, DEQAS has demonstrated that manufacturer data on the specificity of 25(OH)D assays is not always reliable and clinicians should consult their local laboratory. Specifically, there have been reports of vitamin D–deficient patients failing to show a rise in total 25(OH)D despite supplementation with large and increasing doses of vitamin D$_2$. In these circumstances, a change in 25(OH)D assay method may reveal the problem to be analytical.[39]

25-HYDROXYVITAMIN D REFERENCE RANGES

Clinical laboratories provide reference ranges to help clinicians interpret results. Traditionally, reference ("normal") ranges are determined either by using the assay

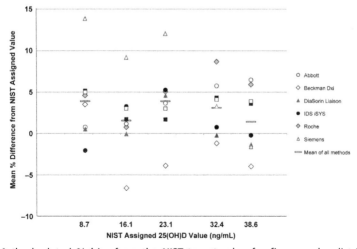

Fig. 7. Method-related % bias from the NIST target value for five samples distributed in October 2016 in DEQAS. Sample variability of nonchomatographic immunoassays is demonstrated at each NIST standard. Method inconsistency is impacted by cross-reactivity with other vitamin D metabolites and matrix effects. The line depicting the mean of all methods reinforces the unpredictability of difference and challenge in using this approach to compare the accuracy of methods.

manufacturer's normal range or from a sample of the local population. When the data are normally distributed, the normal range is defined as two standard deviations above and below the mean and encompasses approximately 95% of normal individuals. Unfortunately, because vitamin D deficiency is so common, such an approach would yield inappropriately low reference ranges and lead to an underdiagnosis of vitamin D deficiency. As such, much effort has gone into attempts to define vitamin D deficiency, inadequacy, and sufficiency using fixed 25(OH)D cutpoints.[3,40] These current guidelines are based on meta-analyses of large clinical and epidemiologic studies that have used a variety of 25(OH)D assays, virtually all of which have not been standardized. As a result the "same" 25(OH)D value has not been used in decisions regarding cutpoint determination and daily vitamin D dose needed. As such, it is unsurprising that controversy continues regarding what constitutes vitamin D sufficiency. It is only by using standardized 25(OH)D results that this controversy can be resolved.

WHAT IS A CLINICIAN TO DO?

Meta-analyses using unstandardized 25(OH)D results are unlikely to allow consensus to be reached. Indeed, it has been suggested that no further meta-analyses using unstandardized 25(OH)D data be performed.[10] Moreover, many clinical trials of vitamin D supplementation performed in the past have flaws, most notably not requiring study subjects to be low in vitamin D before providing additional supplementation. Heaney[41] recently published guidance for design and analysis of studies of nutrients, so there is reason for optimism in the future conduct of clinical trials. Briefly, this guidance includes (1) the necessity that nutrient status must be measured and used as a study inclusion criterion noted in the trial report, (2) that the nutritional intervention be large enough to change nutrient status and also be quantified by appropriate analyses, and (3) that the change in nutrient status be measured and reported.

However, results of yet to be conducted trials following this guidance and meta-analyses limited to use of standardized 25(OH)D data (which currently do not exist) are not helpful to clinical care today. Indeed, clinicians and patients are currently faced with conflicting guidance regarding what vitamin D dose and target 25(OH)D to recommend. Given the challenges with the data available to answer the "how much is enough" question, combined with improving, but ongoing assay variability, it is our opinion that a common sense approach is needed at this time until rigorous randomized longitudinal trials show otherwise.

The Institute of Medicine recommends 600 IU of daily vitamin D for individuals up to age 70 and 800 IU for those aged 71 and older. However, these are public health recommendations that are not necessarily guidelines for care of individual patients, and some individuals may need substantially more than this. Indeed, there is substantial between-individual variability in the 25(OH)D response to implementation of daily vitamin D supplementation. Notably, some people experience little or no increase in serum 25(OH)D following what many would consider high-dose vitamin D supplementation (**Fig. 8**). Clearly, a "one size fits all" approach will not ensure attaining the clinician's target 25(OH)D value.

The mechanisms leading to this variability in 25(OH)D response to supplementation are not clearly defined. However, it is logical that some of this variation reflects differences in absorption, rates of use/degradation (possibly caused by genetic differences), use of medications affecting vitamin D metabolism, high body mass or obesity, and potentially other factors. As a generalization, obese persons require more vitamin D than normal-weight persons to attain the same increase in serum 25(OH)D; it is possible that this simply reflects a larger volume of distribution in

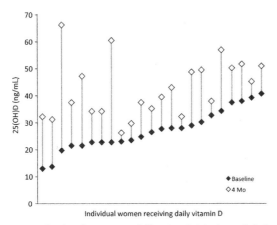

Fig. 8. The increase in 25(OH)D that occurs following initiation of daily supplementation differs between individuals. The 25(OH)D increase following oral vitamin D_3 supplementation varies greatly between people. Presented here are 25(OH)D data from 23 postmenopausal women that received 2300 IU of vitamin D_3 daily for 4 months; all were 95% to 100% compliant with this supplementation. Serum 25(OH)D was measured at baseline and 4 months of follow-up; between-individual variability is apparent.

such individuals. As such, some have suggested that obese persons be given higher doses of vitamin D supplementation (6000–10,000 IU/day) for treatment and prevention of vitamin D deficiency.[40] Vitamin D_3 and D_2 supplements are widely available over-the-counter in doses ranging from 400 to 50,000 IU and are generally well tolerated. Although not all studies agree, there is some evidence that D_3 supplementation produces a greater increment in 25(OH)D than does D_2 supplementation.[42] Finally, given the variation of serum 25(OH)D response following supplementation, it is reasonable to repeat 25(OH)D measurement approximately 4 to 6 months after starting or increasing the vitamin D supplementation dose. It is necessary to wait for several months to determine the new value because 25(OH)D has a half-life of approximately 3 weeks.

The definition of "low" 25(OH)D is extremely controversial. However, virtually all experts and organizations/guidelines agree that 25(OH)D levels lower than 20 ng/mL (50 nmol/L) are "low," whereas some suggest that the ideal target for 25(OH)D is higher than 30 ng/mL (75–80 nmol/L).[40] Based on current clinical assay variability (resulting in inability to know if an individual patient's 25(OH)D value is correct, low, or high), combined with lack of toxicity at modest 25(OH)D levels, we believe it reasonable that clinicians strive for 25(OH)D levels approximately 5 to 10 ng/mL higher than whatever cutpoint value they choose (eg, 20–30 ng/mL if one follows the Institute of Medicine guidance of 20 ng/mL).

Possibly consistent with a target 25(OH)D value of approximately 30 to 40 ng/mL, a recent analysis of more than 26,000 individuals in European cohort studies found the lowest overall mortality in those whose 25(OH)D was 30 to 40 ng/mL.[43] Additionally, but in our opinion importantly, highly sun-exposed individuals have 25(OH)D values that average roughly 35 to 40 ng/mL.[44,45] Previously, no studies of highly sun-exposed people have used standardized 25(OH)D results. Here we report preliminary data in 39 adults from our previously published "surfer study" in which 25(OH)D results were obtained using an LC-MS/MS methodology corrected to the DEQAS assigned NIST values (**Fig. 9**). As noted, none of these highly sun-exposed individuals have a

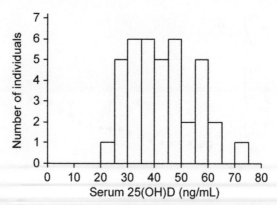

Fig. 9. Serum 25(OH)D in 39 highly sun-exposed white adults as measured using an LC-MS/MS assay traceable to NIST-assigned values in DEQAS. In this cohort of highly sun-exposed individuals, the mean 25(OH)D was 42 ng/mL; no individual's serum 25(OH)D was less than 20 ng/mL.

25(OH)D less than 25 ng/mL, the highest was 71 ng/mL, and the mean was 42 ng/mL. These results are in general similar to the highly sun-exposed hunter-gatherer cohort reported by Luxwolda and colleagues[44] and Afro-Caribbean men from Tobago,[46] which, in our opinion, provide support for clinicians targeting 25(OH)D levels of approximately 30 to 40 ng/mL.

Based on assay variability, combined with lack of toxicity, a reasonable 25(OH)D range of approximately 30 to 40 ng/mL (100 nmol/L) should ensure a "true" 25(OH)D value higher than 20 to 30 ng/mL (50–75 nmol/L) without exposing patients to extremely high levels.

SUMMARY

Use of standardized 25(OH)D data is essential in ongoing and future research studies of vitamin D supplementation. Retrospective standardization of 25(OH)D data from key prior research studies is essential if those studies are to be used in systematic reviews attempting to define low vitamin D status. Without such standardization, efforts to develop guidelines regarding vitamin status are unlikely to reach consensus. Until prospective and retrospective standardized 25(OH)D data are available systematic reviews relating 25(OH)D status to various diseases should be deferred. Thus, in the future, use of standardized 25(OH)D results should provide clinical clarity regarding the definition of vitamin D status. In the interim, based on assay variability, clinicians are advised to target 25(OH)D values of approximately 30 to 40 ng/mL in their patients.

REFERENCES

1. Hollis BW, Wagner CL. Clinical review: the role of the parent compound vitamin D with respect to metabolism and function: why clinical dose intervals can affect clinical outcomes. J Clin Endocrinol Metab 2013;98(12):4619–28.

2. Binkley N, Borchardt G, Siglinsky E, et al. Does vitamin D metabolite measurement help predict 25(OH)D change following vitamin D supplementation? Endocr Pract 2017;23(4):432–41.

3. Ross AC, Taylor CL, Yakine AL, et al. Report on dietary reference intakes for vitamin D and calcium. Washington, DC: Institute of Medicine. The National Academies Press; 2011.

4. Holick MF, Binkley NC, Bischoff-Ferrari HA, et al. Guidelines for preventing and treating vitamin D deficiency and insufficiency revisited. J Clin Endocrinol Metab 2012;97:1153–8.

5. Scientific Advisory Committee on Nutrition (SACN). SACN vitamin D and health report. London: Public Health England; 2016.

6. de la Hunty A, Wallace AM, Gibson S, et al. UK foods standards agency workshop consensus report: the choice of method for measuring 25-hydroxyvitamin D to estimate vitamin D status for the UK National Diet and Nutrition Survey. Br J Nutr 2010;104:612–9.

7. Wallace AM, Gibson S, de la Hunty A, et al. Measurement of 25-hydroxyvitamin D in the clinical laboratory: current procedures, performance characteristics and limitations. Steroids 2010;75:477–88.

8. Carter GD, Carter R, Jones J, et al. How accurate are assays for 25-hydroxyvitamin D? Data from the international vitamin D external quality assessment scheme. Clin Chem 2004;50:2195–7.

9. Binkley N, Krueger D, Cowgill CS, et al. Assay variation confounds the diagnosis of hypovitaminosis D: a call for standardization. J Clin Endocrinol Metab 2004; 89(7):3152–7.

10. Binkley N, Dawson-Hughes B, Durazo-Arvizu R, et al. Vitamin D measurement standardization: the way out of the chaos. J Steroid Biochem Mol Biol 2017; 173:117–21.

11. Le Goff C, Cavalier E, Souberbielle J-C, et al. Measurement of circulating 25-hydroxyvitamin D: a historical review. Pract Lab Med 2015;2:1–14.

12. Sempos CT, Vesper HW, Phinney KW, et al. Vitamin D status as an international issue: National surveys and the problem of standardization. Scand J Clin Lab Invest 2012;72(S243):32–40.

13. Haddad JG, Chyu KJ. Competitive protein-binding radioassay for 25-hydroxycholecalciferol. J Clin Endocrinol Metab 1971;33:992–5.

14. Belsey RE, DeLuca HF, Potts JT. A rapid assay for 25-(OH)vitamin D3 without preparative chromatography. J Clin Endocrinol Metab 1974;38:1046–51.

15. Carter GD, Jones JC, Berry JL. The anomalous behaviour of exogenous 25-hydroxyvitamin D in competitive binding assays. J Steroid Biochem Mol Biol 2007;103(3–5):480–2.

16. Jones GRD, Jackson C. The Joint Committee for Traceability in Laboratory Medicine (JCTLM) - its history and operation. Clin Chim Acta 2016;453:86–94.

17. Anonymous. SRM 972a - Vitamin D metabolites in frozen human serum. Standard reference materials. Available at: https://catalog.data.gov/dataset/srm-972a-vitamin-d-metabolites-in-frozen-human-serum. Accessed March 31, 2017.

18. Tai SS, Nelson MA. Candidate reference measurement procedure for the determination of (24R),25-dihydroxyvitamin D3 in human serum using isotope-dilution liquid chromatography-tandem mass spectrometry. Anal Chem 2015;87(15): 7964–70.

19. Heijboer AC, Blankenstein MA, Kema IP, et al. Accuracy of 6 routine 25-hydroxyvitamin D assays: influence of vitamin D binding protein concentration. Clin Chem 2012;58(3):543–8.

20. Shah I, James R, Barker J, et al. Misleading measures in vitamin D analysis: a novel LC-MS/MS assay to account for epimers and isobars. Nutr J 2011;10:46.

21. Vesper HW, Thienpont LM. Traceability in laboratory medicine. Clin Chem 2009; 55(6):1067–75.
22. Myers GL. Introduction to standardization of laboratory results. Steroids 2008; 73(13):1293–6.
23. Greg Miller W, Myers GL, Lou Gantzer M, et al. Roadmap for harmonization of clinical laboratory measurement procedures. Clin Chem 2011;57(8):1108–17.
24. Tai SSC, Bedner M, Phinney KW. Development of a candidate reference measurement procedure for the determination of 25-hydroxyvitamin D3 and 25-hydroxyvitamin D2 in human serum using isotope-dilution liquid chromatography-tandem mass spectrometry. Anal Chem 2010;82:1942–8.
25. Thienpont LM, Stepman HC, Vesper HW. Standardization of measurements of 25-hydroxyvitamin D3 and D2. Scand J Clin Lab Invest 2012;72(S243):41–9.
26. Mineva EM, Schleicher RL, Chaudhary-Webb M, et al. A candidate reference measurement procedure for quantifying serum concentrations of 25-hydroxyvitamin D(3) and 25-hydroxyvitamin D(2) using isotope-dilution liquid chromatography-tandem mass spectrometry. Anal Bioanal Chem 2015;407(19):5615–24.
27. Stepman HC, Vanderroost A, Van Uytfanghe K, et al. Candidate reference measurement procedures for serum 25-hydroxyvitamin D3 and 25-hydroxyvitamin D2 by using isotope-dilution liquid chromatography-tandem mass spectrometry. Clin Chem 2011;57(3):441–8.
28. Binkley N, Sempos CT. Standardizing vitamin D assays: the way forward. J Bone Miner Res 2014;29(8):1709–14.
29. Sempos CT, Carter GD, Merkel JM, et al. The path to serum total 25-hydroxyvitamin D assay standardization. Austin J Nutr Metab 2016;3(2):1039.
30. College of American Pathologists. Accuracy-based vitmain D (ABVD). Proficiency testing/EQA 2016. Available at: https://estore.cap.org. Accessed February 22, 2016.
31. DEQAS (Vitamin D external quality assessment scheme). Available at: http://www.deqas.org/. Accessed August 9, 2016.
32. Stockl D, Sluss PM, Thienpont LM. Specifications for trueness and precision of a reference measurement system for serum/plasma 25-hydroxyvitamin D analysis. Clin Chim Acta 2009;408(1–2):8–13.
33. Cashman KD, Kiely M, Kinsella M, et al. Evaluation of vitamin D standardization program protocols for standardizing serum 25-hydroxyvitamin D data: a case study of the program's potential for national nutrition and health surveys. Am J Clin Nutr 2013;97(6):1235–42.
34. Sarafin K, Durazo-Arvizu R, Tian L, et al. Standardizing 25-hydroxyvitamin D values from the Canadian health measures survey. Am J Clin Nutr 2015;102(5): 1044–50.
35. Cashman KD, Dowling KG, Skrabakova Z, et al. Standardizing serum 25-hydroxyvitamin D data from four Nordic population samples using the vitamin D standardization program protocols: shedding new light on vitamin D status in Nordic individuals. Scand J Clin Lab Invest 2015;75(7):549–61.
36. Cashman KD, Dowling KG, Skrabakova Z, et al. Vitamin D deficiency in Europe: pandemic? Am J Clin Nutr 2016;103(4):1033–44.
37. Schleicher RL, Sternberg MR, Lacher DA, et al. The vitamin D status of the US population from 1988 to 2010 using standardized serum concentrations of 25-hydroxyvitamin D shows recent modest increases. Am J Clin Nutr 2016;104(2): 454–61.
38. Healy MJR. Outliers in clinical chemistry quality-control schemes. Clin Chem 1979;25:675–7.

39. Leventis P, Garrison L, Sibley M, et al. Underestimation of serum 25-hydroxyvitamin D by the Nichols advantage assay in patients receiving vitamin D replacement therapy. Clin Chem 2005;51(6):1072–4 [author reply: 1074].
40. Holick MF, Binkley N, Bischoff-Ferrari HA, et al. Evaluation, treatment, and prevention of vitamin D deficiency: an endocrine society clinical practice guideline. J Clin Endocrinol Metab 2011;96:1911–30.
41. Heaney RP. Guidelines for optimizing design and analysis of clinical studies of nutrient effects. Nutr Rev 2014;72(1):48–54.
42. Heaney RP, Recker RR, Grote J, et al. Vitamin D_3 is more potent than vitamin D_2 in humans. J Clin Endocrinol Metab 2011. http://dx.doi.org/10.1210/jc.2010-2230.
43. Gaksch M, Jorde R, Grimnes G, et al. Vitamin D and mortality: Individual participant data meta-analysis of standardized 25-hydroxyvitamin D in 26916 individuals from a European consortium. PLoS One 2017;12(2):e0170791.
44. Luxwolda MF, Kuipers RS, Kema IP, et al. Traditionally living populations in East Africa have a mean serum 25-hydroxyvitamin D concentration of 115 nmol/L. Br J Nutr 2012;108:1557–61.
45. Binkley N, Novotny R, Krueger D, et al. Low vitamin D status despite abundant sun exposure. J Clin Endocrinol Metab 2007;92:2130–5.
46. Miljkovic I, Bodnar LM, Cauley JA, et al. Low prevalence of vitamin D deficiency in elderly Afro-Caribbean men. Ethn Dis 2011;21(1):79–84.

Current Controversies

Are Free Vitamin Metabolite Levels a More Accurate Assessment of Vitamin D Status than Total Levels?

Daniel D. Bikle, MD, PhD[a],*, Sofie Malmstroem, MD[b,c], Janice Schwartz, MD[b]

KEYWORDS

- Vitamin D • Free hormone hypothesis • Free vitamin D • Vitamin D metabolism
- Pregnancy • Liver disease

KEY POINTS

- Vitamin D and its metabolites are tightly bound to serum proteins, of which the vitamin D binding protein (DBP) is the most important, such that less than 1% of the total concentration of vitamin D and its metabolites are free in the circulation.
- For most tissues, the vitamin D metabolites enter the cell as the free hormone presumably by diffusion (the free hormone hypothesis), although a few tissues such as the kidney express megalin/cubilin enabling by endocytosis vitamin D metabolites bound to DBP to enter the cell.
- Measuring the free levels of the vitamin D metabolites may provide a better measure of the true vitamin D status than measuring the total levels.
- Early methods to determine the free levels of 25-hydroxyvitamin D (25(OH)D) and 1,25 dihydroxyvitamin D (1,25(OH)$_2$D) demonstrated that the free levels were normal in patients with liver disease despite low total levels and that free levels were elevated in pregnant women in the third trimester more than would be predicted based on total levels.
- Newer methods for measuring free 25(OH)D have been developed that are easier to perform, and their widespread application should help determine the clinical value of determining free 25(OH)D in addition to and/or instead of total 25(OH)D in the evaluation of vitamin D status.

Disclosures: Dr D.D. Bikle is currently or recently funded by grants from the NIH (RO1 AR050023) and VA (IBX001066). Dr S. Malmstroem is supported by a fellowship from the Lundbeck Foundation for Clinical Research. Dr J. Schwartz has received research funds from NIA (R21 AG041660), Future Diagnostics Solutions B.V., and DiaSource and has consulted for Amgen and Pfizer.

[a] Department of Medicine, University of California San Francisco, San Francisco VA Medical Center, 1700 Owens Street, San Francisco, CA 94158, USA; [b] University of California San Francisco, 1700 Owens Street, San Francisco, CA 94158, USA; [c] Department of Endocrinology and Internal Medicine, Aarhus University Hospital, Aarhus, Denmark
* Corresponding author.
E-mail address: Daniel.bikle@ucsf.edu

Endocrinol Metab Clin N Am 46 (2017) 901–918
http://dx.doi.org/10.1016/j.ecl.2017.07.013
0889-8529/17/Published by Elsevier Inc.

INTRODUCTION

Circulating levels of 25-hydroxyvitamin D (25(OH)D) are the most commonly used marker for the assessment of vitamin D nutritional status. The main reason why 25(OH)D levels are used to assess vitamin D nutritional status is because its concentration in blood is higher than all other vitamin D metabolites, making it easier to measure, and because its conversion from vitamin D is substrate dependent with minimal regulation. The liver is the major source of this conversion, performed by several enzymes with 25-hydroxylase activity, the most specific of which is CYP2R1. However, 25OHD is not the most biologically active metabolite of vitamin D. Instead, 25(OH)D must be further metabolized to 1,25 dihydroxyvitamin D (1,25(OH)$_2$D) for vitamin D to achieve its full biologic potential. 1,25(OH)$_2$D is the ligand for a nuclear transcription factor, the vitamin D receptor (VDR), that mediates the genomic and at least some of the nongenomic actions of vitamin D within the cell. Nearly all if not all cells express the VDR at some stage in their development or activation. The kidney produces most of the circulating 1,25(OH)$_2$D through the enzyme CYP27B1, but many cells also express CYP27B1 and so are able to form their own 1,25(OH)$_2$D. As the appreciation that vitamin D and its metabolites affect numerous physiologic processes and not just bone and mineral metabolism, and that these physiologic processes may have different requirements for these vitamin D metabolites,[1] interest in determining optimal levels of the vitamin D metabolites to effect these different biologic processes has grown. Complicating this determination is the fact that all the vitamin D metabolites circulate in blood tightly bound to proteins, of which the vitamin D binding protein (DBP) plays the major role. For most cells, these binding proteins limit the flux of the vitamin D metabolites from blood into the cell, where they exert their biologic activity. This observation raises the issue then of what should be measured to determine vitamin D status: the total levels of these metabolites or the free levels. Before considering this subject directly, a brief review of vitamin D production and metabolism is undertaken by way of introducing the key players in the vitamin D endocrine system.

VITAMIN D PRODUCTION AND METABOLISM
Vitamin D Production

Vitamin D$_3$ (D$_3$) (cholecalciferol) is produced from 7-dehydrocholesterol in the skin through a 2-step process in which the B ring is broken by UV light (UV-B spectrum 280–320 nm), forming pre-D$_3$ that isomerizes to D$_3$ in a thermosensitive but noncatalytic process. Vitamin D is also obtained from the diet. Most foods with the exception of fatty fish contain little vitamin D unless fortified. The vitamin D in fish is D$_3$, whereas that used for fortification is often D$_2$ (ergocalciferol). D$_2$ is produced by UV-B irradiation of ergosterol in plants and fungi (eg, mushrooms). It differs from D$_3$ in having a double bond between C22 and C23 and a methyl group at C24 in the side chain. These differences from D$_3$ in the side chain lower its affinity for DBP, resulting in a higher ratio of free to total vitamin D metabolite concentration as well as faster clearance from the circulation and altered catabolism by the 24-hydroxyase (CYP24A1).[2–4] Moreover, several immunoassays do not recognize the D$_2$ metabolites as well as the D$_3$ metabolites, a problem addressed in later discussion. However, the biologic activity of D$_2$ and D$_3$ metabolites is comparable, and if no subscript is used, both forms are meant.

Vitamin D Metabolism

The 3 main steps in vitamin D metabolism, 25-hydroxylation, 1α-hydroxylation, and 24-hydroxylation, are all performed by cytochrome P450 mixed function oxidases (CYPs) located either in the endoplasmic reticulum (eg, CYP2R1) or in the mitochondrion (eg, CYP27A1, CYP27B1, and CYP24A1).

25-Hydroxylase

The liver is the major if not sole source of 25(OH)D production. There are multiple 25-hydroxyases, but the best studied are CYP27A1 and CYP2R1. CYP27A1 is the only mitochondrial 25-hydroxylase. It was initially identified as a sterol 27-hydroxylase involved in bile acid synthesis and so is not specific for vitamin D. Moreover, it preferentially hydroxylates D_3 versus D_2. It is widely distributed in the body, not just in the liver. Its relevance to vitamin D metabolism is unclear because its deletion in mice results in increased blood levels of 25(OH)D,[5] and inactivating mutations in humans cause cerebrotendinous xanthomatosis, not rickets.[6] CYP2R1 is in the microsomal fraction,[7] with distribution primarily limited to the liver and testes. It 25-hydroxylates both D_2 and D_3 with comparable kinetics. Deletion of CYP2R1 reduces blood levels of 25OHD by 50%, but not to zero,[8] suggesting compensation by other enzymes with 25-hydroxylase activity. However, inactivating mutations in CYP2R1 have been found in humans presenting with rickets.[9] Thus, CYP2R1 is considered the major albeit not the only 25-hydroxylase contributing to circulating levels of 25(OH)D. Regulation of vitamin D 25-hydroxylation is modest at best with production being primarily substrate dependent such that circulating levels of 25(OH)D are a useful marker of vitamin D nutrition.

25-Hydroxyvitamin D 1α-hydroxylase (CYP27B1)

CYP27B1 is the only known 25(OH)D 1-hydroxylase. Although the kidney is the main source of circulating 1,25(OH)$_2$D, several other tissues also express the enzyme. As discussed later, most tissues expressing CYP27B1 rely on the free 25OHD level in blood for their available substrate, whereas the kidney tubule has a mechanism for taking up 25OHD still bound to its major binding protein, DBP. Moreover, regulation of the extrarenal CYP27B1 differs from that of the renal CYP27B1 (review in Ref.[10]). The renal 1α-hydroxylase is tightly regulated primarily by 3 hormones: parathyroid hormone (PTH) (stimulatory), FGF23 (inhibitory), and 1,25(OH)$_2$D itself (inhibitory). CYP27B1 activity in extrarenal tissues is not regulated by PTH and FGF23, but at least in epidermal keratinocytes and cells of the immune system the regulation is by cytokines such as tumor necrosis factor-α and interferon-γ.[11–13] In these tissues as well as in the kidney, 1,25(OH)$_2$D induces CYP24A1, the 24-hydroxylase that catabolizes both 25OHD and 1,25(OH)$_2$D. CYP24A1 is the major mechanism controlling 1,25(OH)$_2$D levels in these cells. As for 25(OH)D, it is anticipated that it is the free concentration of 1,25(OH)$_2$D that enters most cells, the kidney proximal tubule, parathyroid gland, and placenta being likely exceptions as discussed later.

24-Hydroxylase (CYP24A1)

CYP24A1 is the only established 24-hydroxylase involved with vitamin D metabolism. It is strongly induced by 1,25(OH)$_2$D. This enzyme has both 24-hydroxylase and 23-hydroxylase activity, the ratio of which is species dependent[14]; the human enzyme has both capabilities. The 24-hydroxylase pathway results in the biologically inactive calcitroic acid, although 1,24,25(OH)$_3$D, the first step in the pathway for 1,25(OH)$_2$D catabolism, has biological activity, and 24,25(OH)$_2$D, the first step in 25OHD catabolism, may be important for endochondral bone formation.[15] The 23-hydroxylase pathway produces the biologically active 25OHD-26,23-lactone and 1,25(OH)$_2$D-26,23 lactone. Moreover, unlike many other cancers, the expression of CYP24A1 in melanoma is inversely correlated with melanoma progression.[16] Thus, it is incorrect to consider the 24-hydroxylase as purely a catabolic enzyme for 25(OH)D and 1,25(OH)$_2$D. All steps are performed by one enzyme.[17] Regulation of CYP24A1 is the reciprocal of that of CYP27B1 at least in the kidney in that PTH inhibits but FGF23 stimulates its expression.

THE FREE HORMONE HYPOTHESIS
The Hypothesis and Its Modification

The free hormone hypothesis postulates that only the nonbound fraction (the free fraction) of hormones that otherwise circulate in blood bound to their carrier proteins is able to enter cells and exert their biologic effects (**Fig. 1**). Examples include the vitamin D metabolites, which are discussed in this review, sex steroids, cortisol, and thyroid hormone. These molecules are lipophilic hormones assumed to cross the plasma membrane by diffusion and not by an active transport mechanism. However, the free hormone concentration is not the only factor involved with the rate at which the hormone enters the cells. As articulated by Mendel,[18] movement of hormone into the cell in vivo is dependent not only on the free concentration but also on the dissociation of hormone from its binding protein, the rate of blood flow, the rate of uptake into the cell, and the catabolism/sequestration of hormone within the cell. These processes are components of the transport process that Mendel calls the free hormone transport process. Thus, the total concentration of hormone, by affecting the total amount of free hormone available to the cell, does influence the extent of transport of hormone into the cell when the rate of transport is not rate limiting. That said, knowledge of most of those variables is limited, so the focus in this review is on the free hormone itself, its measurement, and what influences this fraction of the total hormone in circulation.

Development of the Hypothesis

One of the earliest articulations of the free hormone hypothesis was published by Recant and Riggs[19] when they examined thyroid function in patients with protein-losing nephropathy. They noted that circulating thyroid hormone (measured as protein-bound iodine) was quite low in these patients along with increased urinary losses but with relatively little evidence for clinical hypothyroidism. They concluded

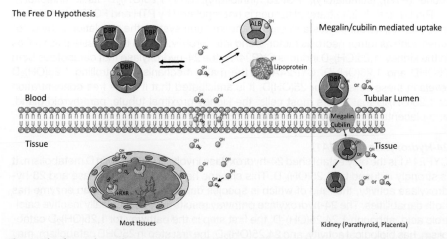

The Free D Hypothesis

Blood — Megalin/cubilin mediated uptake — Lipoprotein — Tubular Lumen — Tissue — Megalin Cubilin — Tissue — Most tissues — Kidney (Parathyroid, Placenta)

Fig. 1. The free D hypothesis. Vitamin D hydroxy metabolites (*blue circles*) in the circulation are primarily bound to DBP and to a lesser extent to albumin (ALB) and possibly to lipoproteins with only the unbound 25(OH)D and 1,25(OH)₂D freely crossing the cell membrane or through the nuclear pore to interact with the VDR. Many tissues express the 1α-25(OH)D-hydroxylase that metabolizes 25(OH)D to the active 1,25(OH)₂D. In several tissues, such as the kidney and potentially the parathyroid and placenta, 25(OH)D and 1,25(OH)₂D bound to DBP may enter cell tissues by endocytosis via megalin/cubulin and are not limited to diffusion by the free hormone.

that "thyroid function and the supply of hormone to the tissues in nephrosis may be normal, and that the low concentration of protein-bound iodine in the plasma is due to the change in concentration or binding capacity of the plasma proteins in nephrosis." Subsequent studies have established the free hormone hypothesis for the thyroid and steroid hormones.[20,21] Similar conclusions regarding the importance of the free levels of vitamin D metabolites came initially from observations that the increase in $1,25(OH)_2D$ levels with administration of oral contraceptives or during the third trimester of pregnancy was not associated with changes in calcium metabolism, at least until the latter stages of pregnancy, but was accompanied by a parallel increase in DBP.[22] This role of DBP as carrier of the vitamin D metabolites was well demonstrated in mice in which the DBP gene was deleted. Although these mice lost substantial amounts of the vitamin D metabolites in the urine, and their circulating levels of 25(OH)D were very low, they did not develop evidence of rickets until put on a low vitamin D diet.[23] These observations parallel the much earlier observations by Recant and Riggs[19] in their nephrotic patients with low thyroid hormone levels in the absence of clinical hypothyroidism. Subsequently, the interest in free 25(OH)D and free $1,25(OH)_2D$ levels has increased substantially because of their relevance to disease states in which the binding proteins are markedly altered such as liver disease and protein-losing nephropathy, normal physiologic states such as pregnancy, and genetic variations in binding proteins that may affect their affinity for the hormone in question.[24]

The Bound, Free, and Bioavailable Fractions in Serum

In serum samples from normal individuals, $\sim 85\%$ of circulating vitamin D metabolites are bound to DBP, whereas albumin with its substantially lower binding affinity binds only $\sim 15\%$ of these metabolites despite its 10-fold higher concentration than DBP. Approximately 0.4% of total $1,25(OH)_2D$ and 0.03% of total 25OHD is free in serum from normal nonpregnant individuals. The fraction of "bioavailable" vitamin D metabolites comprises the fraction of the free vitamin D and the fraction bound to albumin, thus measuring around 15% in normal individuals. At this point, there is little evidence that the albumin fraction is truly bioavailable, although because the albumin-hormone complexes generally dissociate rapidly this fraction may be more bioavailable in a dynamically perfused tissue.[25] That said, this discussion focuses on the free fraction, although data examining the relationship of bioavailable 25(OH)D to clinical outcomes are also considered.

The Megalin/Cubilin Transport System

As noted earlier, the free hormone hypothesis postulates that only the free hormone can cross the plasma membrane. For the vitamin D metabolites, this is not completely accurate. The renal tubule differs from most other tissues in its mechanism for at least 25(OH)D uptake, and likely for all DBP-bound vitamin D metabolites. The DBP-25(OH)D complex is filtered in the glomerulus and reabsorbed in the proximal tubule through endocytosis by the megalin/cubilin complex, thereby providing 25(OH)D for CYP27B1 1α-hydroxylation in the kidney tubule as well as for the rest of the body.[26,27] This complex is not specific for DBP, but when megalin is deleted, the major protein lost in the urine is DBP. In the mice that survive long enough, bone growth is retarded and osteopenic.[26] The impact of cubilin deletion is similar but not as severe.[27] A similar mechanism may operate in the parathyroid gland and placenta, which like the renal tubule express megalin/cubilin,[28] but at this point, experiments to determine the impact of either megalin or cubilin deletion from the parathyroid or gland or placenta have not been reported.

ASSAYS AND METHODS FOR ASSESSING FREE VITAMIN D METABOLITE LEVELS
Centrifugal Ultrafiltration

To test the free hormone hypothesis with respect to vitamin D metabolites, centrifugal ultrafiltration was developed to measure the free fraction of 25(OH)D and 1,25(OH)$_2$D.[29–32] The original motivation was first to determine whether the low vitamin D metabolite levels in patients with liver disease truly indicated vitamin D deficiency. There was good reason to question this in that the authors and others had shown that patients with liver disease develop osteoporosis, not osteomalacia,[33,34] and generally do not respond to vitamin D supplementation[35,36] with respect to their bone disease. In addition, as mentioned earlier, both DBP and 1,25(OH)$_2$D were known to increase during the latter portions of pregnancy, although 25(OH)D levels typically did not, raising the question as to whether the increased 1,25(OH)$_2$D levels were a direct result of the increased DBP levels, or were the free levels also increased disproportionate to that of the total levels.[22] The latter was suggested by the increased intestinal calcium absorption during pregnancy,[37] a well-known physiologic target for 1,25(OH)$_2$D (presumably free).

The centrifugal ultrafiltration assay for the vitamin D metabolites was patterned after the method developed by Hammond and colleagues[38] for the measurement of free sex steroid hormone levels. It consisted of an inner vial capped on one end with dialysis membrane resting on filter pads at the bottom of an outer vial. The serum sample, following incubation with freshly purified ^{3}H-labeled vitamin D metabolite and ^{14}C-labeled glucose as a marker of free water, was placed in the inner vial and centrifuged at 37°C for 45 minutes. The ratio of ^{3}H/^{14}C in the ultrafiltrate to that in the sample determined the % free. The free concentration was then calculated by multiplying the % free times the total metabolite concentration. Although the clinical applications for these measurements are covered subsequently, the initial results demonstrated that indeed patients with liver disease and low DBP and albumin concentrations in parallel with reduced total 25(OH)D and 1,25(OH)$_2$D did have normal free concentrations of these metabolites. This observation supported the concept of using the ratio of total vitamin D metabolite to DBP levels as predictive of the free vitamin D metabolite level, and indeed vitamin D nutritional status. On the other hand, women in their third trimester of pregnancy with elevated DBP and 1,25(OH)$_2$D levels nevertheless had elevated free 1,25(OH)$_2$D disproportionate to the total 1,25(OH)$_2$D, so the ratio of total vitamin D metabolite to DBP levels was not predictive of the free level. Similarly, the directly measured free 25(OH)D (in this case by the enzyme-linked immunosorbent assay [ELISA] method to be described subsequently) was higher than would be expected from the ratio of total 25(OH)D to DBP.[39] Thus, during pregnancy it appears that the body has altered the affinity of DBP for the vitamin D metabolites to increase the free fraction. The mechanism for this is unknown. However, as discussed later, this apparent change in affinity provides a challenge to the use of calculating the free concentration based on the assumption that the affinity constants do not change under physiologic conditions.

Calculating the Free Vitamin D Metabolite Levels

Centrifugal ultrafiltration was used to determine the affinity constants for DBP and albumin binding to 25(OH)D and 1,25(OH)$_2$D. Scatchard analysis indicated that binding of both 1,25(OH)$_2$D and 25(OH)D in serum fit a 2-binding-site model. The high affinity site, shown to be that of DBP, had an affinity constant (Ka) for 1,25(OH)$_2$D of 3.7 to 4.2 × 10^7 M^{-1} and for 25OHD of 7 to 9 × 10^8 M^{-1}. The lower affinity site, corresponding to albumin, was found to have a Ka for 1,25(OH)$_2$D of 5.4 × 10^4 M^{-1} and for 25(OH)

D of 6×10^5 M^{-1}.[30,31] Although differences in the affinity constants for the different DBP alleles have been reported,[24] results from other laboratories have not confirmed these differences.[40]

These affinity constants could then be used in the following formula for calculating the free fraction of the vitamin D metabolite (25(OH)D or 1,25(OH)$_2$D):

$$\frac{1}{F} = 1 + n1Ka(DBP) \times [DBP]_f + n2Ka(alb) \times [alb]_f$$

where F is the free vitamin D metabolite fraction, $[DBP]_f$ is the free DBP concentration, meaning the level of DBP not bound to the vitamin D metabolite, and $[alb]_f$ is the free albumin concentration. $[DBP]_f$ and $[alb]_f$ are essentially equivalent to the total concentrations of these proteins (DBP concentration is approximately 5 μM, albumin 600 μM in normal serum) because the level of saturation of these binding proteins by the vitamin D metabolites is negligible (approximately 1% for DBP and 0.1% for albumin for 25(OH)D, and 3-fold lower for 1,25(OH)$_2$D) under normal circulating levels of the vitamin D metabolites. However, in cases of vitamin D toxicity, this assumption becomes more problematic.[41] $n1$ and $n2$ are the number of sites on DBP and albumin to which the D metabolite binds. $n = 1$ for DBP, but n for albumin is unknown and has been incorporated into the Ka for albumin as a constant. The free fraction is then multiplied by the total levels of the vitamin D metabolite of interest to obtain the free metabolite concentration. The formula has been rearranged since it was first introduced[31] as follows:

$$\text{free vitamin D metabolite} = \frac{\text{total vitamin D metabolite}}{1 + (Ka_{alb} \times albumin) + (Ka_{DBP} \times DBP)}$$

In using this formula, one requires accurate measurement of DBP, albumin, and the vitamin D metabolite of interest. Moreover, the calculation depends on an assumption that the affinity constants are invariant. In the initial studies with serum from normal subjects, in which DBP levels were measured with a polyclonal assay, the calculated values agreed reasonably well with the directly measured values using the centrifugal ultrafiltration method.[29,31] In both cases measurement of the total levels of the vitamin D metabolite was required to go from measurement of the free fraction to that of the free level. However, with the commercial development of assays for DBP using monoclonal antibodies that appear to differ in their ability to detect the different DBP alleles compared with the polyclonal antibody assays,[42,43] and the apparent change in DBP affinities for the vitamin D metabolites under different physiologic/pathologic conditions,[29,32,39] the calculated values diverged substantially from the directly measured levels.[39] Thus, a brief discussion of the DBP and vitamin D metabolite assays in use today is in order before considering the recent development of assays that directly measure the free vitamin D metabolite level and so are not dependent of measurements of total levels or the binding proteins.

Vitamin D Binding Protein and Its Assays

DBP is the major binding and transport protein for vitamin D and its metabolites. DBP is a 51- to 58-kDa multifunctional serum glycoprotein synthesized by hepatic parenchymal cells. DBP is found in plasma, ascites fluid, cerebrospinal fluid, and on the surface of many cell types. DBP is encoded by the single copy *GC* gene located on chromosome 4q12-q13[44] and is a member of a multigene family that includes albumin, α-fetoprotein, and α-albumin/afamin.[45] Initially, isoelectric focusing migration patterns identified phenotypic variants[46] termed Group-Specific Component (Gc)1f, Gcs, and

Gc2 that bound vitamin D.[47] Subsequently, the responsible genetic polymorphisms have been identified. Two common missense point mutations in exon 11 of single-nucleotide polymorphisms (SNPs) rs7041 (G/T single-nucleotide variation) and rs4588 (an A/C single-nucleotide variation) result in 3 common isoforms and different protein products at positions 416 and 420: Gc1F (Asp416, Thr420), Gc1S (Glu 416, Thr420), and Gc2 (Asp416, Lys420).[48] The SNPs are in complete linkage disequilibrium, and only 6 haplotypes are observed with any significant frequency (**Table 1**). Gc2 is the least abundant, and Gc1f is the most abundant. Gc alleles show distinct racial distribution patterns. Black and Asian populations are more likely to carry the Gc1f form, and the Gc2 form is rare, whereas whites more frequently exhibit the Gc1s and the Gc2 form. Gc1f has been stated to have the highest affinity and Gc2 the lowest affinity for vitamin D and its metabolites,[24] but these differences among alleles have not been found by others.[40] In the absence of disease or pregnancy, DBP levels are relatively constant over time in adults.[49] That said, various substances in the blood such as polyunsaturated fatty acids may alter the affinity of DBP for the vitamin D metabolites.[50] Moreover, as noted previously, liver disease leads to reduced levels of DBP[32] as do protein-losing nephropathy[51] and acute illness (DBP is an acute phase reactant),[52,53] whereas DBP levels are elevated during the latter stages of pregnancy and with oral contraceptive use.[22,29]

DBP is generally measured by immunoassays with either monoclonal or polyclonal antibodies. In 2013, Powe and colleagues[54] reported that, compared with white Americans, black Americans had similar levels of calculated bioavailable 25OHD despite lower levels of total 25OHD. Free 25(OH)D levels were not determined. This explanation seemed logical for the observations that although black Americans have lower total 25(OH)D as a group, they do not have obvious evidence of vitamin D deficiency with respect to skeletal BMD, PTH, serum calcium, and phosphate levels. Powe and colleagues used a monoclonal antibody–based ELISA to measure DBP levels and found that those individuals (primarily of African American descent) with the 1f allele had lower DBP levels thus increasing the bioavailable fraction. However, Nielson

Table 1
Vitamin D binding protein characteristics by haplotype

DBP (Gc) Haplotype	Relative Frequency by Race	Sensitivity of Assay for Alleles	
		Monoclonal Antibody	Polyclonal Antibiotic or Proteomic
1f-1f	Black (50%) & Chinese > Hispanic (13%) > white (6%)[a]	Low	High
1f-1s	Unclear[b]	Low	High
1f-2	Unclear[b]	Low	High
1s-1s	White > Chinese > black	High	High
1s-2	White > black	High	High
2-2	Chinese > white > black	High	High

[a] *Data from* Engelman CD, Fingerlin TE, Langefeld CD, et al. Genetic and environmental determinants of 25-hydroxyvitamin D and 1,25-dihydroxyvitamin D levels in Hispanic and African Americans. J Clin Endocrinol Metab 2008;93(9):3381–8; Xu W, Sun J, Wang W, et al. Association of genetic variants of vit D binding protein (DBP/GC) and of the enzyme catalyzing its 25-hydroxylation (DCYP2R1) and serum vit D in postmenopausal women. Hormones (Athens) 2014;13(3):345–52; and Yao P, Sun L, Lu L, et al. Effects of genetic and non-genetic factors on total and bioavailable 25(OH)D responses to vitamin D supplementation. J Clin Endocrinol Metab 2017;102:100–10.
[b] Present in both self-reported black, Chinese, Hispanic, and white.

and colleagues[42,43] subsequently reported their results with measuring DBP levels with 4 different assays: (1) monoclonal antibody-based ELISA, (2) polyclonal antibody-based radial immunodiffusion assay, and (3) 2 different polyclonal antibody–based ELISAs. Moreover, they measured free 25(OH)D directly using ELISA methodology to be described subsequently. The monoclonal antibody–based assay resulted in a 54% lower concentration of DBP in black Americans, compared with white Americans, and, therefore, a significantly higher calculated free 25(OH)D level. In contrast, there were minimal differences in DBP levels using the 3 polyclonal assays, and significantly lower mean concentrations of free 25(OH)D when calculating this parameter using DBP concentrations from the polyclonal antibody–based method or when directly measuring free 25(OH)D by ELISA. Similarly, mass spectrometry (MS) measurements of DBP by Hoofnagle and colleagues[55] have failed to show a difference in DBP levels with the various alleles. Thus, although it is not clear whether the different DBP alleles have different affinities for the vitamin D metabolites, the alleles do affect the results of immunoassays when a monoclonal antibody is used but not when polyclonal antibodies are used.

Vitamin D Metabolite Assays

The different means of measuring the vitamin D metabolite assays have been extensively reviewed.[56] There are 4 general types of assays currently in use today: competitive protein binding assay (CPBA), immunoassays, liquid chromatography (LC)-UV, and LC-tandem mass spectrometry (LC-MS/MS). LC-MS/MS is becoming the gold standard, gradually replacing the CPBA and immunoassays,[57] and is now used as the reference method for measuring 25(OH)D by the National Institute of Standards and Technology and the Centers for Disease Control and Prevention. However, immunoassays still remain the dominant method in use today for both 25(OH)D and 1,25(OH)$_2$D.[58] Each method has its advantages and disadvantages. Immunoassays require less sophisticated equipment and technical expertise to set up, and they are very sensitive. However, they tend to be more variable than LC-MS/MS because they rely on antibodies that may differ in their recognition of both the D$_2$ and the D$_3$ metabolites and may be more affected by interfering substances within the sample than LC-MS/MS. On the other hand, LC-MS/MS is less sensitive than immunoassays, generally requiring concentration of the samples with affinity columns and/or derivatization for metabolites other than 25(OH)D. Moreover, unless high-resolution LC is used, LC-MS/MS fails to detect the 3-epimer of the vitamin D metabolites and is susceptible to ion suppression by interfering substances (so-called matrix effects),[59] and mass spectral overlaps with isobaric compounds with comparable m/z ratios (eg, 7α-hydroxy-4 cholestene-3-one).[60] However, unlike immunoassays, LC-MS/MS can measure multiple vitamin D metabolites in the same sample.

Directly Measured Free 25-Hydroxyvitamin D

Enzyme-linked immunosorbent assay method

A 2-step ELISA that directly measures free 25(OH)D levels has been developed (Future Diagnostics Solutions B.V., Wijchen, The Netherlands) based on patented monoclonal antibodies from DIAsource Immunoassays (Louvain-la-Neuve, Belgium). In the first incubation step, an anti–vitamin D monoclonal antibody immobilized on a microtiter plate binds the free 25(OH)D in the serum sample. After washing away excess serum, the second incubation step is to add biotinylated 25(OH)D in a known amount to react with the unoccupied binding sites on the monoclonal antibody attached to the plate. The nonbound biotinylated 25(OH)D is then removed by a second washing. Thereafter, streptavidin peroxidase conjugate is added followed by the substrate 3,3′,5,5′-tetramethylbenzidine. The bound streptavidin peroxidase can be quantified by measuring the absorbance at 450 nm generated in the reaction spectrophotometrically. The intensity is inversely proportional to the level of free 25(OH)D. The limit of detection is 2.8 pg/mL. This assay is dependent on the quality of the antibody used to bind the free 25(OH)D. The antibody in the current assay does not recognize $25(OH)D_2$ as well as $25(OH)D_3$ (77% of the $25(OH)D_3$ value) so underestimates the free $25(OH)D_2$. However, under most situations where the predominant vitamin D metabolite is $25(OH)D_3$, the data compare quite well to those obtained from similar populations using the centrifugal ultrafiltration assay.[40,61]

Liquid chromatography–tandem mass spectrometry method

LC-MS/MS has been used to detect 25(OH)D in saliva, which is expected to be free of DBP and albumin and so represents free 25(OH)D.[62] In this method, 1 mL of saliva is deproteinized with acetonitrile, purified using a Strata-X cartridge, derivatized with 4-phenyl-1,2,4-triazoline-3,5 dione, ionized by electron spray ionization, and subjected to LC-MS/MS. The limit of detection was reported as 2 pg/mL, comparable with that of the ELISA method described earlier. The range of values obtained in normal controls was between 3 and 15 pg/mL, likewise consistent with the values obtained with the ELISA method[39] and centrifugal ultrafiltration.[32]

Thus, armed with the means to measure free vitamin D metabolite levels, the next section discusses whether measuring free levels provides a better means of assessing vitamin D status clinically than measuring the total levels.

CLINICAL APPLICATIONS

Clinical studies have investigated relationships between calculated and directly measured free or bioavailable 25(OH)D and parathyroid hormone levels (iPTH), bone density, calcium and calcium absorption, inflammatory measures, and the disease states of cirrhosis, nephrotic syndrome, primary hyperparathyroidism, pregnancy, and in relationship to estrogens and birth control pills or race.[40] Results from investigations of calculated free 25(OH)D and directly measured free 25(OH)D have not been in complete agreement primarily because of the challenges and differences in DBP assays, total 25(OH)D assays, uncertainty regarding DBP association constants, use of static equations as discussed earlier, and likely genetic racial admixtures affecting DBP allele distributions in contrast to self-identified race. For this reason, after a brief review of differences of results using the 2 measurement methods (calculated and directly measured free 25(OH)D), the bulk of the following discussion is limited to investigations in humans using directly measured free 25(OH)D.

Comparisons of Directly Measured Free 25-Hydroxyvitamin D to Calculated Free 25-Hydroxyvitamin D

Direct positive statistically significant correlations are found between results with the 2 methods, but the relationship accounts for only 13% of the variation, and calculated free 25(OH)D concentrations are consistently higher than directly measured concentrations in healthy humans of all races.[39,42,43,63,64] Most studies also find weak but statistically significant inverse relationships between iPTH and free 25(OH)D in normal subjects and prediabetics.[39,49,61,65,66] Areas of uncertainty include relationships between free 25(OH)D and race, birth control pills, pregnancy in the second and third trimester, and biomarkers of vitamin D effects on bone.

Findings from Studies of Directly Measured Free 25-Hydroxyvitamin D in Healthy Humans

Directly measured free 25(OH)D concentrations are strongly correlated with total 25(OH)D concentrations and have been reported to be between 0.02% and 0.09% of total 25(OH)D concentrations (**Fig. 2**, **Tables 2** and **3**). Concentrations generally range from 1.2 to 7.9 pg/mL. PTH is negatively correlated with free 25(OH)D as well as total 25(OH)D. Serum C-terminal telopeptide of type I collagen has been reported to have a moderate positive correlation with total and free 25(OH)D.[67] With vitamin D supplementation, free 25(OH)D concentrations increase in concert with total 25(OH)D concentrations,[64,65,67,68] increasing more steeply with D3 supplementation compared with D2.[66] With high-dose D supplementation, the changes in iPTH were significantly related to changes in free 25(OH)D but not to changes in total 25(OH)D or changes in total 1,25(OH)$_2$D.[66] Others have reported that circulating 1,25(OH)$_2$D levels may not correlate with free 25(OH)D.[67]

Effects of Race

There are differences in DBP levels and DBP alleles by race that might predict differences in free 25(OH)D. The results from studies that directly measured free 25(OH)D differ in conclusions regarding racial effects. Two support the

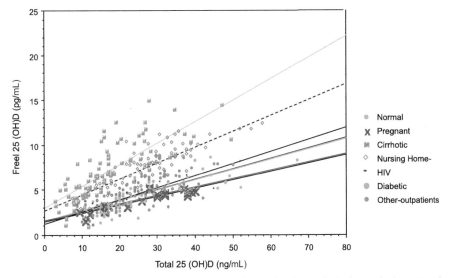

Fig. 2. Relationships between total 25(OH)D and free 25(OH)D in clinical populations. Total 25(OH) vitamin D concentrations are plotted on the x-axis and directly measured free 25(OH)D levels are plotted on the y-axis. Symbols are as follows: X (*red*) represents pregnant women in the second or third trimester; squares (*orange*) represent patients with cirrhosis; open triangles indicate nursing home residents with multimorbidities; solid (*purple*) triangles are HIV-infected patients, and solid circles are normal subjects (*green*), outpatients (*gray*), and diabetics (*blue*). Relationships between total and free 25(OH)D were significantly different for cirrhotics and nursing home residents as compared with the other groups. No differences in relationships between total and free 25(OH)D were detected between normals, pregnant women, diabetics, outpatients, or HIV-infected subjects. (*Data from* Schwartz JB, Lai J, Lizaola B, et al. A comparison of measured and calculated free 25(OH) vitamin D levels in clinical populations. J Clin Endocrinol Metab 2014;99(5):1631–7; and Kane L, Moore K, Lütjohann D, et al. Vitamin D3 effects on lipids differ in statin and non-statin-treated humans: superiority of free 25-OH D levels in detecting relationships. J Clin Endocrinol Metab 2013;98:4400–9.)

Table 2
Free 1,25 dihydroxyvitamin D in alcoholic liver disease and pregnancy compared with controls

Measurement	Alcoholic Liver Disease (n = 25)	Controls (n = 24)	Pregnancy (n = 17)
Total 1,25(OH)$_2$D (pg/mL)[a]	22.6 ± 12.5	41.5 ± 11.5	82 ± 21
Free 1,25(OH)$_2$D (fg/mL)[a]	209 ± 91	174 ± 46	294 ± 98
% Free 1,25(OH)$_2$D	1.098 ± 0.50	0.424 ± 0.07	0.359 ± 0.07
Total 25(OH)D (ng/mL)[c]	9.7 ± 4.5	19.2 ± 6.6	27.8 ± 8.8
DBP (μg/mL)[b]	188 ± 105	404 ± 124 (n = 18)	576 ± 128

[a] Method was centrifugal ultrafiltration.
[b] By rocket immunoelectrophoresis.
[c] By competitive protein-binding radioassay.
Data from Bikle DD, Gee E, Halloran B, et al. Free 1,25-dihydroxyvitamin D levels in serum from normal subjects, pregnant subjects, and subjects with liver disease. J Clin Invest 1984;74(6):1966–71; and Bikle DD, Siiteri PK, Ryzen E, et al. Serum protein binding of 1,25-dihydroxyvitamin D: a reevaluation by direct measurement of free metabolite levels. J Clin Endocrinol Metab 1985;61(5):969–75.

existence of racial differences with measured free 25(OH)D concentrations being lower in blacks than in whites that are related to lower total 25(OH)D. DBP levels by polyclonal assay did not differ between blacks and whites in these studies.[42,43] In contrast, Aloia and colleagues[69] found no difference in free 25(OH)D concentrations between black and white postmenopausal women. Where DBP genotype and phenotype were determined, direct measurement of free 25(OH)D diminished differences between DBP phenotypes as compared with serum total 25(OH)D.[64]

Table 3
Free 25-hydroxyvitamin D in normal subjects compared with patients with cirrhotic liver disease or pregnancy

Measurement	Liver Disease[a] (n = 42)	Controls[a] (n = 22)	Cirrhotics[b] (N = 82)	Pregnancy[c] (n = 20)	Controls[c] (n = 111)
Total 25(OH)D (ng/mL)	10.9 ± 9.5	19.2 ± 6.7	15.5[d] (10.2–23.8)	26.2 ± 11.4[e,f]	26.7 ± 10.[e]
% Free 25(OH)D	0.068 ± 0.029	0.030 ± 0.007	0.043 (0.037–0.053)	0.016 ± 0.004	0.02 ± 0.014
Free 25(OH)D (pg/mL)	6.61 ± 4.61	5.88 ± 2.27	6.8 (5.0–9.1)	4.5 ± 1.6	4.0 ± 1.1
DBP (μg/mL)	178 ± 92	405 ± 128	100.6 (63.3–157.1)	460.3 ± 229.5	220.3 ± 100
Albumin (g/dL)	2.83 ± 0.66	—	3.2 (2.7–3.8)	3.3 ± 0.3	4.2 ± 0.3

[a] Data are from Ref.[31,32] with measurements of free 25(OH)D made by centrifugal ultrafiltration and DBP by rocket immune-electrophoresis.
[b] Data are from Ref.[69]
[c] Data are from Ref.[60] In both studies, measurements of free 25(OH)D were by immunoassay (Future Diagnostics), and DBP was by monoclonal assay (Quantikine Human Vitamin D Binding Protein Immunoassay kit; R&D Systems, Inc), which results in lower DBP levels than the original polyclonal assay employed in Ref.[31]
[d] Data are reported as mean ± SD except for cirrhotics for data not normally distributed; median and range are presented.
[e] Measured by LC MS/MS.
[f] Measured by immunoassay (R&D).
Data from Refs.[31,32,60,69]

Effects of Obesity

Walsh and colleagues[70] studied obese and overweight subjects compared with normal weight subjects in the fall and spring. Body mass index (BMI) was negatively correlated with total 25(OH)D, free 25(OH)D, as well as total 1,25(OH)$_2$D. However, obesity altered the relationship between iPTH with similar iPTH levels in all groups, but lower bone turnover markers and higher bone density in obese subjects.

Effects of Sex, Female Hormones, and Pregnancy

Investigations have not found differences in free levels of 25(OH)D between men and women in those with prediabetes when corrected for total 25(OH)D.[64] Similarly, the authors have found no sex-related differences in free 25(OH)D in normal subjects when corrected for total 25(OH)D (Schwartz and Bikle, unpublished data, 2014 and from refs.[61,71]). One pharmacologic action of estrogen is to increase DBP, and thus one might expect lower free 25(OH)D levels in women receiving estrogen therapy either in oral contraceptives or for postmenopausal hormone replacement. Data on women receiving birth control pills have not been published, and the authors' experience is limited such that definitive statements cannot be made. They have performed an analysis of data from multiple investigations that included information on estrogen administered as hormone replacement therapy to white postmenopausal women and white women of similar age not receiving estrogen. The women receiving estrogen therapy were younger (67 ± 6 years [n = 33] compared with 76.6 ± 13.5 [n = 116], but they had similar BMI [29.6 ± 6.6 compared with 27.9 ± 6.1]). Total 25(OH)D was lower in estrogen-treated women (24.2 ± 10.5 compared 28.1 ± 11 ng/mL), and free 25(OH)D was significantly lower in those on estrogen (4.3 ± 1.9 compared with 5.9 ± 2.8 pg/mL, or 0.015 vs 0.021% of total 25(OH)D). When corrected for total 25(OH)D, the effects of estrogen were no longer significant. DBP was measured in a subgroup (n = 31 estrogen-treated and 41 without estrogen), and no between group differences were detected. These data are cross-sectional, but the clinical interpretation is that estrogen in doses prescribed clinically for postmenopausal hormone replacement does not appear to significantly alter DBP or free 25(OH)D or alter the relationship between total 25(OH)D and free 25(OH)D.

However, directly measured free 25(OH)D tends to be higher, and free 1,25(OH)$_2$D is substantially higher in pregnant women versus comparator groups of women[29,39] (see **Fig. 2**, **Tables 2** and **3**). These results suggest that the affinity of DBP for the vitamin D metabolites appears to be decreased during pregnancy, perhaps compensating for increased DBP concentrations and the needs of both the mother and the fetus for calcium. Whether this reflects the influence of changes in the hormonal milieu during pregnancy on DBP affinity is not known.

Effects of Liver Disease/Cirrhosis

Directly measured free 25(OH)D and 1,25(OH)$_2$D are higher in outpatients with cirrhosis compared with other groups[32,39] despite lower total vitamin D metabolite concentrations (see **Tables 2** and **3**). The relationship between free 25OHD and total 25(OH)D is both steeper and more variable in patients with liver disease than in healthy people (see **Fig. 2**). Findings within cirrhotics vary based on the severity of disease and whether there is a marked protein synthesis dysfunction as characterized by low albumin concentrations (<3.5 mg/dL). Those with the most severe cirrhosis and protein synthesis dysfunction have a higher percentage of free 25(OH)D compared with cirrhotics without protein synthesis dysfunction, but free 25(OH)D concentrations are similar because of the presence of both lower total 25(OH)D concentrations and lower

DBP. Free 25(OH)D concentrations range between 4.5 and 8.1 pg/mL in cirrhotics with low albumin and from 6.4 to 10.6 pg/mL in those with normal albumin. The expected relationships between total or free 25(OH)D and iPTH are present in cirrhotics with normal albumin/serum protein concentrations, but no relationship with iPTH or bone markers is detected in cirrhotic patients with low albumin.

Effects of Multimorbidity

Nursing home residents are older, have more medical problems, receive more medications, and are more likely to have poorer nutrition than younger people or community-dwelling elderly. In vitamin D dose titration studies,[68] free 25(OH)D levels increase in response to increases in total 25(OH)D, but responses appear to be steeper than those of normal subjects, younger outpatients, diabetics, or HIV-infected patients (see **Fig. 2**). It is likely that this reflects impaired protein synthesis and lower DBP and albumin, but this has not been established.

SUMMARY

Direct measurement of free vitamin D metabolite levels avoids potential errors inherent in calculating free or bioavailable metabolite levels and is thus the preferred method for free vitamin D metabolite determinations. Directly measured free 25(OH)D is highly correlated with total 25(OH)D in most subjects and is inversely related to iPTH. However, in disease states such as cirrhosis and in the elderly with multiple comorbid conditions in whom DBP and albumin levels are likely reduced, or during the latter portions of pregnancy when DBP levels are elevated, conclusions regarding D status based on free vitamin D metabolite measurements may differ from those based on measurement of total metabolite levels. Under these circumstances, free vitamin D metabolite levels may represent a better index of vitamin D status. However, experience with direct measurements of the free levels is limited, and firm conclusions cannot be reached regarding the influence of racial differences and the impact of inflammatory or other disease states that may alter the relationship between total and free metabolite levels. Moreover, at present the relationships between free and total vitamin D metabolite levels on markers of vitamin D status such as bone markers and PTH levels do not clearly demonstrate the superiority of free to total measurements. The authors anticipate, however, that free vitamin D measurements will play an increasingly important role in the assessment of vitamin D status, and the availability of a high throughput assay that can be performed by most clinical laboratories to measure the free 25(OH)D should stimulate further evaluation of its role in clinical medicine as well as in the research laboratory.

REFERENCES

1. Bikle DD. Vitamin D: newly discovered actions require reconsideration of physiologic requirements. Trends Endocrinol Metab 2010;21(6):375–84.
2. Houghton LA, Vieth R. The case against ergocalciferol (vitamin D2) as a vitamin supplement. Am J Clin Nutr 2006;84(4):694–7.
3. Hollis BW. Comparison of equilibrium and disequilibrium assay conditions for ergocalciferol, cholecalciferol and their major metabolites. J Steroid Biochem 1984; 21(1):81–6.
4. Horst RL, Reinhardt TA, Ramberg CF, et al. 24-Hydroxylation of 1,25-dihydroxyergocalciferol. An unambiguous deactivation process. J Biol Chem 1986;261(20): 9250–6.

5. Zhu JG, Ochalek JT, Kaufmann M, et al. CYP2R1 is a major, but not exclusive, contributor to 25-hydroxyvitamin D production in vivo. Proc Natl Acad Sci U S A 2013;110(39):15650–5.

6. Moghadasian MH. Cerebrotendinous xanthomatosis: clinical course, genotypes and metabolic backgrounds. Clin Invest Med 2004;27(1):42–50.

7. Cheng JB, Motola DL, Mangelsdorf DJ, et al. De-orphanization of cytochrome P450 2R1: a microsomal vitamin D 25-hydroxilase. J Biol Chem 2003;278(39):38084–93.

8. Bianco SD, Peng JB, Takanaga H, et al. Marked disturbance of calcium homeostasis in mice with targeted disruption of the Trpv6 calcium channel gene. J Bone Miner Res 2007;22(2):274–85.

9. Cheng JB, Levine MA, Bell NH, et al. Genetic evidence that the human CYP2R1 enzyme is a key vitamin D 25-hydroxylase. Proc Natl Acad Sci U S A 2004;101(20):7711–5.

10. Bikle D. Extra renal synthesis of 1,25-dihydroxyvitamin D and its health implications. In: Holick M, editor. Vitamin D: physiology, molecular biology, and clinical applications. New York: Humana Press; 2010. p. 277–95.

11. Bikle DD, Pillai S, Gee E, et al. Tumor necrosis factor-alpha regulation of 1,25-dihydroxyvitamin D production by human keratinocytes. Endocrinology 1991;129(1):33–8.

12. Bikle DD, Pillai S, Gee E, et al. Regulation of 1,25-dihydroxyvitamin D production in human keratinocytes by interferon-gamma. Endocrinology 1989;124(2):655–60.

13. St-Arnaud R, Messerlian S, Moir JM, et al. The 25-hydroxyvitamin D 1-alpha-hydroxylase gene maps to the pseudovitamin D-deficiency rickets (PDDR) disease locus. J Bone Miner Res 1997;12(10):1552–9.

14. Jones G, Prosser DE, Kaufmann M. 25-Hydroxyvitamin D-24-hydroxylase (CYP24A1): its important role in the degradation of vitamin D. Arch Biochem Biophys 2012;523(1):9–18.

15. Plachot JJ, Du Bois MB, Halpern S, et al. In vitro action of 1,25-dihydroxycholecalciferol and 24,25- dihydroxycholecalciferol on matrix organization and mineral distribution in rabbit growth plate. Metab Bone Dis Relat Res 1982;4(2):135–42.

16. Brozyna AA, Jochymski C, Janjetovic Z, et al. CYP24A1 expression inversely correlates with melanoma progression: clinic-pathological studies. Int J Mol Sci 2014;15(10):19000–17.

17. Sakaki T, Sawada N, Komai K, et al. Dual metabolic pathway of 25-hydroxyvitamin D3 catalyzed by human CYP24. Eur J Biochem 2000;267(20):6158–65.

18. Mendel CM. The free hormone hypothesis. Distinction from the free hormone transport hypothesis. J Androl 1992;13(2):107–16.

19. Recant L, Riggs DS. Thyroid function in nephrosis. J Clin Invest 1952;31(8):789–97.

20. Refetoff S. Thyroid hormone serum transport proteins. In: De Groot LJ, Chrousos G, Dungan K, et al, editors. Endotext. South Dartmouth (MA); 2000.

21. Siiteri PK, Murai JT, Hammond GL, et al. The serum transport of steroid hormones. Recent Prog Horm Res 1982;38:457–510.

22. Bouillon R, Van Assche FA, Van Baelen H, et al. Influence of the vitamin D-binding protein on the serum concentration of 1,25-dihydroxyvitamin D3. Significance of the free 1,25-dihydroxyvitamin D3 concentration. J Clin Invest 1981;67(3):589–96.

23. Safadi FF, Thornton P, Magiera H, et al. Osteopathy and resistance to vitamin D toxicity in mice null for vitamin D binding protein. J Clin Invest 1999;103(2): 239–51.

24. Arnaud J, Constans J. Affinity differences for vitamin D metabolites associated with the genetic isoforms of the human serum carrier protein (DBP). Hum Genet 1993;92(2):183–8.

25. Mendel CM. Rates of dissociation of sex steroid hormones from human sex hormone-binding globulin: a reassessment. J Steroid Biochem Mol Biol 1990; 37(2):251–5.

26. Nykjaer A, Dragun D, Walther D, et al. An endocytic pathway essential for renal uptake and activation of the steroid 25-(OH) vitamin D3. Cell 1999;96(4):507–15.

27. Nykjaer A, Fyfe JC, Kozyraki R, et al. Cubilin dysfunction causes abnormal metabolism of the steroid hormone 25(OH) vitamin D(3). Proc Natl Acad Sci U S A 2001;98(24):13895–900.

28. Lundgren S, Carling T, Hjalm G, et al. Tissue distribution of human gp330/megalin, a putative Ca(2+)-sensing protein. J Histochem Cytochem 1997;45(3): 383–92.

29. Bikle DD, Gee E, Halloran B, et al. Free 1,25-dihydroxyvitamin D levels in serum from normal subjects, pregnant subjects, and subjects with liver disease. J Clin Invest 1984;74(6):1966–71.

30. Bikle DD, Siiteri PK, Ryzen E, et al. Serum protein binding of 1,25-dihydroxyvitamin D: a reevaluation by direct measurement of free metabolite levels. J Clin Endocrinol Metab 1985;61(5):969–75.

31. Bikle DD, Gee E, Halloran B, et al. Assessment of the free fraction of 25-hydroxyvitamin D in serum and its regulation by albumin and the vitamin D-binding protein. J Clin Endocrinol Metab 1986;63(4):954–9.

32. Bikle DD, Halloran BP, Gee E, et al. Free 25-hydroxyvitamin D levels are normal in subjects with liver disease and reduced total 25-hydroxyvitamin D levels. J Clin Invest 1986;78(3):748–52.

33. Bikle DD, Genant HK, Cann C, et al. Bone disease in alcohol abuse. Ann Intern Med 1985;103(1):42–8.

34. Guarino M, Loperto I, Camera S, et al. Osteoporosis across chronic liver disease. Osteoporos Int 2016;27(6):1967–77.

35. Herlong HF, Recker RR, Maddrey WC. Bone disease in primary biliary cirrhosis: histologic features and response to 25-hydroxyvitamin D. Gastroenterology 1982; 83(1 Pt 1):103–8.

36. Matloff DS, Kaplan MM, Neer RM, et al. Osteoporosis in primary biliary cirrhosis: effects of 25-hydroxyvitamin D3 treatment. Gastroenterology 1982;83(1 Pt 1): 97–102.

37. Heaney RP, Skillman TG. Calcium metabolism in normal human pregnancy. J Clin Endocrinol Metab 1971;33(4):661–70.

38. Hammond GL, Nisker JA, Jones LA, et al. Estimation of the percentage of free steroid in undiluted serum by centrifugal ultrafiltration-dialysis. J Biol Chem 1980;255(11):5023–6.

39. Schwartz JB, Lai J, Lizaola B, et al. A comparison of measured and calculated free 25(OH) vitamin D levels in clinical populations. J Clin Endocrinol Metab 2014;99(5):1631–7.

40. Bikle D, Bouillon R, Thadhani R, et al. Vitamin D metabolites in captivity? Should we measure free or total 25(OH)D to assess vitamin D status? J Steroid Biochem Mol Biol 2017. http://dx.doi.org/10.1016/j.jsbmb.2017.01.007.

41. Pettifor JM, Bikle DD, Cavaleros M, et al. Serum levels of free 1,25-dihydroxyvitamin D in vitamin D toxicity. Ann Intern Med 1995;122(7):511–3.

42. Nielson CM, Jones KS, Bouillon R, et al. Role of assay type in determining free 25-hydroxyvitamin D levels in diverse populations. N Engl J Med 2016;374(17):1695–6.

43. Nielson CM, Jones KS, Chun RF, et al. Free 25-hydroxyvitamin D: impact of vitamin D binding protein assays on racial-genotypic associations. J Clin Endocrinol Metab 2016;101(5):2226–34.

44. Song YH, Naumova AK, Liebhaber SA, et al. Physical and meiotic mapping of the region of human chromosome 4q11-q13 encompassing the vitamin D binding protein DBP/Gc-globulin and albumin multigene cluster. Genome Res 1999;9(6):581–7.

45. Yang F, Brune JL, Naylor SL, et al. Human group-specific component (Gc) is a member of the albumin family. Proc Natl Acad Sci U S A 1985;82(23):7994–8.

46. Bouillon R, Van Baelen H, Rombauts W, et al. The purification and characterisation of the human-serum binding protein for the 25-hydroxycholecalciferol (trans-calciferin). Identity with group-specific component. Eur J Biochem 1976;66(2):285–91.

47. Daiger SP, Schanfield MS, Cavalli-Sforza LL. Group-specific component (Gc) proteins bind vitamin D and 25-hydroxyvitamin D. Proc Natl Acad Sci U S A 1975;72(6):2076–80.

48. Malik S, Fu L, Juras DJ, et al. Common variants of the vitamin D binding protein gene and adverse health outcomes. Crit Rev Clin Lab Sci 2013;50(1):1–22.

49. Sonderman JS, Munro HM, Blot WJ, et al. Reproducibility of serum 25-hydroxyvitamin D and vitamin D-binding protein levels over time in a prospective cohort study of black and white adults. Am J Epidemiol 2012;176(7):615–21.

50. Bouillon R, Xiang DZ, Convents R, et al. Polyunsaturated fatty acids decrease the apparent affinity of vitamin D metabolites for human vitamin D-binding protein. J Steroid Biochem Mol Biol 1992;42(8):855–61.

51. Marikanty RK, Gupta MK, Cherukuvada SV, et al. Identification of urinary proteins potentially associated with diabetic kidney disease. Indian J Nephrol 2016;26(6):434–45.

52. Madden K, Feldman HA, Chun RF, et al. Critically ill children have low vitamin D-binding protein, influencing bioavailability of vitamin D. Ann Am Thorac Soc 2015;12(11):1654–61.

53. Dahl B, Schiodt FV, Ott P, et al. Plasma concentration of Gc-globulin is associated with organ dysfunction and sepsis after injury. Crit Care Med 2003;31(1):152–6.

54. Powe CE, Evans MK, Wenger J, et al. Vitamin D-binding protein and vitamin D status of black Americans and white Americans. N Engl J Med 2013;369(21):1991–2000.

55. Hoofnagle AN, Eckfeldt JH, Lutsey PL. Vitamin D-binding protein concentrations quantified by mass spectrometry. N Engl J Med 2015;373(15):1480–2.

56. Farrell CJ, Martin S, McWhinney B, et al. State-of-the-art vitamin D assays: a comparison of automated immunoassays with liquid chromatography-tandem mass spectrometry methods. Clin Chem 2012;58(3):531–42.

57. Su Z, Narla SN, Zhu Y. 25-Hydroxyvitamin D: analysis and clinical application. Clin Chim Acta 2014;433:200–5.

58. Muller MJ, Volmer DA. Mass spectrometric profiling of vitamin D metabolites beyond 25-hydroxyvitamin D. Clin Chem 2015;61(8):1033–48.

59. Van Eeckhaut A, Lanckmans K, Sarre S, et al. Validation of bioanalytical LC-MS/MS assays: evaluation of matrix effects. J Chromatogr B Analyt Technol Biomed Life Sci 2009;877(23):2198–207.
60. Shah I, James R, Barker J, et al. Misleading measures in vitamin D analysis: a novel LC-MS/MS assay to account for epimers and isobars. Nutr J 2011;10:46.
61. Schwartz JB, Lai J, Lizaola B, et al. Variability in free 25(OH) vitamin D levels in clinical populations. J Steroid Biochem Mol Biol 2014;144(Pt A):156–8.
62. Higashi T, Shibayama Y, Fuji M, et al. Liquid chromatography-tandem mass spectrometric method for the determination of salivary 25-hydroxyvitamin D3: a noninvasive tool for the assessment of vitamin D status. Anal Bioanal Chem 2008; 391(1):229–38.
63. Lee MJ, Kearns MD, Smith EM, et al. Free 25-hydroxyvitamin D concentrations in cystic fibrosis. Am J Med Sci 2015;350(5):374–9.
64. Sollid ST, Hutchinson MY, Berg V, et al. Effects of vitamin D binding protein phenotypes and vitamin D supplementation on serum total 25(OH)D and directly measured free 25(OH)D. Eur J Endocrinol 2016;174(4):445–52.
65. Alzaman NS, Dawson-Hughes B, Nelson J, et al. Vitamin D status of black and white Americans and changes in vitamin D metabolites after varied doses of vitamin D supplementation. Am J Clin Nutr 2016;104(1):205–14.
66. Shieh A, Chun RF, Ma C, et al. Effects of high-dose vitamin D2 versus D3 on total and free 25-hydroxyvitamin D and markers of calcium balance. J Clin Endocrinol Metab 2016;101(8):3070–8.
67. Aloia J, Dhaliwal R, Mikhail M, et al. Free 25(OH)D and calcium absorption, PTH, and markers of bone turnover. J Clin Endocrinol Metab 2015;100(11):4140–5.
68. Schwartz JB, Kane L, Bikle D. Response of vitamin D concentration to vitamin D3 administration in older adults without sun exposure: a randomized double-blind trial. J Am Geriatr Soc 2016;64(1):65–72.
69. Aloia J, Mikhail M, Dhaliwal R, et al. Free 25(OH)D and the vitamin D paradox in African Americans. J Clin Endocrinol Metab 2015;100(9):3356–63.
70. Walsh JS, Evans AL, Bowles S, et al. Free 25-hydroxyvitamin D is low in obesity, but there are no adverse associations with bone health. Am J Clin Nutr 2016; 103(6):1465–71.
71. Kane L, Moore K, Lütjohann D, et al. Vitamin D3 effects on lipids differ in statin and non-statin-treated humans: superiority of free 25-OH D levels in detecting relationships. J Clin Endocrinol Metab 2013;98:4400–9.

Effect of Vitamin D on Falls and Physical Performance

Ruban Dhaliwal, MD, MPH[a],*, John F. Aloia, MD[b]

KEYWORDS

- Vitamin D • Falls • Fracture • Physical performance • Frailty • Muscle strength

KEY POINTS

- Falls are a major health concern in the elderly because of the high mortality and morbidity associated with consequent fractures and high risk of institutionalization.
- Strategies to prevent falls and decline in physical performance are essential for preservation of quality of life in the aging population.
- Beyond its classic role in bone and mineral metabolism, vitamin D has gained interest for its potential to influence extraskeletal outcomes.
- Emerging evidence suggests an association between vitamin D status and falls and physical performance in older adults, although the mechanisms underlying this relationship have not been completely elucidated.
- The effects of vitamin D on falls remain to be confirmed in a large dose-ranging clinical trial. The effects of vitamin D on physical performance are inconsistent and may depend on the baseline serum 25OHD level.

INTRODUCTION

The classic role of vitamin D in bone and mineral metabolism is well established. Over the last two decades a plethora of literature supports that the role of vitamin D extends far beyond the skeleton. The ubiquitous nature of 1α-hydroxylase enzyme, responsible for converting 25-hydroxyvitamin D to 1,25-dihydroxyvitamin D, and vitamin D receptors (VDR) is now evident. The predominant endocrine function of vitamin D in calcium homeostasis is mediated through conventional, well-known target tissues: intestine, kidneys, bone, and parathyroid gland. Advancements in research have broadened knowledge of the nonclassic role of vitamin D and increased understanding of its extraskeletal target tissues.

Disclosure Statement: The authors have nothing to disclose.
[a] Department of Medicine, Division of Endocrinology, Diabetes and Metabolism, State University of New York Upstate Medical University, 750 East Adams Street, Syracuse, NY 13210, USA;
[b] Bone Mineral Research Center, Winthrop University Hospital, 222 Station Plaza North, Suite 510, Mineola, NY 11501, USA
* Corresponding author.
E-mail address: dhaliwar@upstate.edu

Endocrinol Metab Clin N Am 46 (2017) 919–933
http://dx.doi.org/10.1016/j.ecl.2017.07.004
0889-8529/17/© 2017 Elsevier Inc. All rights reserved.

endo.theclinics.com

Observational data have demonstrated relationships between vitamin D status and infectious, immune, metabolic, degenerative, and neoplastic diseases. Vitamin D may play a role in chronic conditions, including diabetes mellitus, cardiovascular disease, hypertension, pulmonary disease, and osteoarthritis, conditions that are prevalent with aging and lead to physical and functional decline in the elderly.[1,2] Establishing the extraskeletal outcomes of vitamin D can lead to individualized vitamin D recommendations based on functional performance and disease risk in future. Emerging data, although not always congruent, overall support further in-depth exploration of the effect of vitamin D on these tissues, especially the skeletal muscle. This article reviews the epidemiologic data on falls and summarizes the influence of vitamin D status and vitamin D supplementation on falls, postural stability, and physical performance; describes the putative mechanisms underlying this association; and reflects on the controversy surrounding vitamin D recommendations in older adults.

THE BURDEN OF FALLS

Falls are a significant health concern in the aging population. Annual prevalence rate of falls ranges from 30% to 46% and women have a 20% higher rate of falls than men.[3] Falls occur as a result of the interaction between predisposing and precipitating factors.[4] Older age, age-associated decline in sensory and motor function, poor balance, and chronic diseases, particularly neurologic conditions, increase the risk of falls in older adults. Common precipitating factors include dehydration, medications, urinary tract symptoms, acute illnesses, and unfamiliar environment. Approximately 25% to 50% of the older adults who fall experience multiple falls within the same year.[5] After the occurrence of a fall up to 30% of fallers seek medical attention.[6,7] Fall-related hospitalizations are rapidly increasing. In the United States, these hospitalizations almost doubled between 2001 and 2008.[8] Consequently, the direct medical costs of falls in older adults are rising and in 2015 were more than $31 billion to Medicare alone.[9] A World Health Organization report showed that an estimated 500,000 deaths occur annually from falls.[10] Fractures, the most common consequences of falls, are associated with high mortality and morbidity within 1 year. Falls account for more than 90% of hip fractures, which often lead to permanent disability.[11] There is an increased risk of institutionalization following a fall.[12] Furthermore, falls are detrimental to an individual's quality of life with fear of falling limiting activity and inhibiting independent mobility.[13]

The socioeconomic burden of falls coupled with the aging population makes fall prevention a priority. Current recommendations for fall prevention focus on measures to delay the occurrence of falls through identification of modifiable risk factors and customization of interventions directed against these identified factors. Exercise and physical therapy have been shown to be effective in reducing the number of falls by 16% in individuals at high risk.[14] Although these interventions are valuable, they are resource-demanding and labor intensive, strongly dependent on subject compliance, and thus, unsustainable in the long term. Vitamin D supplementation is an appealing population-level strategy recommended for fall prevention in high-risk fallers. Although its efficacy is still debated, vitamin D supplementation is an easily implemented, cost-effective, and well-tolerated approach to reduce the burden of falling in the elderly.

EFFECT OF VITAMIN D ON FALLS

There is conflicting evidence that vitamin D status can influence the incidence of fall. The mechanisms by which vitamin D affects the likelihood of falling are not well understood. The association between vitamin D deficiency, muscle weakness, and poor balance likely is the basis of the relationship between low serum 25OHD levels and increased rates of falls.

Association Studies

A longitudinal study from the Netherlands demonstrated that even after adjusting for covariates (sex, age, education, season, geographic region, smoking, alcohol intake, and physical activity level) serum 25OHD levels less than 10 ng/mL are independently associated with an increased risk for falls.[15] Another study showed no association of the number of falls with serum 25OHD concentrations, but an association with serum parathyroid hormone levels was found.[16] In the Study of Osteoporotic fractures, an increase in falls was noted with increasing serum 25OHD levels (incidence rate ratio, 1.46; 95% confidence interval [CI], 0.95–2.15) in elderly women, although the number of falls and serum 1,25OHD levels were inversely related (incidence rate ratio, 0.70; 95% CI, 0.47–1.05; $P = .039$).[17] In another study, even after adjusting for a previous fracture, cognition, and medications used, serum 25OHD less than 20 ng/mL (50 nmol/L) were independently related to the incidence of first fall (hazard ratio, 0.74; 95% CI, 0.59–0.94).[18] Overall, these data support that low serum 25OHD levels, particularly less than 20 ng/mL (50 nmol/L), are associated with falls.

Vitamin D Supplementation and Falls

The impact of vitamin D on the risk of falls has been evaluated in several randomized controlled trials (RCT). A 1992 study of 3270 elderly nursing home individuals that received 800 IU vitamin D with 1200 mg calcium daily gained interest after showing the decline in incidence of hip fracture by 43% compared with the placebo group, whereas bone mineral density was almost unchanged risk.[19] The antifracture effect of vitamin D and calcium in this study was considered a result of decreased falls. A total of 24 intervention studies have been completed with daily dosing schedule of vitamin D in individuals 60 years or older. Four of these studies in which vitamin D was coadministered with calcium in doses ranging from 700 to 1000 IU daily demonstrated a statistically significant reduction in falls. Several meta-analyses have also reported this effect of vitamin D supplementation on fall risk, but the findings are divergent (**Table 1**).

The US Preventive Services Task Force meta-analysis of vitamin D supplementation and vitamin D metabolites reported a reduction in falls of 17% (but also included studies with calcitriol and alfacalcidol supplementation).[14] In another meta-analysis, a 14% decrease in fall risk was documented with vitamin D supplementation versus placebo.[20] A nonsignificant decrease of 5% was seen in a recent meta-analysis of 20 trials.[21]

The effect of higher doses of vitamin D on risk of falls has also been examined in several studies. In a randomized trial of 173 older patients (mean age, 84 years) with acute hip fracture, the incidence of fallers did not differ in the groups receiving 2000 IU and 800 IU of vitamin D_3 daily over a 12-month follow-up (28%; 95% CI, −4% to 68%).[22] No statistically significant reduction in fall risk has been demonstrated by the studies administering bolus doses of oral vitamin D_3 or parenteral vitamin D_2. A study of 686 women aged 70 years and older randomized to 150,000 IU of oral vitamin D_3 every 3 months showed a null effect on falls and physical function compared with placebo.[23] In another trial of 2256 elderly women at high risk of hip fracture, an increased risk of falling was noted with an annual bolus of 500,000 IU of vitamin D compared with the placebo group (rate ratio, 1.15; 95% CI, 1.02–1.30).[24] Although

Table 1
Meta-analyses of RCTs of vitamin D supplementation and falls and physical performance

Meta-Analysis, Year	Sample Size	Study Population	Intervention	Results
Falls				
Bischoff-Ferrari et al,[6] 2004 (5 RCTs)	11,238	Men and women aged >65 y	Vitamin D[a]	Reduction in fall risk by 22%
Murad et al,[20] 2011 (26 RCTs)	45,782	Men and women of all ages	Vitamin D + calcium	Reduction in fall risk: significant decrease in the number of fallers by 14%
Bolland et al,[21] 2014 (20 RCTs)	29,535	Men and women of all ages	Vitamin D ± calcium	No significant reduction in fall risk (5%)
Physical Performance				
Muir & Montero-Odasso,[rn] 2011 (13 RCTs)	2268	Men and women aged 60 y or older	Vitamin D	Reduction in postural sway Improvement in lower extremity muscle strength
Stockton et al,[57] 2011 (17 RCTs)	5072	Men and women of all ages	Vitamin D	Increase in muscle strength in subjects with baseline 25OHD <25 nmol/L
Beaudart et al,[59] 2014 (30 RCTs)	5615	Men and women of all ages (mean age, 61.1 y)	Vitamin D with or without calcium	Small positive effect on global muscle strength, particularly in those 65 y or older and those with vitamin D deficiency at baseline (<30 nmol/L)

[a] Vitamin D, calcitriol, and alfacalcidol.

data from association studies were positive, the results from intervention studies are mixed and no beneficial effects of bolus doses have been reported.

The efficacy of vitamin D analogues has also been studied in intervention trials, particularly in the elderly with low creatinine clearance. In a double-blind randomized study, 36 weeks of treatment with alfacalcidol (1 μg daily) significantly reduced the number of fallers (OR, 0.26; 95% CI, 0.08–0.80; $P = .019$) and falls (0.29; 95% CI, 0.09–0.88; $P = .028$) in participants with glomerular filtration rate (GFR) less than 65 mL/min compared with placebo.[25] A 3-year RCT demonstrated that calcitriol reduces the rate of falls by 30% (95% CI, −49% to −4%; $P = .027$) in elderly with GFR greater than or equal to 60 mL/min. Calcitriol decreased the rate of falls even better (53%) in the GFR less than 60 mL/min group ($P = .003$).[26]

Postural Stability

Poor postural equilibrium is a known risk factor for falls. Several studies have assessed the effect of vitamin D on postural stability by measuring the degree of sway in the anterior-posterior and medial-lateral planes. A study from London found that individuals (mean age, 76.7 ± 6.1 years) with serum 25OHD levels 12 ng/mL or lower

(≤30 nmol/L) had significantly increased body sway and decreased quadriceps muscle strength.[27] Intramuscular administration of 600,000 IU of vitamin D_2 in these subjects significantly reduced the amplitude of postural sway by 13% in contrast to the 3% increase seen in the placebo group. Two intervention trials compared the effect of 800 IU of vitamin D_3 plus 1000 mg of calcium daily with 1000 mg of calcium alone on sway in older adults.[28,29] In these studies, up to 28% reduction in body sway was seen over periods of 2 and 12 months in the vitamin D groups compared with the calcium groups alone (however, calcium may not be a true placebo because it reduces parathyroid hormone and calcitriol levels). In a more recent RCT, improvement in balance was documented only in older subjects (mean age, 77 years) with severe balance impairment at baseline following administration of 8400 IU weekly of vitamin D_3 for 16 weeks.[30] In the cohort with normal sway at baseline, vitamin D_3 had no effect. Thus, the effect of vitamin D on postural stability may depend on the baseline 25OHD levels.

Overall, the findings of observational and interventional studies on the effect of vitamin D on falls are heterogeneous. This is partially explained by the differences in many aspects of these studies: baseline characteristics of the study populations (25OHD level, age, comorbidities, physical and functional status), cutoff used to define vitamin D deficiency, dose and formulation of vitamin D administered, treatment intervals, final 25OHD level achieved, assay methods for measurement of serum 25OHD, and compliance with vitamin D supplementation. In addition, falls were not the primary outcome in many of these studies. Furthermore, experts suggest that the outcome measure in investigations should be the faller and not the frequency of falls.[31] Although further concrete evidence is needed, accumulating data implicate the role of vitamin D in fall protection (at best 5% risk reduction)[23] in older adults in doses ranging from 700 to 1000 IU daily.

EFFECT OF VITAMIN D ON PHYSICAL PERFORMANCE

A decline in physical performance with concomitant age-related bone loss can lead to an increased risk of falls and fractures in the older population. Although proximal muscle weakness and pain are caused only by severe vitamin D deficiency, mild vitamin D insufficiency also seems to affect muscle performance in older adults.[32] Impaired lower extremity function is a major risk factor for frailty and loss of autonomy.[33,34] In recent years, tools to objectively evaluate specific aspects of lower extremity function have been developed to enhance the ability to quantify physical performance. This typically involves having the individuals perform a prespecified number of standardized tasks simulating activities of daily living of various degrees of difficulty. These standardized instruments vary in terms of validity, reliability, and responsiveness.[35] Common assessments include muscle strength, standing balance, and gait speed.

Cross-sectional Studies

Cross-sectional studies suggest positive association between serum 25OHD and physical performance and strength among older adults.[27,36–42] In 435 men and 531 women (mean age, 74.8 years) of the InCHIANTI study, a significant association between low serum 25OHD levels and poor physical performance was observed.[38] Handgrip strength was higher in subjects with serum 25OHD higher than 20 ng/mL (>50 nmol/L). Subjects with levels lower than 10 ng/mL (<25 nmol/L) performed lower on a short physical performance battery test (chair rises, balance) compared with those with higher 25OHD levels. Positive association between serum 25OHD levels and gait speed among older women has also been reported.[39] In the Pro.V.A study of 2694 community-dwelling elderly men and women (mean age, 74 years), lower serum 25OHD levels were associated with a lower 6-minute-walk test.[40] In another study of elderly men and women with falls, higher serum 25OHD levels were associated with faster time-and-get-up test and sit-to-stand test.[41] In the National Health and Nutrition Examination Survey III (including 4100 ambulatory adults aged 60 years and older), lower extremity muscle performance, measured as the 8-feet-walk test and the repeated sit-to-stand test, was inadequate in subjects with the lowest 25OHD levels and improved increasingly at higher 25OHD levels.[42] These positive associations between vitamin D status and physical performance have also been reported in the younger population.[43,44]

Prospective Studies

Consistent with the National Health and Nutrition Examination Survey III findings, the Longitudinal Aging Study Amsterdam, an epidemiologic study of Dutch men and women aged 65 years and older, found that low baseline serum 25OHD levels (~10–15 ng/mL) were associated with physical performance, but once serum 25OHD exceeded 16 ng/mL there was no further benefit in the multivariate model.[45] Furthermore, low baseline 25OHD concentrations predicted a 3-year decline in physical performance (defined as a loss of handgrip strength more than 40%) in individuals with serum 25OHD levels lower than 10 ng/mL (<25 nmol/L) in comparison with those with levels higher than 20 ng/mL (>50 nmol/L). Another study reported a similar rate of 3-year decline in muscle strength, however at a different 25OHD level.[46] This association between vitamin D status and a decline in physical performance was not seen in the younger cohort of Longitudinal Aging Study Amsterdam aged 55 to 65 years in contrast to those 65 years and older mentioned previously.[47] Similarly, a study of more than 1000 young men (mean age, 47 years), 20% of whom had 25OHD level lower than 20 ng/mL (<50 nmol/L), did not find any relationship between serum 25OHD and physical performance.[48]

Although cross-sectional studies show positive association, data from prospective studies are conflicting. Although some studies showed no relationship, other studies noted greater declines in physical performance with vitamin D deficiency.[17,45,46,49] However, studies that particularly included older participants with vitamin D deficiency at baseline are the ones that indicate vitamin D status as a predictor of decline in physical performance in this population.

Vitamin D Supplementation and Physical Performance

Randomized trials have also found inconsistent results regarding the effect of vitamin D supplementation on physical performance among older adults. In 1991, one study reported no improvement in quadriceps strength with twice a day calcitriol supplementation in adults aged 70[50]; another study of 60 healthy older men showed no statistically significant difference in grip or leg press strength over a 6-month period between the group receiving 1000 IU vitamin D_3 daily and placebo.[51] Even after calcitriol treatment for 3 years, there was no effect on physical performance.[52]

In contrast, another study reported up to 11% improvement in musculoskeletal function after 3 months of treatment with vitamin D_3 plus calcium.[27] These findings were confirmed in a trial of 300 elderly women with a baseline 25OHD level lower than 24 ng/mL (<60 nmol/L). Daily intake of 2000 IU vitamin D showed improvement in muscle strength (faster time-and-get-up test) and those in the lowest quartile showed an additional improvement.[53] Higher muscle mass and lower extremity function with supplementation of vitamin D and leucine-enriched whey protein were observed among older adults with sarcopenia in a recent RCT.[54] Most trials that showed benefit used an average daily dose of 800 IU of vitamin D. Other clinical trials have failed to demonstrate these beneficial effects of vitamin D on physical performance, including two recent trials with 800 IU daily of vitamin D in older women.[55,56] However, some of the trials included subjects with sufficient baseline 25OHD levels (>20 ng/mL as defined by the Institute of Medicine [IOM]) and other trials used lower daily doses of vitamin D, doses likely insufficient to slow the rate of decline in physical performance that occurs with aging.

In a meta-analysis of 17 RCTs with muscle performance as end points, the effect of vitamin D supplementation on lower extremity muscle strength was dependent on baseline 25OHD levels and was present only in subjects with baseline levels lower than 10 ng/mL (<25 nmol/L).[57] This analysis included subjects of all ages. Another meta-analysis of RCTs including elderly men and women (mean age, 78 years) showed beneficial effect of daily vitamin D doses ranging from 800 to 1000 IU on balance and muscle function, but not on gait speed.[58] A more recent meta-analysis also documented this statistically significant effect of vitamin D supplementation on muscle strength, which was more pronounced in subjects aged 65 years and older with baseline 25OHD levels lower than 12 ng/mL (<30 nmol/L; standardized mean difference, 0.25, 95% CI, 0.01–0.48 vs 0.03, 95% CI, −0.08 to 0.14) (see **Table 1**).[59]

The effect of intermittent higher doses of vitamin D on physical performance in the elderly has been studied in one RCT.[23] A total of 689 women with mean age 77 years received 150,000 IU of vitamin D_3 every 3 months for a total of 9 months. No difference in muscle strength was noted in the treatment group compared with the placebo group. These findings suggest that intermittent high doses of vitamin D may not be effective in improving muscular strength.

Findings of these studies of vitamin D effectiveness on physical performance are mixed. The divergent findings are likely a result of multiple confounders similar to those in the studies evaluating falls. In addition, the different tools and methods used to quantify physical performance contribute to the variability in study designs. Nonetheless, collective evidence from intervention trials supports the role of vitamin D supplementation for muscle function improvement in older adults, particularly those deficient in vitamin D (<12 ng/mL as defined by the IOM).

POSTULATED MECHANISMS

The mechanisms by which vitamin D might affect the likelihood of falling and physical function are not fully elucidated. In the past, the role of vitamin D deficiency in increasing the risk of falls and fractures in the elderly was considered an indirect effect on bone remodeling mediated through hyperparathyroidism.[60] Recent findings help explain this association better through an understanding of the direct effect of vitamin D on muscle strength and function.[61] Several mechanisms underlying this association are postulated.

Vitamin D exerts its effect on muscle via the VDR. These VDRs are expressed in skeletal muscle tissue and are activated by 1,25OHD (calcitriol), a mediator of vitamin D–directed gene expression.[61–65] Calcitriol binds to the nuclear VDRs thereby acting as a regulator of calcium uptake by muscle. Aging itself is associated with a decrease in VDR concentration.[66,67] In addition, atrophy of fast twitch muscle fibers (type II) is also known to occur as a function of aging.[68,69] Activation of these fibers is important during a fast reaction (eg, maintaining balance to prevent a fall).[70] Thereby, at a cellular level, age-associated decline in VDRs and atrophy of type II fibers could increase the risk for falling.

Rapid effect on muscle contraction is a nongenomic action of vitamin D mediated through calcium influx. A reversible atrophy of type II fast twitch fibers has been observed in individuals with vitamin D deficiency.[71] Calcitriol-mediated calcium uptake by muscle controls muscle contraction and relaxation, and muscle protein synthesis involved in myocyte proliferation and differentiation.[61] Studies in older adults have confirmed that calcitriol (vitamin D_2) treatment promotes de novo protein synthesis in muscle, particularly of type II fibers.[72] It has also been documented from muscle biopsies in 21 older women that 4-month intake of 4000 IU vitamin D_3 daily increased VDR concentration by 30% and muscle fiber size by 10%.[73] At a clinical level, proximal muscle weakness is a feature of vitamin D deficiency, usually in the lower extremities.[32,71,74] Studies indicate that adequate levels of 25OHD enhance skeletal muscle strength and improve postural stability.

In keeping with the ubiquitous nature of VDRs, an additional effect of vitamin D could be mediated through the nervous system.[75] Impaired cognition and reduced nerve conduction caused by age-related decline in VDR expression could lead to slower reaction time and poor balance.[26,75,76] The extent to which either of these mechanisms explains the association between vitamin D, fall risk, and physical decline in older adults is unknown. Finally, the effect of parathyroid hormone on muscles is also not completely understood. Albeit a catabolic action observed in rodent muscles and the clinical observation of parathyroid hormone as a predictor of falls and muscle strength, the specific roles of vitamin D and parathyroid hormone independent of each other are not yet clear.[77–79] In view of the accumulating data, it is more than likely that a combination of mechanisms underlies the association of vitamin D status and falls and physical performance.

CURRENT CONTROVERSIES

There is a controversy regarding vitamin D supplementation and optimal serum 25OHD levels necessary for preventing adverse extraskeletal health outcomes. In 2010, the IOM report stated that there was insufficient scientific evidence for a basis to make nutritional recommendations for extraskeletal outcomes of vitamin D.[80] The final recommendation was based on bone health outcomes and the recommended daily allowance was set at 20 ng/mL (50 nmol/L). In 2011, the Endocrine Society Clinical Practice Guidelines recommended vitamin D supplementation of 1500 to 2000 IU daily to prevent falls in adults older than 70 years compared with the 800 IU daily dose recommended by the IOM in this population.[80,81] The American Geriatrics Society agreed with the Endocrine Society that a serum 25OHD level of 30 ng/mL (75 nmol/L) should be ensured to benefit older adults and recommended a total daily vitamin D intake of 4000 IU, especially in those with a history of falls.[82] However, given the aforementioned literature, there is limited evidence to support the use of vitamin D supplementation in doses higher than recommended by the IOM for the elderly. Indeed, most of the studies with positive findings used vitamin D doses ranging from 700 to 1000 IU daily. Moreover, some studies suggesting the benefit of vitamin D supplementation on falls and physical performance included older adults with very low serum 25OHD levels at baseline. Lending support to this, a recent study demonstrated the negative effect of higher dose of vitamin D in older adults.[83] In this RCT of 200 men and women, aged 70 years and older, researchers found that a serum 25OHD level of at least 30 ng/mL (75 nmol/L) was effectively achieved with a monthly vitamin D dose of 60,000 IU. However, this group had a significantly higher incidence of falls (66.9%; 95% CI, 54.4–77.5) compared with those receiving 24,000 IU of vitamin

D per month (equivalent to 800 IU/day; 47.9%; 95% CI, 35.8–60.3; P = .048). In addition, higher doses did not improve lower extremity physical performance. The findings of this intervention study, in keeping with the association results of the Study of Osteoporotic fractures,[17] suggest a likelihood of harm with higher serum 25OHD levels in the elderly.

FUTURE CONSIDERATIONS

The recommendations by IOM were based on the knowledge of a U-shaped curve of increasing mortality higher than a 25OHD serum level of 45 to 50 ng/mL (112–125 nmol/L).[80] The reason for detrimental effect of high doses of vitamin D in increasing falls in older adults is unclear. Notwithstanding, definitive evidence regarding beneficial effects of higher doses of vitamin D and threshold response for extraskeletal outcomes is lacking. Therefore, a cautious approach is warranted and higher doses of vitamin D should not be recommended based on putative unproven health benefits. In view of accumulating evidence, a potential adverse effect of falls with higher doses of vitamin D corresponding with serum 25OHD levels exceeding 45 ng/mL (112 nmol/L) should be acknowledged. The tolerable upper limit for vitamin D is based on the known adverse effect of hypercalcemia with an adjustment factor for safety (adjusted from 10,000–4000 IU daily).[80] If confirmed, the new evidence will guide age-specific dietary reference intakes and possible reduction of tolerable upper limit in older population.

Subpopulation Consideration

The incidence of falls is higher among older adults in residential care compared with the general population.[18] Vitamin D deficiency is also more common in institutionalized older adults.[84,85] In this population, it has also been noted that fallers have lower serum vitamin D concentrations than nonfallers.[86] Older age and male gender are independent risk factors for sarcopenia.[87] In addition, vitamin D deficiency in older adults itself is also associated with sarcopenia and disability.[84] A prospective study of 4000 older adults (mean age, 70 years) documented an association between low serum 25OHD, frailty, and all-cause mortality during a 12-year follow-up.[88] Factors including low intake of calcium and vitamin D, reduced cutaneous production of vitamin D, and decreased renal production of 1,25OHD may predispose older institutionalized individuals to proximal myopathy caused by vitamin D deficiency and secondary hyperparathyroidism, thereby increasing falls.[89–91] Hence, this is a specific subpopulation that can avail the benefits of vitamin D supplementation in terms of prevention of fractures, falls, and decline in physical performance.

In a randomized, placebo-controlled double blind study of 625 institutionalized participants (mean age, 83.4 years), vitamin D supplementation over 2 years resulted in reduction of fall incidence (incident rate ratio for falling, 0.73; odds ratio for forever falling, 0.82; odds ratio for forever fracturing, 0.69).[92] Another randomized controlled open label study of 3717 institutionalized adults (76% women; mean age, 85 years) showed no reduction in falls or incidence of fractures with vitamin D supplementation.[93] However, this study administered vitamin D_2 in intermittent doses: ergocalciferol, 2.5 mg every 3 months (equivalent to a daily dose of 1100 IU). Several other RCTs also noted that daily vitamin D supplementation reduces the risk of falling in institutionalized individuals as summarized in the meta-analysis.[94] Notably, the fall prevention effect is dose dependent and only seen with a dose of 700 to 1000 IU of vitamin D, consistent with the IOM recommendations for the elderly. Data on prevention of physical decline from vitamin D supplementation in institutionalized older adults are insufficient. The existing evidence, although limited, is supportive of the potential role of vitamin D in fall prevention in this population, especially those who are deficient in vitamin D. Nevertheless, in addition to other comorbidities, aforementioned risk factors and consequences of vitamin D deficiency also make this population the most vulnerable to harms of overtreatment with higher doses of vitamin D. Clinical trials in this subpopulation may give more precise estimates of vitamin D supplementation doses needed, and levels of 25OHD required to minimize falls.

Future studies should also consider variable dietary intake of vitamin D among populations during participant selection. Food fortification has achieved adequate intakes of vitamin D at a population level. It is really the elderly who are vitamin D deficient that require vitamin D supplementation (800 IU as recommended by the IOM). It is also possible that vitamin D thresholds for skeletal and extraskeletal outcomes are different. All of these considerations can be helpful in designing future clinical trials for conclusive evidence.

SUMMARY

Although, current understanding has highlighted the importance of the extraskeletal role of vitamin D in vitro, the apparent divergent clinical findings in recent observational and interventional studies have intensified the controversy surrounding this role of vitamin D. This article reviews the literature and summarizes the influence of vitamin D status and vitamin D supplementation on falls, postural stability, and physical performance; describes the putative mechanisms underlying this association; and reflects on the controversy surrounding vitamin D recommendations in older adults. Key points are as follows:

- Although the direct effect of vitamin D on muscle tissue is better understood, the mechanisms by which vitamin D affects the likelihood of falling and physical function are not fully elucidated.
- Definitive data are lacking regarding the effectiveness of vitamin D supplementation and dose requirements for reduction in fall risk and improvement in muscle strength.
- No threshold effect of vitamin D status on falls or physical performance has been established in the literature. There is a possibility that the thresholds for skeletal and extraskeletal outcomes of vitamin D are different.
- Heterogeneity in studies (participant characteristics, study designs, assessment tools, falls vs fallers) has contributed to the incongruous clinical findings. Longitudinal, standardized, placebo-controlled, dose studies with uniform end points are needed to determine which vitamin D interventions can influence extraskeletal outcomes.
- Beyond food fortification, vitamin D supplementation is needed to achieve vitamin D sufficiency in certain subpopulations. Until further concrete evidence, it is prudent to follow the IOM recommendations (800 IU of vitamin D daily in adults older than 70 years) to avoid adverse effects in this vulnerable population under the principle *"primum non nocere."*

REFERENCES

1. Holick MF. Vitamin D deficiency. N Engl J Med 2007;357(3):266–81.
2. Fried LP, Guralnik JM. Disability in older adults: evidence regarding significance, etiology, and risk. J Am Geriatr Soc 1997;45(1):92–100.

3. Morrison A, Fan T, Sen SS, et al. Epidemiology of falls and osteoporotic fractures: a systematic review. Clinicoecon Outcomes Res 2013;5:9–18.

4. Berry SD, Miller RR. Falls: epidemiology, pathophysiology, and relationship to fracture. Curr Osteoporos Rep 2008;6(4):149–54.

5. Souberbielle JC, Body JJ, Lappe JM, et al. Vitamin D and musculoskeletal health, cardiovascular disease, autoimmunity and cancer: recommendations for clinical practice. Autoimm Rev 2010;9(11):709–15.

6. Bischoff-Ferrari HA, Dawson-Hughes B, Willett WC, et al. Effect of Vitamin D on falls: a meta-analysis. JAMA 2004;291(16):1999–2006.

7. Peel NM. Epidemiology of falls in older age. Can J Aging 2011;30(1):7–19.

8. Hartholt KA, Stevens JA, Polinder S, et al. Increase in fall-related hospitalizations in the United States, 2001–2008. J Trauma 2011;71(1):255–8.

9. Burns EB, Stevens JA, Lee RL. The direct costs of fatal and non-fatal falls among older adults—United States. J Safety Res 2016;58:99–103.

10. World Health Organization. International statistical classification of diseases and related health problems (10th revision). 2nd edition. Geneva (Switzerland): WHO Press; 2004.

11. Zuckerman JD. Hip fracture. N Engl J Med 1996;334(23):1519–25.

12. Tinetti ME, Williams CS. The effect of falls and fall injuries on functioning in community-dwelling older persons. J Gerontol A Biol Sci Med Sci 1998;53(2):M112–9.

13. Deshpande N, Metter EJ, Lauretani F, et al. Activity restriction induced by fear of falling and objective and subjective measures of physical function: a prospective cohort study. J Am Geriatr Soc 2008;56(4):615–20.

14. Michael YL, Whitlock EP, Lin JS, et al. Primary care-relevant interventions to prevent falling in older adults: a systematic evidence review for the U.S. Preventive Services Task Force. Ann Intern Med 2010;153(12):815–25.

15. Snijder MB, Van Schoor NM, Pluijm SM, et al. Vitamin D status in relation to one-year risk of recurrent falling in older men and women. J Clin Endocrinol Metab 2006;91(8):2980–5.

16. Sambrook PN, Chen JS, March LM, et al. Serum parathyroid hormone predicts time to fall independent of vitamin D status in a frail elderly population. J Clin Endocrinol Metab 2004;89(4):1572–6.

17. Faulkner KA, Cauley JA, Zmuda JM, et al. Higher 1,25-dihydroxyvitamin D3 concentrations associated with lower fall rates in older community-dwelling women. Osteoporos Int 2006;17(9):1318–28.

18. Flicker L, Mead K, MacInnis RJ, et al. Serum vitamin D and falls in older women in residential care in Australia. J Am Geriatr Soc 2003;51(11):1533–8.

19. Chapuy MC, Arlot ME, Duboeuf F, et al. Vitamin D3 and calcium to prevent hip fractures in the elderly women. N Engl J Med 1992;327(23):1637–42.

20. Murad MH, Elamin KB, Abu Elnour NO, et al. The effect of vitamin D on falls: a systematic review and meta-analysis. J Clin Endocrinol Metab 2011;96(10):2997–3006.

21. Bolland MJ, Grey A, Gamble GD, et al. Vitamin D supplementation and falls: a trial sequential meta-analysis. Lancet Diabetes Endocrinol 2014;2(7):573–80.

22. Bischoff-Ferrari HA, Dawson-Hughes B, Platz A, et al. Effect of high-dosage cholecalciferol and extended physiotherapy on complications after hip fracture: a randomized controlled trial. Arch Intern Med 2010;170(9):813–20.

23. Glendenning P, Zhu K, Inderjeeth C, et al. Effects of three-monthly oral 150,000 IU cholecalciferol supplementation on falls, mobility, and muscle strength in older

postmenopausal women: a randomized controlled trial. J Bone Miner Res 2012; 27(1):170–6.

24. Sanders KM, Stuart AL, Williamson EJ, et al. Annual high-dose oral vitamin D and falls and fractures in older women: a randomized controlled trial. JAMA 2010; 303(18):1815–22.

25. Dukas L, Schacht E, Mazor Z, et al. Treatment with alfacalcidol in elderly people significantly decreases the high risk of falls associated with a low creatinine clearance of <65 ml/min. Osteoporos Int 2005;16(2):198–203.

26. Gallagher JC, Rapuri PB, Smith LM. An age related decrease in creatinine clearance is associated with an increase in number of falls in untreated women but not in women receiving calcitriol treatment. J Clin Endocrinol Metab 2007;92(1):51–8.

27. Dhesi JK, Bearne LM, Moniz C, et al. Neuromuscular and psychomotor function in elderly subjects who fall and the relationship with vitamin D status. J Bone Miner Res 2002;17(5):891–7.

28. Pfeifer M, Begerow B, Minne HW, et al. Effects of a short-term vitamin D and calcium supplementation on body sway and secondary hyperparathyroidism in elderly women. J Bone Miner Res 2000;15(6):1113–8.

29. Pfeifer M, Begerow B, Minne HW, et al. Effects of a long-term vitamin D and calcium supplementation on falls and parameters of muscle function in community-dwelling older individuals. Osteoporos Int 2009;20(2):315–22.

30. Lips P, Binkley N, Pfeifer M, et al. Once-weekly dose of 8400 IU vitamin D(3) compared with placebo: effects on neuromuscular function and tolerability in older adults with vitamin D insufficiency. Am J Clin Nutr 2010;91(4):985–91.

31. Gallagher JC. Vitamin D and falls: the dosage conundrum. Nat Rev Endocrinol 2016;12(11):680–4.

32. Glerup H, Mikkelsen K, Poulsen L, et al. Hypovitaminosis D myopathy without biochemical signs of osteomalacic bone involvement. Calcif Tissue Int 2000; 66(6):419–24.

33. Cummings SR, Nevitt MC. Non-skeletal determinants of fractures: the potential importance of the mechanics of falls. Study of Osteoporotic Fractures Research Group. Osteoporos Int 1994;4(Suppl 1):67–70.

34. Fried LP, Tangen CM, Walston J, et al. Frailty in older adults: evidence for a phenotype. J Gerontol A Biol Sci Med Sci 2001;56(3):M146–56.

35. Freiberger E, de Vreede P, Schoene D, et al. Performance-based physical function in older community-dwelling persons: a systematic review of instruments. Age Ageing 2012;41(6):712–21.

36. Mowé M, Haug E, Bøhmer T. Low serum calcidiol concentration in older adults with reduced muscular function. J Am Geriatr Soc 1999;47(2):220–6.

37. Zamboni M, Zoico E, Tosoni P, et al. Relation between vitamin D, physical performance, and disability in elderly persons. J Gerontol A Biol Sci Med Sci 2002; 57(1):M7–11.

38. Houston DK, Cesari M, Ferrucci L, et al. Association between vitamin D status and physical performance: the InCHIANTI study. J Gerontol A Biol Sci Med Sci 2007;62(4):440–6.

39. Annweiler C, Schott AM, Montero-Odasso M, et al. Cross-sectional association between serum vitamin D concentration and walking speed measured at usual and fast pace among older women: the EPIDOS study. J Bone Miner Res 2010;25(8):1858–66.

40. Toffanello ED, Perissinotto E, Sergi G, et al. Vitamin D and physical performance in elderly subjects: the Pro.V.A study. PLoS One 2012;7(4):e34950.

41. Boyé ND, Oudshoorn C, van der Velde N, et al. Vitamin D and physical performance in older men and women visiting the emergency department because of a fall: data from the improving medication prescribing to reduce risk of falls (IMPROveFALL) study. J Am Geriatr Soc 2013;61(11):1948–52.

42. Bischoff-Ferrari HA, Dietrich T, Orav EJ, et al. Higher 25-hydroxyvitamin D concentrations are associated with better lower-extremity function in both active and inactive persons aged ≥60 y. Am J Clin Nutr 2004;80(3):752–8.

43. Valtueña J, Gracia-Marco L, Huybrechts I, et al. Cardiorespiratory fitness in males, and upper limbs muscular strength in females, are positively related with 25-hydroxyvitamin D plasma concentrations in European adolescents: the HELENA Study. QJM 2013;106(9):809–21.

44. von Hurst PR, Conlon C, Foskett A. Vitamin D status predicts hand-grip strength in young adult women living in Auckland, New Zealand. J Steroid Biochem Mol Biol 2013;136(1):330–2.

45. Wicherts IS, Van Schoor NM, Boeke AJ, et al. Vitamin D status predicts physical performance and its decline in older persons. J Clin Endocrinol Metab 2007; 92(6):2058–65.

46. Verreault R, Semba RD, Volpato S, et al. Low serum vitamin d does not predict new disability or loss of muscle strength in older women. J Am Geriatr Soc 2002;50(5):912–7.

47. Sohl E, de Jongh RT, Heijboer AC, et al. Vitamin D status is associated with physical performance: the results of three independent cohorts. Osteoporos Int 2013; 24(1):187–96.

48. Ceglia L, Chiu GR, Harris SS, et al. Serum 25-hydroxyvitamin D concentration and physical function in adult men. Clin Endocrinol (Oxf) 2011;74(3):370–6.

49. Dam TT, von Mühlen D, Barrett-Connor EL. Sex-specific association of serum vitamin D levels with physical function in older adults. Osteoporos Int 2009; 20(5):751–60.

50. Grady D, Halloran B, Cummings S, et al. 1,25-Dihydroxyvitamin D3 and muscle strength in the elderly: a randomized controlled trial. J Clin Endocrinol Metab 1991;73(5):1111–7.

51. Kenny AM, Biskup B, Robbins B, et al. Effects of vitamin D supplementation on strength, physical function, and health perception in older, community-dwelling men. J Am Geriatr Soc 2003;51(12):1762–7.

52. Gallagher JC. The effects of calcitriol on falls and fractures and physical performance tests. J Steroid Biochem Mol Biol 2004;89-90(1–5):497–501.

53. Zhu K, Austin N, Devine A, et al. A randomized controlled trial of the effects of vitamin D on muscle strength and mobility in older women with vitamin D insufficiency. J Am Geriatr Soc 2010;58(11):2063–8.

54. Bauer JM, Verlaan S, Bautmans I, et al. Effects of a vitamin D and leucine-enriched whey protein nutritional supplement on measures of sarcopenia in older adults, the PROVIDE study: a randomized, double-blind, placebo-controlled trial. J Am Med Dir Assoc 2015;16(9):740–7.

55. Hansen KE, Johnson RE, Chambers KR, et al. Treatment of vitamin D insufficiency in postmenopausal women: a randomized clinical trial. JAMA Intern Med 2015; 175(10):1612–21.

56. Uusi-Rasi K, Patil R, Karinkanta S, et al. Exercise and vitamin D in fall prevention among older women: a randomized clinical trial. JAMA Intern Med 2015;175(5): 703–11.

57. Stockton KA, Mengersen K, Paratz JD, et al. Effect of vitamin D supplementation on muscle strength: a systematic review and meta-analysis. Osteoporos Int 2011; 22(3):859–71.
58. Muir SW, Montero-Odasso M. Effect of vitamin D supplementation on muscle strength, gait and balance in older adults: a systematic review and meta-analysis. J Am Geriatr Soc 2011;59(12):2291–300.
59. Beaudart C, Buckinx F, Rabenda V, et al. The effects of vitamin D on skeletal muscle strength, muscle mass, and muscle power: a systematic review and meta-analysis of randomized controlled trials. J Clin Endocrinol Metab 2014;99(11): 4300–45.
60. Brazier M, Kamel S, Maamer M, et al. Markers of bone remodeling in the elderly subject: effects of vitamin D insufficiency and its correction. J Bone Miner Res 1995;10(11):1753–61.
61. Ceglia L, Harris SS. Vitamin D and its role in skeletal muscle. Calcif Tissue Int 2013;92(2):151–62.
62. Bischoff HA, Borchers M, Gudat F, et al. In situ detection of 1,25-dihydroxyvitamin D3 receptor in human skeletal muscle tissue. Histochem J 2001;33(1):19–24.
63. Zehnder D, Bland R, Williams MC, et al. Extrarenal expression of 25 hydroxyvitamin D3-1a-hydroxylase 1. J Clin Endocrinol Metab 2001;86(2):888–94.
64. Hewison M, Burke F, Evans KN, et al. Extra-renal 25-hydroxyvitamin D 3-1a-hydroxylase in human health and disease. J Steroid Biochem Mol Biol 2007; 103(3):316–21.
65. Rosen CJ, Adams JS, Bikle DD, et al. The nonskeletal effects of vitamin D: an Endocrine Society scientific statement. Endocr Rev 2012;33(3):456–92.
66. Bischoff-Ferrari HA, Borchers M, Gudat F, et al. Vitamin D receptor expression in human muscle tissue decreases with age. J Bone Miner Res 2004;19(2):265–9.
67. Geng S, Zhou S, Glowacki J. Age-related decline in osteoblastogenesis and 1-hydroxylase/CYP27B1 in human mesenchymal stem cells: stimulation by parathyroid hormone. Aging Cell 2011;10(6):962–71.
68. Lexell J, Henriksson-Larsen K, Wimblod B, et al. Distribution of different fiber types in human skeletal muscles: effects of aging studied in whole muscle cross sections. Muscle Nerve 1983;6(8):588–95.
69. Larsson L. Histochemical characteristics of human skeletal muscle during aging. Acat Physiol Scand 1983;117(3):469–71.
70. Domingues-Faria C, Chanet A, Salles J, et al. Vitamin D deficiency downregulates Notch pathway contributing to skeletal muscle atrophy in old Wistar rats. Nutr Metab (Lond) 2014;11(1):47.
71. Ziambaras K, Dagogo-Jack S. Reversible muscle weakness in patients with vitamin D deficiency. West J Med 1997;167(6):435–9.
72. Sorensen OH, Lund B, Saltin B, et al. Myopathy in bone loss of ageing: improvement by treatment with 1 alpha-hydroxycholecalciferol and calcium. Clin Sci (Lond) 1979;56(2):157–61.
73. Ceglia L, Niramitmahapanya S, da Silva Morais M, et al. A randomized study on the effect of vitamin D3 supplementation on skeletal muscle morphology and vitamin D receptor concentration in older women. J Clin Endocrinol Metab 2013;98(12):E1927–35.
74. Al-Shoha A, Qiu S, Palnitkar S, et al. Osteomalacia with bone marrow fibrosis due to severe vitamin D deficiency after a gastrointestinal bypass operation for severe obesity. Endocr Pract 2009;15(6):528–33.
75. Annweiler C, Schott AM, Berrut G, et al. Vitamin D and ageing: neurological issues. Neuropsychobiology 2010;62(3):139–50.

76. Menant JC, Close JCT, Delbaere K, et al. Relationships between serum vitamin D levels, neuromuscular and neuropsychological function and falls in older men and women. Osteoporos Int 2012;23(3):981–9.
77. Garber AJ. Effects of parathyroid hormone on skeletal muscle protein and amino acid metabolism in the rat. J Clin Invest 1983;71(6):1806–21.
78. Stein MS, Wark JD, Scherer SC, et al. Falls relate to vitamin D and parathyroid hormone in an Australian nursing home and hostel. J Am Geriatr Soc 1999; 47(10):1195–201.
79. Campbell PM, Allain TJ. Muscle strength and vitamin D in older people. Gerontology 2006;52(6):335–8.
80. Institute of Medicine & Food and Nutrition Board Institute. Dietary reference intakes for calcium and vitamin D. Washington, DC: National Academies Press; 2011.
81. Holick M, Binkley N, Bischoff-Ferrari HA, et al. Evaluation, treatment, and prevention of vitamin D deficiency: an Endocrine Society clinical practice guideline. J Clin Endocrinol Metab 2011;96(7):1911–30.
82. American Geriatrics Society Workgroup on Vitamin D Supplementation for Older Adults. Recommendations abstracted from the American Geriatrics Society Consensus Statement on vitamin D for prevention of falls and their consequences. J Am Geriatr Soc 2014;62(1):147–52.
83. Bischoff-Ferrari HA, Dawson-Hughes B, Orva EJ, et al. Monthly high-dose vitamin D treatment for the prevention of functional decline: a randomized clinical trial. JAMA Intern Med 2016;176(2):175–83.
84. Girgis CM, Clifton-Bligh RJ, Turner N, et al. Effects of vitamin D in skeletal muscle: falls, strength, athletic performance and insulin sensitivity. Clin Endocrinol (Oxf) 2014;80(2):169–81.
85. Visser M, Deeg DJ, Puts MT, et al. Low serum concentrations of 25-hydroxyvitamin D in older persons and the risk of nursing home admission. Am J Clin Nutr 2006;84(3):616–22.
86. Thomas MK, Lloyd-Jones MD, Thadhadi RI, et al. Hypovitaminosis D in medical inpatients. N Engl J Med 1998;338(12):777–83.
87. Landi F, Liperoti R, Fusco D, et al. Prevalence and risk factors of sarcopenia among nursing home older residents. J Gerontol A Biol Sci Med Sci 2012;67(1):48–55.
88. Smit E, Crespo CJ, Michael Y, et al. The effect of vitamin D and frailty on mortality among non-institutionalized US older adults. Eur J Clin Nutr 2012;66(9):1024–8.
89. Lips P. Vitamin D deficiency and secondary hyperparathyroidism in the elderly: consequences for bone loss and fractures and therapeutic implications. Endocr Rev 2001;22(4):477–501.
90. Bischoff HA, Stahelin HB, Tyndall A, et al. Relationship between muscle strength and vitamin D metabolites: are there therapeutic possibilities in the elderly? Z Rheumatol 2000;59(Suppl 1):39–41.
91. Dawson-Hughes B. Serum 25-hydroxyvitamin D and muscle atrophy in the elderly. Proc Nutr Soc 2012;71(1):46–9.
92. Flicker L, MacInnis RJ, Stein MS, et al. Should older people in residential care receive vitamin D to prevent falls? Results of a randomized trial. J Am Geriatr Soc 2005;53(11):1881–8.
93. Law M, Withers H, Morris J, et al. Vitamin D supplementation and the prevention of fractures and falls: results of a randomized trial in elderly people in residential accommodation. Age Ageing 2006;35(5):482–6.
94. Cranney A, Horsley T, O'Donnell S, et al. Effectiveness and safety of vitamin D in relation to bone health. Evid Rep Technol Assess (Full Rep) 2007;(158):1–235.

Vitamin D Effect on Bone Mineral Density and Fractures

Ian R. Reid, MD, FRACP[a,b,*]

KEYWORDS

- Vitamin D • Osteoporosis • Osteomalacia • Calcium • Fracture • Bone density

KEY POINTS

- Vitamin D was identified as the cause and cure of osteomalacia.
- Vitamin D influences skeletal mineralization principally through the regulation of intestinal calcium absorption.
- Meta-analyses of vitamin D trials show no effects on bone density or fracture risk when the baseline 25-hydroxyvitamin D is greater than 40 nmol/L.
- Provision of vitamin D supplements to those at risk of 25-hydroxyvitamin D levels less than 40 nmol/L is supported by current evidence, but untargeted supplementation is not.
- A daily dose of 400 to 800 IU vitamin D_3 is usually adequate.

INTRODUCTION

Although the syndrome of rickets has been recognized for hundreds of years, the role of vitamin D in its genesis and treatment was only documented in the early twentieth century, when both sunlight exposure and cod liver oil supplements were found to be curative.[1] These discoveries suggested that vitamin D was good for bone, and it has been regarded by some as a skeletal tonic since that time. However, more recent investigations have demonstrated that this is an oversimplification, and that the primary role of the vitamin D endocrine system is to maintain normocalcemia and normophosphatemia, thus permitting normal skeletal mineralization. The principal way in which vitamin D does this is through regulation of intestinal absorption of these minerals.

Disclosure Statement: The author's research is supported by the Health Research Council of New Zealand (15/576).
[a] Department of Medicine, Faculty of Medical and Health Sciences, University of Auckland, Private Bag 92019, Auckland, New Zealand; [b] Department of Endocrinology, Auckland District Health Board, Auckland, New Zealand
* Faculty of Medical and Health Sciences, University of Auckland, Private Bag 92019, Auckland, New Zealand.
E-mail address: i.reid@auckland.ac.nz

The most striking abnormality in vitamin D receptor (VDR) knockout mice is the presence of osteomalacia.[2] This osteomalacia can be reversed either by provision of high intakes of calcium and phosphate sufficient to normalize serum concentrations[3] or by the selective expression of the VDR in enterocytes alone.[4,5] These findings are complemented by the demonstration that selective knockout of VDR in enterocytes reproduces the skeletal abnormalities seen in the systemic knockout.[6] Thus, enterocytic VDR expression is necessary and adequate to maintain normal skeletal mineralization.

VDR is expressed in bone, mainly in osteoblasts and osteocytes, where its main role is to stimulate bone resorption, consistent with the function of the vitamin D endocrine system in the maintenance of circulating calcium levels. VDR in osteoblastic cells does this by regulating RANKL and osteoprotegerin to promote osteoclastogenesis.[7,8] Selective knockout of VDR in bone results in increases in bone mass.[6,8,9] These findings are corroborated by a study in which femora from either wild-type or VDR knockout mice were transplanted into normal mice.[9] VDR-knockout bone in a wild-type environment had a 40% higher bone mineral density (BMD) than the wild-type bone in the same environment. Further corroboration comes from human studies showing that single large doses of vitamin D increase bone resorption markers,[10–12] that vitamin D intoxication is associated with sustained increases in bone resorption,[13] and that correction of vitamin D intoxication is associated with increases in BMD.[14] A second direct effect of vitamin D on bone is to increase local pyrophosphate levels resulting in inhibition of mineralization.[6] This vitamin D effect is also consistent with vitamin D being a procalcemic factor rather than a direct stimulator of bone growth and mineralization, as many clinicians have tended to regard it. The finding that high levels of vitamin D or its metabolites can increase bone resorption and impair mineralization suggests that incautious use of vitamin D or its metabolites could adversely affect bone, and there are studies of high-dose calciferol or vitamin D metabolites that show increased bone loss[15] or fractures.[16,17]

WHAT IS VITAMIN D DEFICIENCY?

Profound loss of vitamin D signaling results in hypocalcemia and osteomalacia. Partial loss of signaling (eg, from vitamin D deficiency) stimulates parathyroid hormone (PTH) secretion leading to increased bone resorption and increased renal retention of calcium, but with maintenance of serum calcium levels within the normal range. In this situation, bone mineralization is maintained, but at the expense of bone mass. Preventing such secondary hyperparathyroidism is the principal rationale for using vitamin D in the management of osteoporosis. Interestingly, many individuals with markedly reduced levels of 25-hydroxyvitamin D (eg, <25 nmol/L) do not develop secondary hyperparathyroidism,[18,19] for reasons that are unclear. Arabi and colleagues[20] have demonstrated that accelerated loss of BMD is only observed in vitamin D–deficient older adults who also have secondary hyperparathyroidism, and Sayed-Hassan and colleagues[19] report that BMD is not related to 25-hydroxyvitamin D in a D-deficient cohort, but is related to PTH. Similarly, in a bone biopsy study of sudden death subjects, at serum 25OHD levels less than 12 ng/mL (30 nmol/L), more than half of the population studied failed to demonstrate osteoid accumulation, indicating that factors other than low 25OHD contribute to osteomalacia.[21] Thus, many individuals do not appear to suffer adverse effects from levels of 25-hydroxyvitamin D that are associated with bone loss or undermineralization in others. Whether this is related to their diet (eg, intake of calcium or of calcium binders such as phytates) or to other factors (such as the efficiency of renal calcium conservation) is unclear. This variability between individuals may contribute to the variability seen in the outcomes of trials of vitamin D as an intervention.

Cross-sectional data can be used to identify levels of 25-hydroxyvitamin D that are associated with adverse clinical outcomes or with surrogates thought to be associated with such outcomes. In a study of older adults, Need and colleagues[22] found that circulating 25(OH)D levels less than 15 nmol/L were associated with lower 1,25(OH)$_2$D and reduced intestinal calcium absorption, and with higher serum alkaline phosphatase activity. Using a similar cross-sectional approach, Lips and van Schoor[23] found that 25(OH)D and PTH were inversely related over a wide range of values, but with a steeper increase in PTH levels once 25(OH)D was less than 50 nmol/L. However, the 25-hydroxyvitamin D threshold for an increase in bone turnover markers was about 30 nmol/L. Sai and colleagues[24] found a similar dissociation of the relationships of 25(OH)D with PTH and with bone turnover markers. These findings suggest a window between 30 and 50 nmol/L within which PTH compensates for low vitamin D levels (eg, by increasing both 1,25-hydroxyvitamin D production and renal tubular reabsorption of calcium) without increasing bone resorption. Thus, both the Need and the Lips studies suggest that adverse biochemical consequences of vitamin D deficiency arise when 25-hydroxyvitamin D is in the region of 15 to 30 nmol/L.

The most convincing way to identify the threshold for vitamin D deficiency is to use clinical trials to determine at what baseline 25-hydroxyvitamin D level beneficial effects become evident. Two studies with mean baseline 25-hydroxyvitamin D levels of 34[25] and 40[26] nmol/L, respectively, have shown no increase in intestinal calcium absorption following vitamin D supplementation, suggesting that the threshold for deficiency is lower than this. Two trials have indicated that vitamin D supplements reduce PTH levels when baseline 25-hydroxyvitamin D is less than 50 nmol/L, but not when it is above this level.[27,28] The more marked the D deficiency, the greater the PTH change after supplementation.[27] Similar threshold data are needed for trials assessing vitamin D effects on BMD and fracture.

EFFECTS ON BONE MINERAL DENSITY

Some trials assessing the effects of vitamin D on bone administer vitamin D alone as the intervention, and others use a combined intervention of calcium plus vitamin D. Because calcium is biologically active, these 2 groups of trials must be considered separately in order to determine whether effects are attributable to calcium, vitamin D, or to their combination.

Vitamin D Monotherapy

In 2014, the author published a systematic review of trials assessing the effects of vitamin D supplementation alone on BMD in adults.[29] The study identified data from 23 trials, details of which are shown in **Table 1**. These trials had a mean duration of 23.5 months and involved 4082 participants, 92% women, with an average age of 59 years. In these studies, BMD was measured at between 1 and 5 skeletal sites, so 70 tests of statistical significance were carried out across the studies. Six of these found significant benefit; 2 found significant detriment, and the rest were nonsignificant. Only one study showed significant benefit at more than one measurement site, both of which were in the femur.

When the trial results were meta-analyzed (**Fig. 1**), there was no significant effect in the lumbar spine, there were nonsignificant negative effects in the total body and forearm, but in the femoral neck there was a positive treatment effect of 0.8% (95% confidence interval 0.2% to 1.4%, $P = .005$). The femoral neck data showed evidence of heterogeneity among the trials and also of publication bias. When the trials were grouped by mean baseline 25-hydroxyvitamin D (**Fig. 2**), those with starting

Table 1
Randomized controlled trials of vitamin D on bone mineral density in adults not included in Fig. 1

Study	t (m)	N	Mean Age (Range)	Baseline 25OHD (nmol/L)	Spine	Total Hip	Femoral Neck	Forearm	Total Body
Iuliano-Burns et al,[33] 2012	12	110	41 (24–65)	60	NS	NS	NS	...	...
Wamberg et al,[31] 2013	6	52	40 (18–50)	35	NS	NS	NS	+/NS[a]	NS
Macdonald et al,[30] 2013	12	305	(60–70)	34	NS	+/NS[b]	...	...	...
Hansen et al,[32] 2015	12	230	61 (PM and <75)	52	NS	NS	+	...	NS

BMD results are shown in the right-hand columns.

Abbreviations: N, number of participants randomized; NS, no significant effect at that skeletal site in that study; PM, postmenopausal (>5 y since last period); t, trial duration in months; +, a positive effect of vitamin D.

[a] Significant effect at ultradistal forearm, but not in total forearm.
[b] Benefit in 1000 IU/d group, not in 400 IU/d group.

levels less than 50 nmol/L showed a significant increase in femoral neck BMD, whereas those above did not. Treatment effects also differed by vitamin D dose: a supplement of less than 800 units per day was associated with significant increases in both lumbar spine and femoral neck BMD (0·4% [0·0–0·8] and 1·4% [0·4–2·4], respectively) but higher doses were not (−0·1% [−0·4–0·2] and 0·3% [−0·2–0·8]). Trial duration did not impact the between-groups differences, suggesting that if there is a benefit it does not cumulate over time. The coadministration of calcium to both groups in a study tended to reduce the treatment effect, consistent with

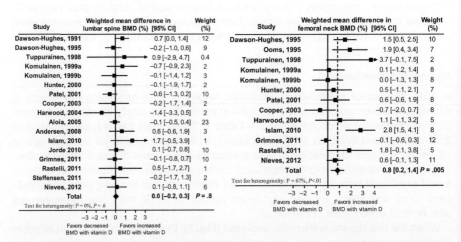

Fig. 1. Meta-analyses of the effects of vitamin D supplementation on BMD at the lumbar spine and femoral neck. Data are weighted mean differences in BMD between the vitamin D and control groups in each study. CI, confidence interval. (*From* Reid IR, Bolland MJ, Grey A. Effects of vitamin D supplements on bone mineral density: a systematic review and meta-analysis. Lancet 2014;383:149; with permission.)

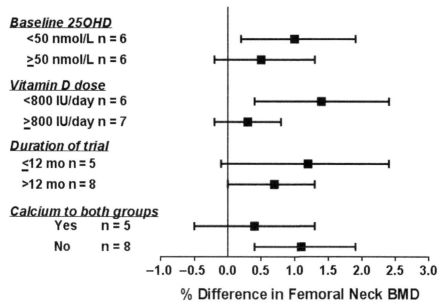

Fig. 2. Meta-analysis of vitamin D effects on femoral neck BMD in subgroups of trials classified by trial characteristics. Vitamin D effects tended to be greater in studies where participants had lower baseline 25-hydroxyvitamin D (25OHD), were given smaller vitamin D doses, and were not given calcium. (*Data from* Reid IR, Bolland MJ, Grey A. Effects of vitamin D supplements on bone mineral density: a systematic review and meta-analysis. Lancet 2014;383:151.)

other evidence that a higher calcium intake can partially compensate for low vitamin D levels.

Since that meta-analysis, 4 further trials have been published, and these are shown in **Table 1**. Their results are broadly consistent with those of the meta-analysis. Thus, a study of Scottish postmenopausal women randomized to vitamin D 1000 IU/d, vitamin D 400 IU/d, or placebo over 1 year showed a 0.5% difference in BMD at the total hip with the higher dose, but nothing at the spine.[30] A 6-month Danish study of 52 obese adults found no effect of vitamin D 7000 IU/d on BMD of the hip, spine, or total body, but a benefit at one forearm site.[31] An American study of postmenopausal women with baseline 25-hydroxyvitamin D greater than 35 nmol/L found no effect of either 800 IU/d or 50,000 IU twice a month on spine, total hip, or total body BMD, although there was an effect at the femoral neck that was no longer significant after correcting for multiple statistical testing.[32] The fourth study was carried out in 110 healthy adults in Antarctica and had uniformly negative results.[33]

The suggestion from the meta-analysis that baseline 25-hydroxyvitamin D influences trial outcome is borne out by examination of the individual trials in **Table 1**. With 2 exceptions, significant benefit at any skeletal site was only seen in trials where the mean baseline 25(OH)D was in the range 25 to 40 nmol/L. The exceptions are the 2 Dawson-Hughes studies, which were carried out in sequence in the same cohort of women who had dietary calcium intakes of less than 400 mg/ d. It appears that the 25-hydroxyvitamin D assays used were poorly calibrated,[34] substantially overestimating baseline analyte concentrations. Thus, there is a consistent body of evidence from these 27 trials involving 4779 participants that vitamin D supplements do not influence BMD when baseline levels are greater than 40 nmol/L, and the author has recently completed a further large study that is consistent with this.[35] A daily dose of 400 to 800 IU vitamin D_3 is usually adequate to correct such deficiency.[36]

Vitamin D Plus Calcium

Unlike vitamin D supplements, calcium given as a supplement or as part of a modified diet does consistently increase BMD, by about 1%.[37] This change is detectable at 1 year and does not increase with longer-term supplement use.[37] A recent comprehensive meta-analysis of calcium trials, either as a monotherapy or together with vitamin D, showed no further benefit to BMD from the addition of vitamin D to a calcium supplement.[37] Thus, at 1 year, calcium alone produced a benefit to spine BMD of 1.3 (0.8–1.7)% compared with placebo (21 trials) and calcium plus vitamin D (7 trials) produced a benefit of 1.1 (0.2–2.1)% (between groups comparison, $P = .81$). Results were similar at the femoral neck ($P = .86$). Therefore, it is very important not to simply pool studies of vitamin D alone with those of calcium plus vitamin D, just as one would not pool data from any other pharmaceuticals and attribute effects caused by one to the other. The absence of any additional benefit from adding vitamin D to calcium is completely consistent with the evidence reviewed herein indicating that vitamin D alone does not impact on BMD.

EFFECTS ON FRACTURE

As for BMD, interpretation of trials of fracture prevention is complicated by coadministration of calcium in many cases. Therefore, these 2 interventions are considered separately.

Vitamin D Monotherapy

These studies have recently been systematically reviewed and meta-analyzed by Bolland and colleagues.[38] In trials involving greater than 28,000 participants, there were no demonstrable benefits in terms of either total fracture (relative risk 0·97 [0·88–1·08]) or hip fracture (relative risk 1·11 [0·97–1·27]; **Fig. 3**). Using the novel technique of trial sequential analysis, Bolland demonstrated that the available trials provide a sufficiently large cohort to rule out a clinically significant benefit from vitamin D in the prevention of these fracture types. Thus, further studies of this intervention in comparable populations are most unlikely to produce a significant change in the meta-analytic outcome, so investment in such studies is not justifiable.

The findings of the Bolland meta-analysis are completely consistent with the results of the DIPART individual patient meta-analysis.[39] In 3 trials involving a total of 14,024 participants, there was no effect of vitamin D alone on either total fracture numbers (hazard ratio 1.01 [0.92–1.12]) or on hip fractures (hazard ratio 1.09 [0.92–1.29]). When they pooled these findings with trial level data from 4 other studies, the combined hazard ratio for hip fracture was 1.11 (0.96–1.29). The recent *Cochrane Review* agrees with these findings, concluding that "there is high quality evidence that vitamin D alone … is unlikely to be effective in preventing hip fracture (11 trials, 27,693 participants; risk ratio 1.12 [0.98–1.29]) or any new fracture (15 trials, 28,271 participants; risk ratio 1.03 [0.96–1.11])."[40]

There are 2 trials that merit specific mention in that they each showed statistically significant *increases* in fractures, either in the hip[41] or for total fractures.[16] Each study used annual administration of a high-dose supplement, so many investigators have since concluded that infrequent bolus dosing is unsafe. Interestingly, the Sanders

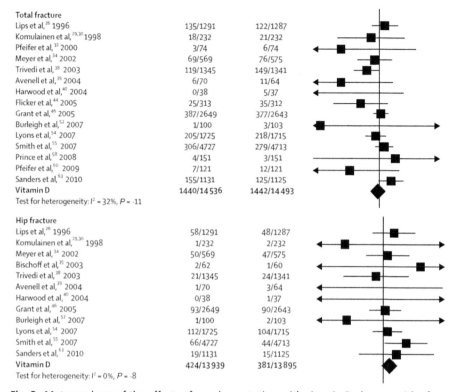

Fig. 3. Meta-analyses of the effects of supplementation with vitamin D alone on risk of any fracture or of hip fracture. The meta-analytic relative risks were 0·97 (0·88–1·08) for any fracture and 1·11 (0·97–1·27) for hip fracture. (*From* Bolland MJ, Grey A, Gamble GD, et al. The effect of vitamin D supplementation on skeletal, vascular, or cancer outcomes: a trial sequential meta-analysis. Lancet Diabetes Endocrinol 2014;2:313; with permission.)

study also showed an increase in falls in those receiving this vitamin D regimen, an adverse effect that has also been observed with high doses of vitamin D given monthly[42] or daily.[43] These findings emphasize that hypercalcemia is not the only potential toxicity from vitamin D supplements, and the falls data suggest that it is not dose frequency that creates the risk but the absolute levels of 25-hydroxyvitamin D that are achieved.

Vitamin D Plus Calcium

In the Bolland meta-analysis referred to in the previous section,[38] randomization to vitamin D plus calcium reduced total fracture (relative risk 0·92 [0·85–0·99]) and hip fracture (relative risk 0·84 [0·74–0·96]). DIPART and Cochrane have also found that vitamin D with calcium reduces both total fractures and hip fractures by similar amounts. The marked difference between these findings and those with vitamin D alone suggests that it is the calcium supplement that is critical to these benefits, or the characteristics of those trials using the combination.

The key role of calcium is supported by consideration of a complementary group of meta-analyses that assess the antifracture efficacy of calcium alone and of calcium plus vitamin D. Both Bolland and colleagues[44] and Tang and colleagues[45] found no evidence that trials of calcium plus vitamin D produced more positive effects on total fractures than those of calcium alone, suggesting that vitamin D supplements do not affect total fracture risk whether or not calcium supplements are used. For hip fracture, however, calcium alone (relative risk 1.51 [0.93–2.48]) and calcium plus vitamin D (relative risk 0.84 [0.74–0.96]) appear to have very different effects (P = .02).[44] This difference appears to be substantially attributable to the impact of the study of Chapuy and colleagues,[46] which was carried out in institutionalized, frail, elderly women with severe vitamin D deficiency; serum 25-hydroxyvitamin D levels in the placebo group during the study were about 14 nmol/L (after correction for errors in assay calibration[34]). Thus, many of these trial participants probably had osteomalacia, and it is therefore inappropriate to pool that study with others that assessed supplements in individuals with much higher baseline 25-hydroxyvitamin D levels. The likelihood that these women had osteomalacia is supported by the finding of a 7% increase in total hip BMD in the Chapuy study, a change much greater than is seen with any osteoporosis treatment, but quite consistent with the increases reported after treatment of osteomalacia (eg, +16% at the hip and +51% at the spine[47]). Parenthetically, it should be noted that antifracture efficacy of calcium with or without vitamin D has not been seen in the large trials published in the last decade, and the finding depends on older studies of less rigorous design.[44]

In contrast to these findings, an analysis by Bischoff-Ferrari and colleagues[48] concluded that "high-dose vitamin D supplementation (≥800 IU daily) was somewhat favorable in the prevention of hip fracture and any nonvertebral fracture in persons 65 years of age or older." This analysis used participant-level data from 11 trials of oral vitamin D supplementation with or without calcium and compared quartiles of actual intake of vitamin D in the treatment groups (including each participant's adherence to the treatment and supplement use outside the study protocol) with data from the control groups. Fracture prevention was found in participants identified as having vitamin D intakes greater than 800 IU/d, who were the more adherent subjects in the vitamin D groups and those self-administering supplements. Both medication adherence and supplement use have been shown previously to be associated with better health outcomes, so to select for these characteristics in the treatment group but not in the placebo group destroys the baseline comparability of these groups established by randomization. Thus, the analysis effectively produces a cohort study and is subject to all the biases that that design entails. A detailed critique of this study has been published elsewhere.[49]

FUTURE CONSIDERATIONS/SUMMARY

It is frequently stated that the role of vitamin D in managing bone conditions, particularly osteoporosis, is controversial and that the evidence is conflicting. Most of these conflicts in the clinical trial data can be resolved if the outcomes are interpreted in the light of the trial participants' baseline 25-hydroxyvitamin D. Thus, in the recent large studies in which vitamin D (with or without calcium) has been administered, positive effects on BMD or fracture rates have not been observed. In contrast, these interventions in the Chapuy trial, where baseline 25-hydroxyvitamin D levels were less than 25 nmol/L, had substantial beneficial effects on both BMD and fracture. Vitamin D was discovered a century ago as the factor that could cure osteomalacia, and that remains its principal therapeutic role. Treatment of the secondary hyperparathyroidism that is associated with incipient osteomalacia may also be of benefit, at least in terms of rates of bone loss. In humans, vitamin D is not a simple tonic for bone, which will progressively increase bone density and reduce fracture risk whatever the prevailing vitamin D status.

It is time to move past the simplistic concept that vitamin D (and calcium) is good for bone and that the more we provide the better. Both are substrates: vitamin D for a regulatory endocrine system and calcium for the mineralization of the skeleton. Their status as substrates implies that there is a minimum requirement for each, but once this is met and optimal circulating concentrations of minerals are achieved, then homeostatic regulation ensures that surplus vitamin D and calcium are disposed of to prevent extraskeletal calcification. There are specific regulatory systems to prevent soft tissue calcification, but overenthusiastic use of supplements runs the risk of overwhelming these defenses and producing adverse outcomes.

The key research agenda moving forward is to define more precisely the level of 25-hydroxyvitamin D at which adverse skeletal effects on the skeleton become apparent, and to determine whether levels optimal for bone are also optimal for extraskeletal tissues. These data will determine who is vitamin D deficient and likely to benefit from supplementation, and the form such supplementation should take.

REFERENCES

1. DeLuca HF. History of the discovery of vitamin D and its active metabolites. Bonekey Rep 2014;3:479.
2. Bouillon R, Carmeliet G, Verlinden L, et al. Vitamin D and human health: lessons from vitamin D receptor null mice. Endocr Rev 2008;29:726–76.
3. Masuyama R, Nakaya Y, Katsumata S, et al. Dietary calcium and phosphorus ratio regulates bone mineralization and turnover in vitamin D receptor knockout mice by affecting intestinal calcium and phosphorus absorption. J Bone Miner Res 2003;18:1217–26.
4. Marks HD, Fleet JC, Peleg S. Transgenic expression of the human vitamin D receptor (hVDR) in the duodenum of VDR-null mice attenuates the age-dependent decline in calcium absorption. J Steroid Biochem Mol Biol 2007;103:513–6.
5. Xue Y, Fleet JC. Intestinal vitamin D receptor is required for normal calcium and bone metabolism in mice. Gastroenterology 2009;136:1317–27.
6. Lieben L, Masuyama R, Torrekens S, et al. Normocalcemia is maintained in mice under conditions of calcium malabsorption by vitamin D-induced inhibition of bone mineralization. J Clin Invest 2012;122:1803–15.
7. Haussler MR, Haussler CA, Whitfield GK, et al. The nuclear vitamin D receptor controls the expression of genes encoding factors which feed the "Fountain of Youth" to mediate healthful aging. J Steroid Biochem Mol Biol 2010;121:88–97.
8. Yamamoto Y, Yoshizawa T, Fukuda T, et al. Vitamin D receptor in osteoblasts is a negative regulator of bone mass control. Endocrinology 2013;154:1008–20.
9. Tanaka H, Seino Y. Direct action of 1,25-dihydroxyvitamin D on bone: VDRKO bone shows excessive bone formation in normal mineral condition. J Steroid Biochem Mol Biol 2004;89–90:343–5.
10. Rossini M, Gatti D, Viapiana O, et al. Short-term effects on bone turnover markers of a single high dose of oral vitamin D3. J Clin Endocrinol Metab 2012;97:E622–6.
11. Sanders KM, Nicholson GC, Ebeling PR. Is high dose vitamin D harmful? Calcif Tissue Int 2013;92:191–206.
12. Rossini M, Adami S, Viapiana O, et al. Dose-dependent short-term effects of single high doses of oral vitamin D3 on bone turnover markers. Calcif Tissue Int 2012;91:365–9.

13. Selby PL, Davies M, Marks JS, et al. Vitamin D intoxication causes hypercalcaemia by increased bone resorption which responds to pamidronate. Clin Endocrinol 1995;43:531–6.
14. Adams JS, Lee G. Gains in bone mineral density with resolution of vitamin d intoxication. Ann Intern Med 1997;127:203–6.
15. Ott SM, Chesnut CH. Calcitriol treatment is not effective in postmenopausal osteoporosis. Ann Intern Med 1989;110:267–74.
16. Sanders KM, Stuart AL, Williamson EJ, et al. Annual high-dose oral vitamin D and falls and fractures in older women: a randomized controlled trial. JAMA 2010;303:1815–22.
17. Ebeling PR, Wark JD, Yeung S, et al. Effects of calcitriol or calcium on bone mineral density, bone turnover, and fractures in men with primary osteoporosis: a two-year randomized, double blind, double placebo study. J Clin Endocrinol Metab 2001;86:4098–103.
18. Isaia G, Giorgino R, Rini GB, et al. Prevalence of hypovitaminosis D in elderly women in Italy: clinical consequences and risk factors. Osteoporos Int 2003;14:577–82.
19. Sayed-Hassan R, Abazid N, Koudsi A, et al. Vitamin D status and parathyroid hormone levels in relation to bone mineral density in apparently healthy Syrian adults. Arch Osteoporos 2016;11:18.
20. Arabi A, Baddoura R, El-Rassi R, et al. PTH level but not 25 (OH) vitamin D level predicts bone loss rates in the elderly. Osteoporos Int 2012;23:971–80.
21. Priemel M, von Domarus C, Klatte TO, et al. Bone mineralization defects and vitamin D deficiency: histomorphometric analysis of iliac crest bone biopsies and circulating 25-hydroxyvitamin D in 675 patients. J Bone Miner Res 2010;25:305–12.
22. Need AG, O'Loughlin PD, Morris HA, et al. Vitamin D metabolites and calcium absorption in severe vitamin D deficiency. J Bone Miner Res 2008;23:1859–63.
23. Lips P, van Schoor NM. The effect of vitamin D on bone and osteoporosis. Best Pract Res Clin Endocrinol Metab 2011;25:585–91.
24. Sai AJ, Walters RW, Fang X, et al. Relationship between vitamin D, parathyroid hormone, and bone health. J Clin Endocrinol Metab 2011;96:E436–46.
25. Gallagher CJ, Jindal PS, Lynette MS. Vitamin D does not increase calcium absorption in young women: a randomized clinical trial. J Bone Miner Res 2014;29(5):1081–7.
26. Gallagher JC, Yalamanchili V, Smith LM. The effect of vitamin D on calcium absorption in older women. J Clin Endocrinol Metab 2012;97:3550–6.
27. Bacon CJ, Gamble GD, Horne AM, et al. High-dose oral vitamin D3 supplementation in the elderly. Osteoporos Int 2009;20:1407–15.
28. Malabanan A, Veronikis IE, Holick MF. Redefining vitamin D insufficiency. Lancet 1998;351:805–6.
29. Reid IR, Bolland MJ, Grey A. Effects of vitamin D supplements on bone mineral density: a systematic review and meta-analysis. Lancet 2014;383:146–55.
30. Macdonald HM, Wood AD, Aucott LS, et al. Hip bone loss is attenuated with 1000 IU but not 400 IU daily vitamin D3: a 1-year double-blind RCT in postmenopausal women. J Bone Miner Res 2013;28:2202–13.
31. Wamberg L, Pedersen SB, Richelsen B, et al. The effect of high-dose vitamin D supplementation on calciotropic hormones and bone mineral density in obese subjects with low levels of circulating 25-hydroxyvitamin D: results from a randomized controlled study. Calcif Tissue Int 2013;93:69–77.

32. Hansen KE, Johnson RE, Chambers KR, et al. Treatment of vitamin D insufficiency in postmenopausal women: a randomized clinical trial. JAMA Intern Med 2015; 175:1612–21.

33. Iuliano-Burns S, Ayton J, Hillam S, et al. Skeletal and hormonal responses to vitamin D supplementation during sunlight deprivation in Antarctic expeditioners. Osteoporos Int 2012;23:2461–7.

34. Lips P, Chapuy MC, Dawson-Hughes B, et al. An international comparison of serum 25-hydroxyvitamin D measurements. Osteoporos Int 1999;9:394–7.

35. Reid IR, Horne A, Mihov B, et al. Effect of monthly high-dose vitamin D on bone density in community-dwelling older adults sub-study of a randomized controlled trial. J Int Med, in press.

36. Gallagher JC, Sai A, Templin T, et al. Dose response to vitamin D supplementation in postmenopausal women a randomized trial. Ann Intern Med 2012;156:425–37.

37. Tai V, Leung W, Grey A, et al. Calcium intake and bone mineral density: systematic review and meta-analysis. BMJ 2015;351:h4183.

38. Bolland MJ, Grey A, Gamble GD, et al. The effect of vitamin D supplementation on skeletal, vascular, or cancer outcomes: a trial sequential meta-analysis. Lancet Diabetes Endocrinol 2014;2:307–20.

39. Abrahamsen B, Masud T, Avenell A, et al. Patient level pooled analysis of 68 500 patients from seven major vitamin D fracture trials in US and Europe. BMJ 2010; 340:B5463.

40. Avenell A, Mak JCS, O'Connell D. Vitamin D and vitamin D analogues for preventing fractures in post-menopausal women and older men. Cochrane Database Syst Rev 2014;(4):CD000227.

41. Smith H, Anderson F, Raphael H, et al. Effect of annual intramuscular vitamin D on fracture risk in elderly men and women. A population-based, randomized, double-blind, placebo-controlled trial. Rheumatology 2007;46:1852–7.

42. Bischoff-Ferrari HA, Dawson-Hughes B, John Orav E, et al. Monthly high-dose vitamin D treatment for the prevention of functional decline a randomized clinical trial. JAMA Intern Med 2016;176:175–83.

43. Smith LM, Gallagher JC, Suiter C. Medium doses of vitamin D decrease falls and higher doses of daily vitamin D3 increase falls: a randomized clinical trial. J Steroid Biochem Mol Bio 2017;173:317–22.

44. Bolland MJ, Leung W, Tai V, et al. Calcium intake and risk of fracture: systematic review. BMJ 2015;351:h4580.

45. Tang BMP, Eslick GD, Nowson C, et al. Use of calcium or calcium in combination with vitamin D supplementation to prevent fractures and bone loss in people aged 50 years and older: a meta-analysis. Lancet 2007;370:657–66.

46. Chapuy MC, Arlot ME, Duboeuf F, et al. Vitamin D3 and calcium to prevent hip fractures in the elderly women. N Engl J Med 1992;327:1637–42.

47. El-Desouki MI, Othman SM, Fouda MA. Bone mineral density and bone scintigraphy in adult Saudi female patients with osteomalacia. Saudi Med J 2004;25: 355–8.

48. Bischoff-Ferrari HA, Willett WC, Orav EJ, et al. A pooled analysis of vitamin D dose requirements for fracture prevention. N Engl J Med 2012;367:40–9.

49. Abrahamsen B, Avenell A, Bolland M, et al. A pooled analysis of vitamin D dose requirements for fracture prevention. IBMS BoneKEy 2013;10. http://dx.doi.org/10.1038/bonekey.2012.1256.

Vitamin D Metabolism in Bariatric Surgery

Marlene Chakhtoura, MD, MSc*, Maya Rahme, MSc, Ghada El-Hajj Fuleihan, MD, MPH

KEYWORDS

- Vitamin D • Obesity • Bariatric surgery • RYGB • SG • Guidelines

KEY POINTS

- Vitamin D deficiency is common before and after bariatric surgery, and is more severe after roux-en-Y gastric bypass than after sleeve gastrectomy, because of decreased vitamin D absorption.
- The increase in serum 25-hydroxyvitamin D [25(OH)D] level (ng/100 IU) after vitamin D seems dose dependent and decreases at high doses.
- Based on limited evidence, vitamin D replacement doses of 3000 IU/d to 50,000 IU 1 to 3 times per week are recommended by various organizations.
- Dose-ranging randomized trials according to the type of surgery will help define the recommended daily allowance for vitamin D to achieve a serum 25(OH)D level greater than 20 ng/mL.
- The desirable 25(OH)D level to optimize musculoskeletal health in the bariatric population is unknown.

BACKGROUND

Obesity, defined as a body mass index (BMI) greater than or equal to 30 kg/m², is a major risk factor for cancer and noncommunicable diseases, and is associated with a 50% to 100% increase risk of premature death. The World Health Organization (WHO) projected that, by 2015, around 2.3 billion adults will be overweight (BMI ≥25 kg/m²) and more than 700 million will be obese.[1] The US Centers for Disease Control and Prevention (CDC) estimates that 78 million Americans are obese,[2] and 24 million are severely or morbidly obese.[3] The prevalence of obesity in the United States tripled between 1960 and 2010,[4] and is still steadily increasing. The National Health

Disclosure: The authors have nothing to disclose.

Department of Internal Medicine, Division of Endocrinology, Calcium Metabolism and Osteoporosis Program, WHO Collaborating Center for Metabolic Bone Disorders, American University of Beirut Medical Center, Riad El Solh, Beirut, Lebanon

* Corresponding author. Calcium Metabolism and Osteoporosis Program, WHO Collaborating Center for Metabolic Bone Disorders, American University of Beirut Medical Center, PO Box: 113-6044/C8, Beirut, Lebanon.

E-mail address: mc39@aub.edu.lb

Endocrinol Metab Clin N Am 46 (2017) 947–982
http://dx.doi.org/10.1016/j.ecl.2017.07.006
0889-8529/17/© 2017 Elsevier Inc. All rights reserved.

endo.theclinics.com

and Nutrition Examination Survey (NHANES) study revealed that one-third of Americans adults were obese, 35.7% in 2009 to 2010, and 36.5% in 2011 to 2014.[5,6] This epidemic has not spared the youth. One-third of children and adolescents aged 6 to 19 years are considered overweight or obese, and more than 1 in 6 are obese.[7]

Hypovitaminosis D is prevalent worldwide, and across all age groups.[8–13] Skin is the major source of vitamin D and its synthesis requires ultraviolet B (UVB) rays, but small amounts (100–200 IU) are obtained from the diet.[13] Serum 25-hydroxyvitamin D [25(OH)D] concentration is the preferred indicator of vitamin D nutritional status, because of its fat solubility and long half-life. Obesity is a major risk factor for low 25(OH)D levels.[13–17] This association was also established in a meta-analysis of 23 studies, in adults/elderly as well as children and adolescents, and was independent of latitude, vitamin D cutoffs used, and human development index of the study location.[18] The cause for this association is not clear, but may in part be explained by decreased outdoor activities and poor dietary habits.[17–19] Other possibilities include decreased skin synthesis in response to a given UVB dose, decreased ability of the skin to release vitamin D into the circulation, alterations in the synthetic pathway in the liver from nonalcoholic fatty liver disease (NAFLD), enhanced degradation of 25(OH)D caused by increased cytochrome P (CYP) 24A1 activity, decreased synthesis of 1,25-dihydroxyvitamin D [1,25(OH)$_2$ D] caused by altered 1-alpha hydroxylase activity and negative feedback caused by increased parathyroid hormone (PTH) and calcitriol levels.[17,20] In addition, dilution caused by large body size, and decreased bioavailability and/or sequestration of 25(OH)D in fat, both visceral and subcutaneous, have been proposed.[14,16,17,21,22] This possibility was further examined in a study that directly measured vitamin D content in various adipose tissue compartments in 27 obese and 26 control subjects. Vitamin D total body stores were higher in the obese group, and serum 25(OH)D level was directly related to adipose tissue in both study groups.[16] However, the 2 groups did not differ in visceral or subcutaneous vitamin D stores, and the comparable mean serum 25(OH)D levels at entry were a major study limitation.[16]

Diet therapy and medical management have limited success in the treatment of morbid obesity, and bariatric surgery, therefore, prevails as the only effective long-term treatment option for weight reduction.[23] It results in substantial improvements or complete remission of associated comorbidities and reduced mortality.[24–26] A meta-analysis that included 22,904 patients showed that bariatric surgery resulted in a mean weight loss of 61%, with substantial improvement in diabetes, hyperlipidemia, hypertension, and obstructive sleep apnea,[27] and a reduction in the risk of premature death by 30% to 40%.[28,29] The Swedish Obese Subjects trial showed prevention of incident diabetes and cardiovascular events, and reduced mortality, on long-term follow-up.[28,30]

The estimated number of bariatric surgery procedures in the United States has increased from 158,000 in 2011 to 196,000 in 2015.[31] Although roux-en-Y gastric bypass (RYGB) was the commonest procedure worldwide,[32] it is fast being replaced by sleeve gastrectomy (SG) because of a good efficacy and a lower complication rate. Gastric banding (GB) is the least effective, with inferior efficacy that further decreases on long-term follow-up. To-date, these procedures are almost exclusively performed through a laparoscopic approach, and the most recent estimates from the American Society of Metabolic and Bariatric Surgery (ASMBS) reveal that 54% of these procedures are laparoscopic SG, 23% are laparoscopic RYGB, 14% are revisions, and 6.7% are laparoscopic GB.[33] Although GB (**Fig. 1**C) is a purely restrictive procedure that reduces the amount of food (thus energy consumed), SG (see **Fig. 1**A) and RYGB (see **Fig. 1**B) have additional components incurred from alterations in the secretion of gut

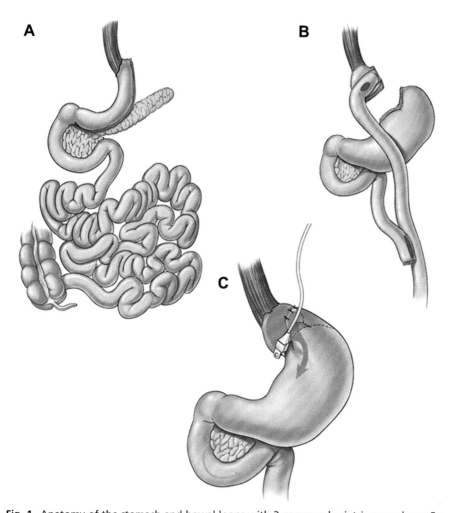

Fig. 1. Anatomy of the stomach and bowel loops with 3 common bariatric procedures. For additional details regarding the procedures please see the Web site of the American Society of Metabolic and Bariatric Surgery page https://asmbs.org/patients/bariatric-surgery-procedures. Reprinted with permission, Cleveland Clinic Center for Medical Art & Photography © 2006 to 2017 All rights reserved. (*A*) SG: more than three-quarters of the stomach are removed, and the remaining tubular pouch holds a considerably smaller volume, and thus less food and fewer calories are consumed, compared with the normal stomach. The greater impact on weight loss seems to be the effect this surgery has on gut hormones that affect hunger, satiety, and glycemic control. (*B*) RYGB: a small stomach pouch, approximately 30 mL (1 fluid ounce), is created by dividing the top of the stomach from the rest of the stomach, the bottom end of the divided small intestine is brought up and connected to this pouch, and its top portion is connected further down the intestine, to allow the bypassed stomach acids and digestive enzymes to eventually mix with the food. The mechanism of action for weight loss is similar to SG and in addition results from a malabsorptive element resulting from the bypassed small intestine (75–150 cm). (*C*) GB: an inflatable band is placed around the upper portion of the stomach, creating a small stomach pouch above the band, and the rest of the stomach below the band. The feeling of fullness depends on the size of the opening between the pouch and the remainder of the stomach. The size of the opening is adjustable by filling the band with sterile saline, injected through a port placed under the skin.

and satiety hormones. RYGB also bypasses large portions (75–150 cm) of the small intestine, causing delays and reduction in the timing allowed for the mixing of food with gastric and pancreatic juices, and thus further reductions in energy absorption. This anatomic change is also seen in SG with duodenal switch and biliopancreatic diversion, procedures that cause the most malabsorption.[32,34–36]

Despite its substantial advantages, bariatric surgery is accompanied by several complications, such as leaks (0.5%), bleeds (1%), pulmonary embolism (0.5%), strictures (3%–4%),[37] and deficiencies in various macronutrients and micronutrients, including water-soluble nutrients and the fat-soluble vitamins A and D, iron, vitamin B_{12}, and folate in 20% to 50% of patients.[36,38–41] Vitamin D plays a key role in mineral and musculoskeletal metabolism across the lifecycle.[13,42–45] In obese patients undergoing bariatric surgery, vitamin D is also implicated in bone and mineral metabolism.[32,35,46,47]

This article reviews studies describing vitamin D nutritional status before and after surgery, vitamin D replacement (including observational studies and randomized trials), and vitamin D guidelines issued by several organizations, in adult patients undergoing bariatric surgery. Studies that investigate the impact of vitamin D on skeletal and nonskeletal outcomes in patients undergoing bariatric surgery are beyond the scope of this article, and therefore are only briefly discussed.

SEARCH METHODOLOGY
Vitamin D Randomized Controlled Trials in Bariatric Surgery

The authors conducted a literature search for an ongoing systematic review of randomized controlled trials (RCTs) on the topic for the Cochrane Library in 5 databases (Medline, Cochrane, PubMed, Embase, LILACS), updated in March 2017, through automatic Ovid alerts. The search strategy was designed as described previously.[48] The authors used MeSH (Medical Subject Headings) terms and keywords relevant to vitamin D, bariatric surgery, and RCTs, with different combinations, to ensure a comprehensive search methodology.

Vitamin D Replacement Guidelines in Bariatric Surgery

The authors conducted a systematic literature search to identify guidelines on vitamin D replacement following bariatric surgery in Medline, PubMed, Embase, and the National Guideline Clearinghouse, updated in March 2017, through automatic Ovid alerts. MeSH terms and keywords relevant to vitamin D, bariatric surgery, and guidelines were used. Details of the original search methodology are published elsewhere.[49]

We also conducted a PubMed search using MeSH terms and keywords relevant to vitamin D and bariatric surgery from 2015 to March 2017, and screened the reference list of the relevant retrieved articles and of articles available in the authors' library. For the identification of ongoing prospective studies and randomized trials, we searched the ClinicalTrials.gov (https://clinicaltrials.gov/) and the WHO International Clinical Trials Registry Platform (ICTRP) (http://www.who.int/ictrp/en/), in March 2017, using MeSH terms and keywords relevant to vitamin D and bariatric surgery.

HYPOVITAMINOSIS D IN BARIATRIC SURGERY AND ASSOCIATIONS WITH OUTCOMES

The cause of vitamin D deficiency after bariatric surgery is multifactorial. In addition to altered vitamin D metabolism preoperatively and low sun exposure, there is poor adherence to dietary and supplement recommendations. Bypass of the duodenum and proximal ileum, which are sites of vitamin D absorption, further reduce the dietary vitamin D intake from diet.

Generalized absorption problems occur from vomiting, the reduced time available for food digestion, and bacterial overgrowth.[36,38,40,41,50] The RYGB procedure circumvents the duodenum and proximal jejunum, thus bypassing the transport pathways for iron, calcium, and the fat-soluble vitamins A and D.[18] The reported prevalence of low vitamin D levels depends on factors discussed earlier, the definition of vitamin D deficiency, and the type of surgery performed. It is most extensively reported and characterized in RYGB, the commonest procedure until recently, and one that incurs significant malabsorption. Both osteomalacia and osteitis fibrosa cystica have been described in patients post-RYGB.[32] Concomitant vitamin D deficiency and increased PTH levels are associated with increased bone remodeling and bone loss. These abnormalities in calciotropic hormones persist or could even be exacerbated by the malabsorptive state and nutritional deficiencies that often ensue from bariatric surgery. In addition, although high BMI has long been considered a protective factor against osteoporosis, concerns regarding an increased risk, incurred from the inflammatory state and increased marrow adiposity commonly seen in obesity, have emerged.[51,52]

Mineral and Skeletal Metabolism

A recent systematic review of 14 observational studies reported on findings from 2688 patients following RYGB, all followed for 24 months and half of whom received calcium and/or vitamin D, at doses of up to 1100 IU/d.[53] Hypovitaminosis D and secondary hyperparathyroidism were common up to 5 years after bypass. The weighted mean serum 25(OH)D level initially increased from 18.3 (3.6) ng/mL to 24.7 (2.3) ng/mL at 2 years, then decreased to 20.5 (4.4) ng/mL and 20.8 (3.8) ng/mL at 2 to 5 years and 5 years postoperatively.[53] The adjusted mean PTH level increased progressively from 53.7 (11.3) pg/mL preoperatively to 60.3 (7.5) pg/mL at 2 years, 71.7 (6.6) pg/mL at 2 to 5 years, and 78.3 (13.2) pg/mL at more than 5 years.[53] Two studies have compared vitamin D status and hyperparathyroidism rate before and after laparoscopic SG and laparoscopic RYGB, using the same supplementation regimen in both groups.[54,55] The first did not present baseline mineral parameters but showed a significantly higher prevalence of hypovitaminosis D and secondary hyperparathyroidism at 3 to 36 months postoperatively in the laparoscopic RYGB group, compared with the laparoscopic SG group.[54] The other study reported comparable 25(OH)D and PTH levels in laparoscopic RYGB and laparoscopic SG groups, before and 1 and 2 years postoperatively.[55]

Hypovitaminosis D was inversely correlated with PTH levels postoperatively both in prospective and retrospective studies, and was associated with osteoporosis.[56–58] Serum 25(OH)D level was one of the significant predictors of bone density following weight loss surgery.[47,59–61] However, a causative effect of vitamin D on bone loss has been put into question in light of studies performed in patients post-RYGB who showed an increase in bone remodeling[62] and a decrease in dual-energy x-ray absorptiometry (DXA) bone mineral density (BMD) at multiple skeletal sites, not related to changes in serum 25(OH)D and PTH levels.[62,63] Increased bone remodeling may be related to the concomitant calcium malabsorption, rather than to vitamin D.[20] DXA-derived bone density measurements are limited by logistic and technical considerations. These considerations include artifacts from overlying soft tissue for axial sites (spine and hip), in addition to accuracy errors caused by changes in body composition, secondary to drastic weight loss following bypass procedures, panniculus fat pad overlying the hip region, and so forth.[32,35] However, post–bariatric surgery true bone loss has been validated by concomitant volumetric bone density assessment using quantitative computed tomography at the lumbar spine,[64] and ultrasonography measurements of the peripheral skeleton.[62]

In addition to secondary hyperparathyroidism after RYGB surgery, other mechanisms contribute to alterations in bone metabolism.[32,35,46] These mechanisms include decreased mechanical loading, an increase in adiponectin level, a decrease in leptin level, and changes in the levels of gut-derived hormones, all of which favor bone loss, with the exception of serotonin and glucagonlike peptide-1.[46] In addition, there is a decrease in gonadal steroid levels.[46]

Fracture risk following bariatric surgery is a matter of debate. Results were inconsistent between several observational studies, secondary to the heterogeneity in study design; data collection methods; and, importantly, type of surgical procedure.[65–69] However, there may be a more consistent increase in fracture risk following malabsorptive procedures, such as RYGB and the less commonly used biliopancreatic diversion (BPD).[67,70,71] In the last 3 studies, fracture risk increased by 40% to 200%, depending on the fracture site, the surgical procedure, and the comparator group (community population, obese control patients, or obese patients undergoing a restrictive procedure).[67,70,71] In the most recent study, by Yu and colleagues,[70] analysis of claims from a US health care plan, with 12,482 RYGB and 8922 GB patients, there was a significant increase in fracture risk of hip (relative risk [RR] = 1.54) and radius (RR = 1.45) in patients post-RYGB compared with GB, that occurred 2.3 (1.9) years postoperatively (propensity matched analyses). None of the studies provided 25(OH)D levels and therefore the contribution of vitamin D to fracture risk is unclear. However, reported vitamin D deficiency in one retrospective study was identified as a significant risk factor, and it was associated with a doubled risk of fracture, after adjustment for age and type of surgery.[67]

For detailed reviews on bone disease following bariatric surgery, please refer to dedicated reviews and systematic reviews on the topic.[32,35,47,72,73]

Nonskeletal Outcomes

A serum 25(OH)D level less than 30 ng/mL was linked to a 3-fold increase in the risk of infections, after controlling for several covariates, demographics, and comorbidities, in a study of 770 obese patients (70% female), with a mean baseline BMI of 46 to 48 kg/m^2 undergoing RYGB.[74] In a retrospective study from France that enrolled 258 obese patients, 87% female, with a mean baseline BMI of 40.90 kg/m^2, there was no association between vitamin D deficiency and complication rate post-RYGB.[75] In unadjusted analyses from the same study, subjects who were vitamin D replete at baseline (serum 25(OH)D level >30 ng/mL) had a 10% higher excess weight loss at 2 years postsurgery, compared with those with vitamin D insufficiency or deficiency.[75] However, RCTs have not shown an effect of vitamin D on weight loss post–bariatric surgery (discussed later). Serum 25(OH)D level was also associated with resolution of hypertension 1 year post-RYGB in 196 obese patients, with a baseline BMI of 32 to 33 kg/m^2. In an unadjusted analysis, hypertension resolution rate was significantly lower in patients with serum 25(OH)D less than or equal to 20 ng/mL (42%) compared with patients with serum 25(OH)D level greater than 20 ng/mL (61%).[76] The association between vitamin D and cardiovascular morbidity and mortality, and all-cause mortality, post–bariatric surgery, has not been evaluated.

Findings from these observational studies remain limited by the retrospective study design, the small sample size, and confounders that were only adjusted for in 1 study.[74]

VITAMIN D STATUS AND REPLACEMENT IN PATIENTS UNDERGOING BARIATRIC SURGERY

A vitamin D intake that is body weight specific may be needed to achieve target 25(OH) D levels in obese individuals. A systematic review of 144 cohorts reported in 94 independent studies that included 11,566 subjects who received 200 to 10,000 IU/d of vitamin D, and 9766 controls, reported that baseline BMI is a strong predictor of response to vitamin D supplementation in obese individuals.[77] Other predictors included age, calcium intake from diet or supplements, baseline 25(OH)D level,[77] and possibly polymorphisms in the vitamin D receptor, vitamin D binding protein, and CYP enzymes.[17] Weight loss is accompanied by increments in serum 25(OH)D levels caused by mobilization of vitamin D from fat stores,[78–80] and patients who lose more weight experience a greater increase in serum 25(OH)D level.[81]

Special considerations when interpreting serum 25(OH)D levels in patients after bypass gastric surgery include the type of surgery incurred and the regimen prescribed, whether a loading dose for a certain period preoperatively or postoperatively was administered, and patient adherence. A 25% decrease in the absorption of cholecalciferol was shown in 14 morbidly obese premenopausal women 4 weeks after RYGB.[82] All of these covariates explain the wide variability in 25(OH)D levels achieved, at varying time points, in response to varying vitamin D regimens post–gastric bypass.

Observational Studies

Before bariatric surgery

The prevalence of hypovitaminosis D in obese patients undergoing bariatric surgery was reported to vary widely between studies conducted in Western populations, ranging from 13% to 92%.[83] Similarly, a single-center study from the Middle East (N = 257) showed that 91% of the obese patients presenting for bariatric surgery had a 25(OH)D level less than 30 ng/mL, and 69% were vitamin D deficient [25(OH) D level <20 ng/mL].[84] In a recent systematic review of observational studies, the authors identified 51 studies, each with at least 50 participants, describing vitamin D status before and/or after bariatric surgery.[85] All studies were conducted in Western populations, 7 studies were cross-sectional and 44 longitudinal, with retrospective or prospective designs. Thirty-eight studies were conducted in patients undergoing malabsorptive/combination procedures, 5 studies were conducted in laparoscopic SG patients, and 8 studies included both types of procedures.[85] The mean serum 25(OH)D level was less than 30 ng/mL preoperatively in 29 studies and less than 20 ng/mL in more than half of them (N = 17 studies).[85] Serum 25(OH)D levels did not differ between the BMI categories with weighted means (standard deviations [SDs]) of 43.6 (8.2), 47.6 (15.5), and 52.8 (9.9) kg/m^2.[85] Similar results were described in a 2017 systematic review of 15 observational studies conducted in patients undergoing SG, in Europe and the United States.[60] All studies reported a mean serum 25(OH)D level less than 30 ng/mL, and 8 studies a mean 25(OH)D level less than 20 ng/mL.[60] Ethnic differences in vitamin D levels, similar to those reported in the general population, were observed in a study from the United States. White people had the highest mean 25(OH)D level, with a mean of 25.5 ng/mL, compared with 12.9 ng/mL in African Americans, and 14.9 ng/mL in Hispanic people.[86] Therefore, the prevalence of hypovitaminosis D in Western and non-Western countries is comparable, if the ranges reported in individual studies are considered.[53,83,84] Systematic reviews that report mean serum 25(OH) levels also consistently yield comparable but more conservative estimates.[60,85]

After bariatric surgery

Despite various vitamin D supplementation regimens, our systematic review of observational studies revealed that only 13% of the included studies reported a mean post-replacement 25(OH)D level greater than 30 ng/mL, measured 3 months to 10 years postoperatively.[85] Several studies administering a low dose of vitamin D, 200 to 800 IU/d, showed no change or a decrease in 25(OH)D level.[85] In vitamin D–deficient patients, a significant increase in 25(OH)D level, of 9 to 13 ng/mL, was shown only in studies that used loading doses of vitamin D (1100–7100 IU/d) followed by a maintenance dose (400–2000 IU/d).[85] However, these increments in 25(OH)D level remained lower than increments observed with similar doses in the general nonobese population.[87,88] These indirect comparisons suggest that higher doses of vitamin D are needed to correct vitamin D deficiency in obese patients undergoing bariatric surgery. The proportion of patients reaching a 25(OH)D level greater than or equal to 20 ng/mL, the target set by the Institute of Medicine (IOM) for a normal population,[89] increased from 25% to 55% at baseline to 70% to 93% at follow-up, depending on the replacement dose and type of surgery.[85] Another systematic review and meta-analysis of prospective studies in patients undergoing gastric bypass, of at least 6 months' duration, revealed no significant change in serum 25(OH)D level with vitamin D doses less than or equal to 1200 IU/d.[90] The mean difference in serum 25(OH)D level was 1.35 (−1.12; 3.83, unit not provided; $P = .28$), and the high heterogeneity (I^2 84%) could be explained by the wide range of vitamin D doses used (from none to 1200 IU/d), follow-up duration (6–36 months), and baseline BMI.[90]

It is noteworthy that the few studies that did not include any supplementation following laparoscopic SG showed a significant improvement in serum 25(OH)D level at early (6 months)[91] and late (1–2 years) follow-up.[92,93] In one study, 25(OH)D level increased from 23.6 (14.2) to 32.2 (16.5) ng/mL, at 6 months postoperatively.[91] In 2 studies, 25(OH)D levels at baseline were 13.5 (8.1) and 17.4 (8) ng/mL, and increased to 26.3(7.6) and 42.1(10.2), at 1 year after surgery, respectively[92,93] and 1 of them reported a 25(OH)D level of 49.4 (14.4) at 2 years.[93] The increase in serum 25(OH)D in the early postoperative period could be explained by the lack of a malabsorptive element in this type of procedure, coupled with vitamin D mobilization from adipose tissue,[94] whereas the long-term improvement may be related to lifestyle changes, sun exposure, and other factors.

Such differences by type of surgery were not readily detectable in our systematic review.[85] We identified 5 studies that included more than 50 participants per arm, each comparing RYGB with SG (N = 2) or GB (N = 3), and only 2 studies showed that subjects undergoing RYGB procedures may require a higher dose of vitamin D, compared with those having SG or GB procedures, in unadjusted analyses.[85]

There was a large variability in the 25(OH)D assays used, which by itself may account for differences between studies,[13,95] and time points at which vitamin D status was assessed in the studies discussed earlier.[85] Furthermore, the type of vitamin D used, duration of supplementation, and compliance rates were poorly reported. These limitations explain the wide heterogeneity of results obtained and underscore the need for high-quality randomized trials to define the vitamin D dose response in this specific population.

Randomized Controlled Trials

Eight trials investigated vitamin D replacement in obese patients undergoing bariatric surgery, all from Western countries (**Table 1**).[96–103] The number of participants was fewer than 50 per arm in all but 2 studies (Dogan and colleagues[102] [n = 75/arm], Muschitz and colleagues[103] [n = 110/arm]). With 1 exception,[99] all were conducted

Table 1

Randomized controlled trials and controlled clinical trials of vitamin D replacement in bariatric surgery

Author, Year Country	Intervention Equivalent Daily Dose	N Randomized	N Completers	Gender % Women	Age (y) Mean (SD)	BMI Baseline (kg/m²) Mean (SD)	BMI Follow-up (kg/m²) Mean (SD)	Type of Surgery	Vitamin D Assay	Duration (mo)	Cointervention Ca (mg/d)	Baseline 25(OH)D Level (ng/mL) Mean (SD)	Postintervention 25(OH)D Level Mean (SD)	Change in 25(OH)D Level (ng/mL) Mean (SD)	Comorbidities (%)	Adverse Events
Intervention ≤ 3 months:																
Stein et al,[96] 2009 United States[a]	D₃ 1143 IU/d	12	12	75.0	39	47.5	NR	NR	LCMS Rochester, MN	2	NR	15.1 (6.9)	23.6 (6.9)	NR	NR	None
	D₂ 7143 IU/d	13	13	75.0								13.6 (4.3)	31.3 (7.2)			
Sundbom et al,[99] 2016 Sweden[d]	UVB (for 4 wk) +D₃ 600 IU/d	31	NR	70	40.5 (5.7)	42.7 (5.2)	31.3 (5.4)	RYGB	HPLC	3	NR	27.3 (11.9)	28.7 (9.9)	NR	NR	NR
	D₃ 600,000 IU IM once + 600 IU/d	21		75	38.2 (5.3)	42.7 (5)	30.2 (5.9)					22.3 (7.2)	31.2 (6.3)			
	Control + D₃ 600 IU/d	27		65.0	40.6 (6.3)	42.4 (4.3)	29.9 (4.6)					20.2 (6.7)	19.5 (6.3)			
Wolf et al,[98] 2016 Germany[c]	Placebo + D₃ 200 IU/d	47	41	61.7	43 (11)	50 (46.3; 58.8)	NR	SG	ELISA kit IDS, Frankfurt/Main, Germany	3	NR	23.2 (10.3)	NR	0	HTN: 66 DM: 29.8 Arthrosis: 6.4 Depression: 8.5 OSA: 40.4 Degenerative alteration 59.6	NR
	D₃ 3200 IU/d + 200 IU/d	47	38	66.0	43 (10)	46.7 (44.6; 57.4)						24 (7.4)	NR	Estimated change 12.8	HTN: 61.7 DM: 25.5 Arthrosis: 6.4 Depression: 14.9 OSA: 31.9 Degenerative alteration: 57.4	

(continued on next page)

Table 1 (continued)

Author, Year Country	Intervention Equivalent Daily Dose	N Randomized	N Completers	Gender % Women	Age (y) Mean (SD)	BMI Baseline (kg/m²) Mean (SD)	BMI Follow-up (kg/m²) Mean (SD)	Type of Surgery	Vitamin D Assay	Duration (mo)	Cointervention Ca mg/d	Baseline 25(OH)D Level (ng/mL) Mean (SD)	Postintervention 25(OH)D Level (ng/mL) Mean (SD)	Change in 25(OH)D Level (ng/mL) Mean (SD)	Comorbidities (%)	Adverse Events
Luger et al,[97] 2017 Austria[b]	D3 100,000 IU every 2 wk for 3 doses then 3420 IU/d	25	21	80.0	43 (12.6)	44.6 (4.2)	33.1 (3.9)	Omega loop gastric bypass	NR	6	NR	15.5 (5.7)	27	NR	Liver fibrosis: 36	In the whole study Myocardial infarct (n = 1)
	Placebo (3 doses) then D3 3420 IU/d	25	22	80.0	41.8 (13)	42.9 (4.3)	31.1 (3.5)					15.7 (5.9)	21		Liver fibrosis: 20	Liver hepatoma (n = 1)
Intervention ≥ 12 months:																
Carlin et al,[100] 2009 United States[e]	Control + D 800 IU/d	30	29	100	42.9 (11.3)	50.9 (6.6)	32.7 (4.6)	RYGB	CLIA Liaison Platform DiaSorin, Stillwater, MN	12	Ca ≥1500	19.7 (8.5)	NR	-4.4 (11.4)	NR	Death (n = 1) in the high dose group
	D 7143 + 800 IU/d	30	24	100	43.0 (11.9)	50.3 (4.9)	32.5 (5.1)				Ca ≥1500	18.5 (9.4)		16.3 (15.7)		
Goldner et al,[101] 2009 United States[f]	D3 800 IU/d	13	9	NR	48.2 (11.8)	52.5 (9)	Change in weight (kg) -52.2 (18)	RYGB	CLIA Salt Lake City, UT	12	Ca 2000	19.1 (9.9)	NR	11 (12.4)	NR	Hypercalciuria (n = 1) in the high dose group
	D3 2000 IU/d	13	9		48.3 (6.6)	60.4 (14.2)	-41.7 (19)				Ca 2000	15 (9.3)		24.1 (15)		
	D3 5000 IU/d	15	10		44.6 (10.9)	56.2 (10.3)	-45.7 (13)				Ca 2000	22.9 (10.3)		26.4 (16.9)		
Dogan et al,[102] 2014 Holland[g]	D 160 + 1200 IU/d	75	74	68.0	43.4 (10)	44.8 (4.8)	Weight at follow-up (kg) 90.6 (17.4)	RYGB	NR	12	Ca 1500	17 (7.2)	30.7 (9.8)	13.2 (10.9)	DM: 32 HTN: 44 DL: 13.3 OSA: 14.7	No adverse events related to intervention
	D 500 + 1200 IU/d	75	74	71.0	45.3 (10.2)	44.8 (6.4)	93.8 (16.9)				Ca 1500	17.7 (8.2)	28.2 (10.2)	10 (10.8)	DM: 33.3 HTN: 37.3 DL: 26.7 OSA: 18.7	

						Change in BMI (kg/m²)								
Muschitz et al,[103] 2016 Austria[h]	D₃ 4000 IU/d for 8 wk then 2286 IU/d + D 200 IU/d	110	94	60.0	41 (34–45)	44.3 (41.1; 47.9)	−5.5 (−9.4; −3.2)	RYGB and SG	Chemiluminescence on the IDS-iSYS System, Boldon, United Kingdom	24	Calcium and lifestyle changes	17.4 (13.4; 22.6)	44.6 (34.9;52.8)	NR	NR	NR
	Control + D 200 IU/d	110	97	55.5	40 (35–45.8)	44.2 (40.7; 47.7)	−7.3 (−9.4; −1.7)				NR	17.7 (13; 21.9)	18 (15; 22.1)	NR	NR	NR

Abbreviations: CLIA, chemiluminescent immunoassay; DL, dyslipidemia; DM, diabetes mellitus; ELISA, enzyme-linked immunosorbent assay; HPLC, high-pressure liquid chromatography; HTN, hypertension; IDS, Iduronate-2-Sulfatase; LCMS, liquid chromatography mass spectrometry; NR, not reported; OSA, obstructive sleep apnea.

a Longitudinal pilot study: intervention was D₂ 50,000 IU weekly versus D₃ 8000 IU weekly for 8 weeks; participants with vitamin D deficiency in the cross-sectional study were included in the trial; baseline characteristics for the pilot study were same as for the cross-sectional study; results on demographics included here are for all the participants in the cross-sectional study.

b Intervention was given as a loading dose of 100,000 IU at 0, 2 weeks, and 4 weeks, but the study duration was 6 months.

c Study compared 3200 IU/d versus placebo; two-thirds of all participants received an additional 200 IU/d and one-third of participants received an additional 10 to 20 IU/d. Medians (range) of BMI at baseline are provided.

d Study was conducted at 4.1 (1.1) years after bariatric surgery; as per the authors, "although no hypercalcemia or other toxic symptoms, for example, poor appetite and constipation to severe thirst and failure, were seen in the kidney present study, the risk cannot be ignored." All participants received 600 IU/d.

e Open-label study comparing 50,000 IU weekly versus no vitamin D; all participants received 800 IU/d; one of the limitations of the trial was noncompliance, but further details were not provided.

f The investigators describe that they had difficulty in compliance, but no further details were provided. Data on 6, 12, and 24 months are available.

g All participants received vitamin D 1200 IU/d and Ca 1500 mg/d; all participants received other multivitamins and minerals, in 2 different doses. These vitamins and minerals were: biotin, calcium, chloride, chrome, copper, folic acid, iodine, iron, manganese, magnesium, molybdenum, selenium, vitamins (A, B₁, B₂, B₃, B₅, B₆, B₁₂, C, D, E, K₁), and zinc. No significant difference in 25(OH)D level was detected between the 2 arms. Vitamin D deficiency before surgery was corrected with a mean loading dose of 226,087 (±60,442) IU with a maintenance dose of 25,000 IU/mo, and stopped 2 months before surgery.

h The intervention group received 28,000 IU cholecalciferol per week for 8 weeks before bariatric surgery, 16,000 IU/wk after surgery, the control group did not receive any loading nor maintenance vitamin D; in addition to vitamin D, the intervention consisted of 1000 mg of calcium monocitrate per day, daily BMI-adjusted protein supplementation, and physical exercise. All participants received vitamin D 200 IU/d.

in the immediate postoperative phase. The surgical procedures were RYGB,[99–102] omega loop bypass,[97] SG,[98] or one of the 2 procedures, RYGB or SG,[103] and not specified in 1 study.[96] Vitamin D supplementation was given for a period greater than or equal to 12 months in 4 studies,[100–103] 3 months in 1 study,[98] and less than 3 months in the other 3 studies.[96,97,99] We did not identify any study in which supplementation was started immediately postsurgery and given for a duration of between 3 and 12 months postsurgery, a period during which the most rapid weight loss occurs, and during which vitamin D levels may increase because of mobilization from fat. The vitamin D doses were given daily (3 studies),[98,101,102] weekly (3 studies),[96,100,103] or biweekly (1 study),[97] and consisted of D_3 in a liquid form,[97,98] a sublingual tablet,[103] or as a single intramuscular (IM) high dose of vitamin D compared with UVB (and no supplementation).[99] The daily equivalent vitamin D doses varied from 200 to 7940 IU/d. Five studies gave, in addition to the intervention, vitamin D as part of multivitamins for all participants, at a dose of 200 to 1200 IU/d.[98–100,102,103] All studies had a preponderance of women, in their 40s, with a mean BMI at the start of the intervention less than or equal to 50 kg/m^2 in 6 studies,[96–99,102,103] and between 50 and 60 kg/m^2 in 2 studies.[100,101] Only 2 studies used high-pressure liquid chromatography[99] and liquid chromatography mass spectrometry[96] to measure serum 25(OH)D levels, which is an important consideration in studies that may have used use D_2 instead of D_3, and platform assays that do not detect 100% of this D_2 metabolite.[104] Baseline 25(OH)D levels ranged between 15 and 20 ng/mL in 6 studies,[96,97,100–103] and 20 and 30 ng/mL in 2 studies.[98,99] Three studies gave concomitant calcium supplementation, at a dose of 1500 to 2000 mg daily, to all treatment arms,[100–102] and cointervention differed between arms in 2 studies.[102,103] In 1 of them, the intervention consisted of vitamin D_3 in addition to exercise and high-protein diet versus no intervention.[103] In the other, cointervention included calcium, iron, and other vitamins and minerals, at different doses between arms.[102] Comorbidities such as diabetes mellitus, hypertension, obstructive sleep apnea, and dyslipidemia were discussed in only 2 studies[98,102] (see **Table 1** for details). Adherence with supplementation was reported in only 2 studies and exceeded 80% in both.[96,98]

Effect of Vitamin D Supplementation for at Least 12 Months

Four RCTs[100–103] administered vitamin D as D_3 in 2 studies,[101,103] whereas no details were provided in the other 2 (**Fig. 2**, see **Table 1**).[100,102] The same cointervention was used in all study arms in 2 studies.[100,101] The first study compared a vitamin D (type not specified) dose of 50,000 IU/wk with controls in an open-label study design in 60 women who had RYGB. However, all participants received multivitamins postoperatively.[100] Therefore, the equivalent vitamin D doses were 7943 IU/d versus 800 IU/d.[100] The baseline 25(OH)D level was 18 to 19 ng/mL, decreased by 4.4 (11.4) ng/mL in the control arm, but increased by 16.3 (15.7) ng/mL in the high-dose arm at 12 months.[100] The authors calculated an increase in serum 25(OH)D of 0.2 ng/mL per 100 IU of vitamin D.[100] The second was a pilot study, comparing 3 different cholecalciferol doses in patients undergoing RYGB: 800 IU/d (n = 13), 2000 IU/d (n = 13), and 5000 IU/d (n = 15). Despite the imbalance in the baseline characteristics between treatment arms, including serum 25(OH)D level (see **Table 1**), the absolute increase in serum 25(OH)D was 24 ng/mL on the intermediate dose, 26 ng/mL on the high dose, and 11 ng/mL on the low dose.[101] The increase in serum 25(OH)D per 100 IU vitamin D was calculated to be 1.4 ng/mL in the low dose, 1.2 ng/mL in the intermediate dose, and 0.5 ng/mL in the high dose.

In 2 other studies, the cointervention differed between study arms.[102,103] In the largest trial, from Austria, there was a significant increase in mean serum 25(OH)D level

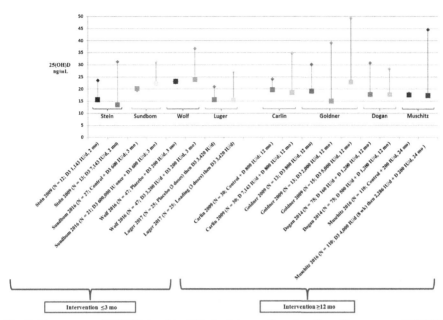

Fig. 2. Mean serum 25(OH)D level in RCTs, by intervention duration. Mean serum 25(OH)D levels in studies grouped by the duration of the intervention (≤3 months and ≥12 months) before and after vitamin D supplementation, in patients undergoing RYGB,[97,99–102] SG,[98] SG or RYGB.[103] One study did not specify the surgical procedure type.[96] Each color represents 1 study; dark colors represent low dose or controls, and light colors represent high dose. (*Data from* Refs.[97–103])

from 17.4 ng/mL to 44.6 ng/mL in response to vitamin D_3 doses of 4000 IU/d for 8 weeks followed by 2286 IU/d (n = 110), and no change in the control arm (n = 110) in patients undergoing RYGB or SG.[103] However, cointervention with 200 IU/d, high-protein diet, and other lifestyle changes could have affected the response to vitamin D supplementation.[103] Another trial compared 2 doses of vitamin D [160 IU/d (n = 75) versus 500 IU/d (n = 75)] in 2 supplements, containing differing concentrations of calcium, iron, and other minerals and vitamins (see footnote to **Table 1**).[102] There was no significant difference in serum 25(OH)D level 12 months post-RYGB; these findings could be explained by the small difference in the vitamin D dose between the 2 arms, the 1200 IU in the cointervention, and/or nutrient interference in vitamin D absorption, specifically calcium and iron supplementation.[102]

Effect of Vitamin D Supplementation for Less Than or Equal to 3 Months

The authors identified 4 studies administering vitamin D for a duration of 3 months or less (see **Fig. 2**, see **Table 1**). The effect of a cholecalciferol dose of 3200 IU/d (n = 47), was compared with placebo (n = 47) in patients undergoing SG, with baseline serum 25(OH)D level of 23 to 24 ng/mL, and all participants received 200 IU/d, as part of post-operative multivitamins.[98] Although there was no change in serum 25(OH)D level in the placebo group, an estimated increase of 12.8 ng/mL was reported with the high dose.[98] The authors calculate the increase in 25(OH)D level to be 0.4 ng/mL/100 IU of vitamin D. A study that extended over 6 months compared the effect of a loading vitamin D dose, cholecalciferol 100,000 IU for 3 doses, at 0, 2, and 4 weeks, followed by a maintenance dose (3420 IU/d) (n = 25), with placebo loading followed by the same maintenance dose (3420 IU/d) (n = 25)[97] in omega loop gastric bypass (includes 200 cm of jejunal bypass).[97] The mean serum 25(OH)D level increased from a baseline of 15 ng/mL to 27 ng/mL in the group receiving a loading/maintenance dose and to 21 ng/mL in the maintenance arm.[97] However, the study results cannot be generalized because a subset of patients had liver fibrosis.[97] In addition, 1 study compared parenteral vitamin D supplementation (single IM dose of 600,000 IU once) versus placebo or UVB in patients undergoing RYGB.[99] All subjects received cholecalciferol 600 IU/d as part of a multivitamin.[99] There was a significant increase in serum 25(OH)D level, from 22.3 (7.2) to 31.2 (6.3) ng/mL, only in the intervention arm, 3 months postintervention.[99] However, a single high loading dose of vitamin D may not be sufficient to maintain a steady state in the long term, both in normal-weight and obese patients.[105] Similarly, treatment with vitamin D for a period of less than 2 to 3 months may not be sufficient to reach a steady state in vitamin D levels.[87] Therefore, with the exception of Wolf and colleagues,[98] the effect of vitamin D supplementation cannot be accurately evaluated in these studies, secondary to the short study duration.

Based on the studies of at least 3 months' duration, with the same cointervention across study arms, the absolute serum 25(OH)D levels achieved were higher in response to higher vitamin D doses. The increments, expressed in ng/mL per 100 IU daily equivalent of vitamin D, were inversely proportional to the vitamin D doses administered. They are similar to changes in the general population but lower in magnitude for comparable vitamin D doses.[88,106,107]

Despite the use of high-vitamin-D doses, the mean 25(OH)D level achieved in the studies described earlier remained less than 40 ng/mL (see **Table 1**), with the exception of 2 studies, both of which lasted 12 months (see **Fig. 2**, see **Table 1**). One used a loading dose of 4000 IU/d for 8 weeks followed by a maintenance dose of 2286 IU/d, and the mean 25(OH)D level reached was 44.6 ng/mL.[103] The study that used a high dose of 5000 IU/d led to an estimated 25(OH)D level of 49 ng/mL.[101] In that study, baseline 25(OH)D levels differed, but the mean change in 25(OH)D was comparable for the 2000 IU/d and the 5000 IU/d doses, an observation worthy of follow-up in larger blinded randomized trials. The findings in 3 randomized trials are limited by the low quality of the studies, related to the lack of description of allocation concealment (3 studies),[98,100,101] the high attrition rate and lack of blinding (2 studies),[100,101] the imbalance in baseline characteristics (1 study),[101] in addition to the small sample size. None of the studies reported an increase in 25(OH)D level to a toxic level, toxicity being defined as a 25(OH)D level greater than 100 to 150 ng/mL in association with hypercalcemia.[13] The reporting of adverse events in the individual studies was poor (see **Table 1**). Notoriously, information regarding kidney stones was lacking, which is an important consideration in view of the increased risk of kidney stones post-RYGB.[108,109]

Effect of Vitamin D Supplementation on Other Bone and Mineral Parameters

Serum and urine calcium level

None of the studies reported a significant change in mean serum calcium level in the intervention arms, and hypercalcemia was not reported. There were no data on 24-hour urine calcium excretion.

Parathyroid hormone level

All the identified studies evaluated the effect of vitamin D supplementation on PTH level. In 1 study, PTH levels were significantly different at baseline, 88.1 (42.0), 106.4 (51.6), and 70.8 (63.3) pg/mL in the 800 IU/d, the 2000 IU/d, and the 5000 IU/d arms, respectively (P = .03). At 12 months, PTH level decreased by 17.0

(42.6) pg/mL, 32.4 (62.3) pg/mL, and 25.3 (82.1) pg/mL, in the low, intermediate, and high doses, respectively (P = nonsignificant).[101] Two other studies with an intervention for less than 3 months showed significant decreases in PTH levels (17%–21%) only in the intervention arms, whereas they remained increased in the controls.[97,103]

In a pilot study comparing vitamin D_2 50,000 IU weekly with vitamin D_3 8000 IU weekly over 8 weeks, the mean PTH level decreased from 91 (10) pg/mL to 76 (6) ng/mL in the cholecalciferol group, and from 77 (10) to 72 (6) pg/mL in the ergocalciferol group (P>.05).[96] These findings raise questions as to whether D_3 is more potent than D_2 in suppressing PTH levels,[96] as has been debated for normal individuals. The other trials did not report significant changes in PTH levels within or between arms throughout the study period. The variable findings with regard to PTH levels may be related to the small sample size, the differences in baseline 25(OH)D level, the variability in the vitamin D dose, and the 25(OH)D levels achieved in the individual studies.

Bone density, bone markers, and fracture

Two RCTs assessed the effect of vitamin D supplementation on BMD following bariatric surgery.[100,103] One study showed a nonsignificant decrease in bone density of spine and radius at 12 months post-RYGB but a significant change in hip BMD, in favor of a protective effect of the high vitamin D dose of 50,000 IU weekly (high dose, 0.08 (0.05) g/cm^2; low dose, 0.12 (0.06) g/cm^2; P = .043). This finding was paralleled by a significant increase in bone turnover markers in both study arms.[100] The serum 25(OH)D level achieved with the high dose was 34.8 ng/mL.[100] In the second study, which combined RYGB and SG, the intervention group received vitamin D_3 4000 IU/d for 8 weeks, followed by 2286 IU/d for a total of 24 months, and reached a mean serum 25(OH)D level of 44.6 ng/mL.[103] There was a significant decrease in total hip and total body BMD, but to a lesser extent in the intervention group compared with the control group.[103] In contrast, lumbar spine BMD did not change in the intervention group, whereas it decreased in the control group.[103] The increase in bone turnover markers was also significant in both groups, but to a lesser extent in the intervention group, following the same pattern as changes in bone density.[103] This study is the only one that collected data on fracture and reported a traumatic rib fracture in the intervention group and 2 atraumatic fractures (radius, humerus) in the control group.[103]

These findings suggest a potential protective effect of a high vitamin D dose against bone loss following bariatric surgery. However, the optimal 25(OH)D level and/or vitamin D dose that result in improved skeletal outcomes could not be defined, and procedure-specific conclusions could not be drawn.

Effect of Vitamin D Supplementation on Weight and Cardiometabolic Parameters

None of the randomized trials showed any vitamin D dose–dependent weight loss following bariatric surgery. One study showed a significant improvement in lipid parameters over time, after 12 weeks, in subjects who received 200 IU/d and 3400 IU/d of D_3, but there were no significant differences between the 2 arms.[98] In contrast, the decrease in glycemic and inflammatory indices was only significant in the placebo arm.[98] Another study showed a higher hypertension resolution rate: 75% in the high-dose group versus 32% in the low-dose group (P = .029).[100]

Comparison of Vitamin D Replacement in Sleeve Gastrectomy Versus Roux-en-Y Gastric Bypass

Two small studies assessed the impact of the surgical procedure on bone and vitamin D metabolism, using the same vitamin D replacement dose in both study arms.[110,111] The first compared the effect of RYGB (n = 7) or SG (n = 8) on bone loss at 1 year after surgery in participants who received cholecalciferol 600 IU/d.[111] Although participants had comparable BMIs at study entry (RYGB, 43.1 (3.9) kg/m^2; SG, 43.5 (3.2) kg/m^2), as expected, RYGB patients lost more weight compared with SG patients (follow-up BMI, 26.2 (2.7) kg/m^2, and 30.5 (2.6) kg/m^2, respectively).[111] Serum 25(OH)D level increased significantly in the SG group, whereas it remained unchanged in the RYGB group.[111] Another study compared the effect of monthly cholecalciferol 100,000 IU (daily equivalent dose of 3333 IU/d) in 45 subjects undergoing RYGB and 55 who had SG.[110] Vitamin D deficiency was similar in both groups at baseline, but there was a significant reduction in the prevalence of vitamin D deficiency (from 84% to 48%) in the SG group.[110]

Although limited by the small number of studies and the restricted sample size, these findings possibly suggest a better response to vitamin D supplementation in SG compared with RYGB. Assuming adherence in the reported RCTs, and a normal distribution for serum 25(OH)D levels, our findings confirm that, as anticipated, vitamin D requirements post–bariatric surgery are higher than those of the normal population, of 600 to 800 IU/d.[89] Considering studies that lasted at least 12 months (see **Fig. 2**), a dose of 800 IU/d would not enable > 97.5% of the patients who undergo RYGB to achieve a serum 25(OH)D level above 20 ng/mL. Based on the Goldner dose ranging study, it may be closer to 2000 IU/d, but the sample size consisted of only 41 subjects.[101] There is no clear evidence of a need for a loading dose. The limited evidence from RCTs for patients undergoing SG does not allow any solid conclusions regarding dosing in this population.

Ongoing Vitamin D Studies in Bariatric Surgery

The authors identified 5 observational studies, all with a sample size less than 50, being conducted in Europe and the United States (Appendix 1 provides details on outcomes of interest). The authors also identified 6 ongoing RCTs, mostly using cholecalciferol, at doses ranging between a daily equivalent of 3333 and 10,000 IU, most being of short duration (<12 weeks), and the longest follow-up of 12 months. Four studies are being conducted in Western countries and 2 in the Middle East (see Appendix 1). The sample size is less than 100 in 4 studies, and greater than 100 in 2 studies. The target population as specified is obese adults undergoing RYGB or SG (3 studies) or bariatric surgery in general (3 studies). The primary outcomes are serum 25(OH)D level (3 studies), PTH level (1 study), and BMD (1 study), and 25(OH)D level is a secondary outcome in 1 study (see Appendix 1).

VITAMIN D REPLACEMENT GUIDELINES FOR PATIENTS UNDERGOING BARIATRIC SURGERY

Several guidelines on the postoperative care of obese patients undergoing bariatric surgery are summarized in **Table 2**.[112–117] The Endocrine Society (ES)[112] and the National Health Service (NHS) England Obesity Clinical Reference Group[116] used the Grading of Recommendations Assessment, Development and Evaluation (GRADE) approach to derive their recommendations, whereas the American Association of Clinical Endocrinologists (AACE), American Association of Metabolic and Bariatric Surgery (ASMBS), and The Obesity Society (TOS) guidelines used the AACE Protocol for Standardized Production of Clinical Practice Guidelines methodology.[113] The British Obesity and Metabolic Surgery Society (BOMSS) report was based on a review of the available guidelines (AACE/TOS/ASMBS, ES, Interdisciplinary European guidelines, ASMBS Position Statement, and the Canadian Agency for Drugs and

Table 2
Guidelines on vitamin D screening, monitoring, and replacement in bariatric surgery

Society	Screening and Monitoring	Replacement Dose	Case of Severe Malabsorption
Endocrine Society 2010[112]	Checking 25(OH)D level before, all types of bariatric surgery, and after RYGB, BPD, and BPD/DS, at 6, 12, 18, 24 mo and annually thereafter	First phase (weeks 1–2, liquids): oral vitamin D 50,000 IU daily. Second phase (weeks 3–6, soft food): calcitriol D 1000 IU daily. Vitamin D can be provided with ergocalciferol, 50,000 IU 1 to 3 times per week; no grading[a] Malabsorptive surgical procedures: *Vitamin D supplementation is recommended postoperatively for malabsorptive obesity surgical procedures and the doses be adjusted by a qualified medical professional based on serum markers and measures of bone density.* Strong recommendation with moderate quality of evidence	*50,000 IU vitamin D 1–3 times daily - No grading*
American Association of Clinical Endocrinologists, American Association of Metabolic and Bariatric Surgery and The Obesity Society[113]	Checking 25(OH)D level before any bariatric surgery, and after RYGB and BPDDS, at 1, 3 and 6–12 mo thereafter	RYGB and LSG: *Vitamin D at least 3000 IU daily, titrate to >30 ng/mL grade A, BEL 1[b]* LAGB: *At least 3000 IU of vitamin D daily (titrated to therapeutic 25-dihydroxyvitamin D levels)* RYGB, BPD, BPD/DS: *Treatment with oral calcium citrate and vitamin D2 or D3 is indicated to prevent or minimize secondary hyperparathyroidism without inducing frank hypercalciuria: grade C, BEL 3*	*Oral D2 or D3 may need to be as high as 50,000 units 1–3 times weekly to daily, more recalcitrant cases may require concurrent oral calcitriol (1,25(OH)$_2$ D): grade D*
British Obesity and Metabolic Surgery Society 2014[114]	*Vitamin D level should be monitored following SG, gastric bypass and BPDI DS. If vitamin D supplementation is adjusted, the serum 25OHD levels should be rechecked after a minimum of three months*	Gastric bypass and SG: *Usual practice is in the region of a minimum of 800–1200 mg calcium and 20 mcg [µg] (800 IU) vitamin D per day. Additional vitamin D supplementation will also be needed following the BPD/DS* Preparations may be given as: • 50,000 IU capsules, one given weekly for 6 wk (300,000 IU) • 20,000 IU capsules, two given weekly for 7 wk (280,000 IU) • 800 IU capsules, five a day given for 10 wk (280,000 IU) *This may then be followed by maintenance regimens 1 mo after loading with doses equivalent to 800 to 2000 IU daily*	NA

(continued on next page)

Table 2
(continued)

Society	Screening and Monitoring	Replacement Dose	Case of Severe Malabsorption
		(occasionally up to 4000 IU daily), given either daily or intermittently at a higher equivalent dose: no grading	
Interdisciplinary European 2014[115]	*A metabolic and bone evaluation before surgery, and follow up after surgery was suggested (details on type of surgery and timing not provided)*	AGB and RYGB: *Vitamin and micronutrient supplements (oral) should routinely be prescribed to compensate for their possible reduced intake and absorption.* BPD: *Lifelong daily vitamin and micronutrient supplementation (vitamins should be administered in a water-soluble form): Vitamins A, D, E and K: no grading*	NA
National Health Service England Obesity Clinical Reference Group 2016[116]	*All patients should have their vitamin D status assessed and treated prior to surgery and should have replacement prescribed after surgery: grade B*[a]	NA	NA
Ontario Bariatric Network 2016[117]	25(OH)D level at baseline and at 3, 6, 12 mo and then annually thereafter	NA	NA

In the presence of several guidelines versions, the latest version is included in this table. Sentences in italic are taken verbatim from the original guidelines document.

Abbreviations: AGB, adjustable gastric banding; BEL, best evidence level; BPD, bilio-pancreatic diversion; BPD/DS, BPD and duodenal switch; LAGB, laparoscopic adjustable gastric banding; LSG, laparoscopic SG; NA, not available.

[a] GRADE approach was used for the rating of the quality of evidence and the strength of the recommendations.

[b] The American Association of Clinical Endocrinologists protocol for standardized production of clinical practice guidelines methodology was used for the rating of the quality of evidence and the strength of the recommendations.

Technologies in Health Technical Report [Ottawa, Canada]), in addition to recent publications on the topic.[114] The other guidelines did not provide details on the methodology used or any quality rating of their recommendations (see **Table 2**).[115,117]

A critical appraisal of the ES, AACE/ASBMS/TOS and Interdisciplinary European guidelines is available elsewhere.[49]

Screening and Monitoring for Hypovitaminosis D

Although screening for vitamin D deficiency is not recommended for the general healthy population, it is recommended for obese patients undergoing bariatric surgery.[118–120] In 2009, a review of European and US guidelines and expert recommendations available at that time suggested monitoring serum 25(OH)D level for gastric bypass every 3 months during the first year, twice yearly in the second year, and yearly thereafter, and for SG and adjustable gastric banding (AGB), once yearly after surgery.[121] The ES (2010) and the AACE/ASMBS/TOS guidelines (2013) both recommend screening with serum 25(OH)D level before all types of bariatric surgery and then periodically every 3 to 6 months for a duration of 1 to 2 years, in patients having RYGB, BPD, and BPD and duodenal switch (BPDDS).[112,113] The Interdisciplinary European Guidelines (2014) recommend a metabolic and bone evaluation before surgery and at follow-up, without specifying when and what tests should be performed. The BOMSS guidelines (2014) recommend monitoring serum 25(OH)D level in patients on supplementation after SG, GB, and BPDDS,[114] and to check serum 25(OH)D level and adjust the dose 3 months postprocedure.[114] The NHS England Obesity Clinical Reference Group recommends the evaluation of vitamin D status before bariatric surgery (SG, RYGB, and BPDDS) but is silent on monitoring postoperatively.[116] The Ontario Bariatric Network Task Force document provides a summary table on the laboratory investigations required following bariatric surgery and for monitoring of vitamin D status at baseline, 3 months, 6 months, 12 months, and then annually, without any specification of the type of bariatric surgery.[117]

Recommended Replacement Doses

The ES guidelines recommend vitamin D supplementation for malabsorptive procedures, adjusting the dose based on serum and bone parameters (strong recommendation with moderate quality of evidence). They suggest a vitamin D dose of 50,000 IU 1 to 3 times per week, increasing to 50,000 IU 1 to 3 times per day in cases of severe malabsorption (no grading).[112] The AACE/TOS/ASMBS guidelines recommend 3000 IU of vitamin D daily for RYGB, laparoscopic SG, and laparoscopic AGB to reach a 25(OH)D level of greater than or equal to 30 ng/mL (grade A; best level of evidence, 1).[113] Similar to ES guidelines, a vitamin D dose of 50,000 IU 1 to 3 times weekly, with increments to daily doses is recommended in cases of severe malabsorption (grade D).[113] Both guidelines suggested that active vitamin D can be used in refractory cases.[112,113] The BOMSS guidelines suggest a minimum of 800 IU/d, and additional doses for BPD procedures, such as a loading dose of 50,000 IU weekly for 6 weeks, or 40,000 IU weekly for 7 weeks, or 4000 IU daily for 10 weeks, followed by 800 to 2000 IU/d vitamin D (no grading).[114] The other guidelines do not provide any recommendations/suggestions regarding the doses needed (see **Table 2**).

In summary, the guidelines available to date differed between societies in terms of dosing, had comparable monitoring intervals when specified, and only AACE/TOS/ASMBS specified a desirable 25(OH)D level of 30 ng/mL, based on their recommended desirable levels in the general population.[113] The guidelines do not fulfill optimal guidance development criteria, in part because of limited resources, and are mostly based on expert opinion because of the scarcity of high-quality evidence available.

SUMMARY, KNOWLEDGE GAPS, AND FUTURE CONSIDERATIONS

Hypovitaminosis D [mean serum 25(OH)D level ≤20 ng/mL] before and after bariatric surgery is common, with the exception of a few observational studies using a loading dose followed by a maintenance dose of vitamin D postoperatively. The data are most abundant post-RYGB. Results of randomized trials of similar nature were not always consistent, possibly because of small sample size, confounding by various predictors, type and vitamin D regimen used, cointervention with calcium and other supplements, variability in follow-up, and patient adherence.

Low 25(OH)D levels are often accompanied by secondary hyperparathyroidism postoperatively, and this may be more severe after RYGB. High remodeling and bone loss has been observed, but it is not clear that vitamin D and PTH levels are the main regulators of these changes in bone metabolism postoperatively. Data on fractures are scarce and conflicting and there is no clear evidence for a role of a low vitamin D level in causing these fractures.

Several replacement regimens are available to date, and some are recommended in guidelines issued from relevant scientific societies. However, the quality of the evidence for the dosing and regimens recommended is limited, and the efficacy and effectiveness of recommended doses in increasing 25(OH)D level and improving major outcomes have not been shown.

A desirable serum 25(OH)D level is one that prevents secondary hyperparathyroidism and osteomalacia, improves calcium balance and BMD, and decreases fracture risk. Such data in patients undergoing bariatric surgery are for the most part lacking, and the desirable vitamin D level in this population remains unknown. It is likely that regimens differ by type of surgery because of the additional decreased absorption of vitamin D in RYGB procedures. Vitamin D dose-ranging trials will help define the optimal regimen (dose, frequency, and vehicle [liquid, sublingual tablet, capsule, or injection]) by type of surgery, to reach a 25(OH)D level greater than 20 ng/mL (a putative desirable level extrapolating from the general population). Assessment of surrogate markers of calcium balance and mineral metabolism will help define the desirable level in this population. This assessment is best complemented by systematic reviews of high-quality randomized trials that investigate the effect of bariatric surgery on bone density, bone quality in the various skeletal compartments, muscle mass, falls, and fractures as end points. Adequate reporting on adherence and adverse events is also essential.

The number of vitamin D randomized trials, identified from 2 major trial registries, currently being conducted in bariatric surgery patients, and their duration, are suboptimal to investigate the changes in vitamin D levels that occur within the first year post-surgery. It is hoped that several more are in progress. Although some data are gathered from Western countries, data from non-Western countries, where obesity is fastest growing, is almost inexistent. The obesity epidemic and its implications for health in general and skeletal health in particular in the pediatric population are also of great concern, in view of the potential deleterious impact of hypovitaminosis D, and other nutritional deficiencies, on the growing skeleton at a critical time for bone mass accretion.

Awaiting high-quality evidence studies, the authors suggest starting with regimens of 2000 to 4000 IU of vitamin D_3 per day, selecting the higher end of this range for patients undergoing RYGB. Loading does not seem necessary unless patients have severe vitamin D deficiency preoperatively. The sublingual and injectable forms, which bypass the gastrointestinal tract, may be particularly attractive. Recommendations regarding adequate hydration are important to minimize the risk of stone precipitation. In consideration of the large variations in serum 25(OH)D levels achieved, and the number of confounders, periodic monitoring of such levels at 1, 3, 6, and 12 months postoperatively, and annually thereafter, allows therapy to be tailored to individual patients' risk profiles.

ACKNOWLEDGMENTS

The work and research reported in this article were supported in part by the Fogarty International Center and the Office of Dietary Supplements of the National Institutes of Health under award number D43 TW009118. The content is solely the responsibility of the authors and does not necessarily represent the official views of the National Institutes of Health. The authors thank Mr Ali Hammoudi for his help with tables and figures, and Ms Aida Farha, Medical Information Specialist, Saab Medical Library, at the American University of Beirut, for her advice and assistance in designing comprehensive and complex searches of the various medical literature resources, and retrieval of select articles.

REFERENCES

1. World Health Organization. Obesity and overweight statistics. Available at: http://www.who.int/mediacentre/factsheets/fs311/en/. Accessed August, 2017.
2. Ogden CL, Carroll MD, Kit BK, et al. Prevalence of obesity among adults: United States, 2011–2012. NCHS Data Brief 2013;131:1–8. Available at: http://www.cdc.gov/nchs/data/databriefs/db131.htm. Accessed August, 2017.
3. American Society for Metabolic and Bariatric Surgery (ASMBS).Obesity in America. Available at: https://asmbs.org/wp/uploads/2014/06/Obesity-in-America-1.pdf. Accessed August, 2017.
4. American Heart Association. Overweight & obesity. Statistical fact sheet 2013 Update. Available at: http://www.heart.org/idc/groups/heart-public/@wcm/@sop/@smd/documents/downloadable/ucm_319588.pdf. Accessed August, 2017.
5. Flegal KM, Carroll MD, Kit BK, et al. Prevalence of obesity and trends in the distribution of body mass index among US adults, 1999-2010. JAMA 2012;307(5):491–7.
6. Ogden CL, Carroll MD, Fryar CD, et al. Prevalence of obesity among adults and youth: United States, 2011-2014. NCHS Data Brief 2015;(219):1–8.
7. National Institute of Health. Overweight and obesity statistics. Available at: https://www.niddk.nih.gov/health-information/health-statistics/Pages/overweight-obesity-statistics.aspx#b. Accessed August, 2017.
8. Holick MF. Vitamin D deficiency. N Engl J Med 2007;357(3):266–81.
9. Lips P. Worldwide status of vitamin D nutrition. J Steroid Biochem Mol Biol 2010;121(1–2):297–300.
10. Wahl DA, Cooper C, Ebeling PR, et al. A global representation of vitamin D status in healthy populations. Arch Osteoporos 2012;7:155–72.
11. Looker AC, Johnson CL, Lacher DA, et al. Vitamin D status: United States, 2001–2006. NCHS Data Brief 2011;(59):1–8.
12. Hilger J, Friedel A, Herr R, et al. A systematic review of vitamin D status in populations worldwide. Br J Nutr 2014;111(1):23–45.

13. El-Hajj Fuleihan G, Bouillon R, Clarke B, et al. Serum 25-hydroxyvitamin D levels: variability, knowledge gaps, and the concept of a desirable range. J Bone Miner Res 2015;30(7):1119–33.
14. Bell NH, Epstein S, Greene A, et al. Evidence for alteration of the vitamin D-endocrine system in obese subjects. J Clin Invest 1985;76(1):370–3.
15. Samuel L, Borrell LN. The effect of body mass index on adequacy of serum 25-hydroxyvitamin D levels in US adults: the National Health and Nutrition Examination Survey 2001 to 2006. Ann Epidemiol 2014;24(10):781–4.
16. Carrelli A, Bucovsky M, Horst R, et al. Vitamin D storage in adipose tissue of obese and normal weight women. J Bone Miner Res 2017;32(2):237–42.
17. Shapses SA, Pop LC, Schneider SH. Vitamin D in obesity and weight loss. In nutritional influences on bone health. London: Springer International Publishing; 2016. p. 185–96.
18. Pereira-Santos M, Costa PR, Assis AM, et al. Obesity and vitamin D deficiency: a systematic review and meta-analysis. Obes Rev 2015;16(4):341–9.
19. Hyppönen E, Power C. Hypovitaminosis D in British adults at age 45 y: nationwide cohort study of dietary and lifestyle predictors. Am J Clin Nutr 2007;85(3): 860–8.
20. Schafer AL. Vitamin D and intestinal calcium transport after bariatric surgery. J Steroid Biochem Mol Biol 2017;173:202–10.
21. Wortsman J, Matsuoka LY, Chen TC, et al. Decreased bioavailability of vitamin D in obesity. Am J Clin Nutr 2000;72(3):690–3.
22. Drincic AT, Armas LA, Van Diest EE, et al. Volumetric dilution, rather than sequestration best explains the low vitamin D status of obesity. Obesity (Silver Spring) 2012;20(7):1444–8.
23. Weiner RA. Indications and principles of metabolic surgery. U.S. National Library of Medicine. Chirurg 2010;81(4):379–94.
24. Chikunguw S, Dodson P, Meador J, et al. Durable resolution of diabetes after Roux-en-Y gastric bypass associated with maintenance of weight loss. Surg Obes Relat Dis 2009;5(3):S1.
25. Kaplan LM. Body weight regulation and obesity. J Gastrointest Surg 2003;7(4): 443–51.
26. Kokkinos A, Alexiadou K, Liaskos C, et al. Improvement in cardiovascular indices after Roux-en-Y gastric bypass or sleeve gastrectomy for morbid obesity. Obes Surg 2013;23(1):31–8.
27. Buchwald H, Avidor Y, Braunwald E, et al. Bariatric surgery: a systematic review and meta-analysis. JAMA 2004;292:1724–37.
28. Sjöström L, Narbro K, Sjöström CD, et al. Effects of bariatric surgery on mortality in Swedish obese subjects. N Engl J Med 2007;357(8):741–52.
29. Adams TD, Gress RE, Smith SC, et al. Long-term mortality after gastric bypass surgery. N Engl J Med 2007;357(8):753–61.
30. Sjöström L, Peltonen M, Jacobson P, et al. Bariatric surgery and long-term cardiovascular events. JAMA 2012;307(1):56–65.
31. American Society for Metabolic and Bariatric Surgery (ASMBS). Estimate of bariatric surgery numbers, 2011-2015. Available at: https://asmbs.org/resources/estimate-of-bariatric-surgery-numbers. Accessed August, 2017.
32. Yu EW. Bone metabolism after bariatric surgery. J Bone Miner Res 2014;29(7): 1507–18.
33. American Society for Metabolic and Bariatric Surgery (ASMBS). Metabolic and bariatric surgery. Available at: https://asmbs.org/wp/uploads/2014/05/Metabolic+Bariatric-Surgery.pdf. Accessed August, 2017.

34. American Society for Metabolic and Bariatric Surgery (ASMBS). Bariatric surgery procedures. Available at: https://asmbs.org/patients/bariatric-surgery-procedures. Accessed August, 2017.

35. Stein EM, Silverberg SJ. Bone loss after bariatric surgery: causes, consequences, and management. Lancet Diabetes Endocrinol 2014;2(2):165–74.

36. Bal BS, Finelli FC, Shope TR, et al. Nutritional deficiencies after bariatric surgery. Nat Rev Endocrinol 2012;8(9):544–56.

37. Elms L, Moon RC, Varnadore S, et al. Causes of small bowel obstruction after Roux-en-Y gastric bypass: a review of 2,395 cases at a single institution. Surg Endosc 2014;28(5):1624–8.

38. Saltzman E, Karl JP. Nutrient deficiencies after gastric bypass surgery. Annu Rev Nutr 2013;33:183–203.

39. Devi P, Palanivelu PR. Calcium and vitamin D deficiencies in bariatric surgery. In bariatric surgical practice guide. Singapore: Springer; 2017. p. 289–95.

40. Gillon S, Jeanes YM, Andersen JR, et al. Micronutrient status in morbidly obese patients prior to laparoscopic sleeve gastrectomy and micronutrient changes 5 years post-surgery. Obes Surg 2017;27(3):606–12.

41. Dogan K, Homan J, Aarts EO, et al. Long-term nutritional status in patients following Roux-en-Y gastric bypass surgery. Clin Nutr 2017, in press.

42. Wacker M, Holick MF. Vitamin D - effects on skeletal and extraskeletal health and the need for supplementation. Nutrients 2013;5(1):111–48.

43. Schwartz JB, Kane L, Bikle D. Response of vitamin D concentration to vitamin D3 administration in older adults without sun exposure: a randomized double-blind trial. J Am Geriatr Soc 2016;64(1):65–72.

44. Gallagher JC. Vitamin D and falls - the dosage conundrum. Nat Rev Endocrinol 2016;12(11):680–4.

45. Bikle DD. Vitamin D and bone. Curr Osteoporos Rep 2012;10(2):151–9.

46. Hage MP, El-Hajj Fuleihan G. Bone and mineral metabolism in patients undergoing Roux-en-Y gastric bypass. Osteoporos Int 2014;25(2):423–39.

47. Gregory NS. The effects of bariatric surgery on bone metabolism. Endocrinol Metab Clin North Am 2017;46(1):105–16.

48. Chakhtoura MT, Nakhoul NF, Akl EA, et al. Vitamin D supplementation for obese adults undergoing bariatric surgery. Cochrane Database Syst Rev 2015;(7):CD011800.

49. Chakhtoura MT, Nakhoul N, Akl EA, et al. Guidelines on vitamin D replacement in bariatric surgery: identification and systematic appraisal. Metabolism 2016; 65(4):586–97.

50. Bazuin I, Pouwels S, Houterman S, et al. Improved and more effective algorithms to screen for nutrient deficiencies after bariatric surgery. Eur J Clin Nutr 2017;71(2):198–202.

51. Zhao LJ, Jiang H, Papasian CJ, et al. Correlation of obesity and osteoporosis: effect of fat mass on the determination of osteoporosis. J Bone Miner Res 2008;23(1):17–29.

52. Devlin MJ, Rosen CJ. The bone-fat interface: basic and clinical implications of marrow adiposity. Lancet Diabetes Endocrinol 2015;3(2):141–7.

53. Switzer NJ, Marcil G, Prasad S, et al. Long-term hypovitaminosis D and secondary hyperparathyroidism outcomes of the Roux-en-Y gastric bypass: a systematic review. Obes Rev 2017;18(5):560–6.

54. Gehrer S, Kern B, Peters T, et al. Fewer nutrient deficiencies after laparoscopic sleeve gastrectomy (LSG) than after laparoscopic Roux-Y-gastric bypass (LRYGB) - a prospective study. Obes Surg 2010;20(4):447–53.

55. Lanzarini E, Nogués X, Goday A, et al. High-dose vitamin D supplementation is necessary after bariatric surgery: a prospective 2-year follow-up study. Obes Surg 2015;25(9):1633–8.

56. Chapin BL, LeMar HJ Jr, Knodel DH, et al. Secondary hyperparathyroidism following biliopancreatic diversion. Arch Surg 1996;131(10):1048–52.

57. De Prisco C, Levine SN. Metabolic bone disease after gastric bypass surgery for obesity. Am J Med Sci 2005;329(2):57–61.

58. White MG, Ward M, Applewhite MK, et al. Rates of secondary hyperparathyroidism after bypass operation for super-morbid obesity: an overlooked phenomenon. Surgery 2017;161(3):720–6.

59. Costa TL, Paganotto M, Radominski RB, et al. Calcium metabolism, vitamin D and bone mineral density after bariatric surgery. Osteoporos Int 2015;26(2):757–64.

60. Dix CF, Bauer JD, Wright OR. A systematic review: vitamin D status and sleeve gastrectomy. Obes Surg 2017;27(1):215–25.

61. Folli F, Sabowitz BN, Schwesinger W, et al. Bariatric surgery and bone disease: from clinical perspective to molecular insights. Int J Obes (Lond) 2012;36(11):1373–9.

62. Coates PS, Fernstrom JD, Fernstrom MH, et al. Gastric bypass surgery for morbid obesity leads to an increase in bone turnover and a decrease in bone mass. J Clin Endocrinol Metab 2004;89(3):1061–5.

63. Yu EW, Wewalka M, Ding SA, et al. Effects of gastric bypass and gastric banding on bone remodeling in obese patients with type 2 diabetes. J Clin Endocrinol Metab 2016;101(2):714–22.

64. Yu EW, Bouxsein ML, Roy AE, et al. Bone loss after bariatric surgery: discordant results between DXA and QCT bone density. J Bone Miner Res 2014;29(3):542–50.

65. Berarducci A, Haines K, Murr MM. Incidence of bone loss, falls, and fractures after Roux-en-Y gastric bypass for morbid obesity. Appl Nurs Res 2009;22(1):35–41.

66. Lalmohamed A, de Vries F, Bazelier MT, et al. Risk of fracture after bariatric surgery in the United Kingdom: population based, retrospective cohort study. BMJ 2012;345:e5085.

67. Nakamura KM, Haglind EG, Clowes JA, et al. Fracture risk following bariatric surgery: a population-based study. Osteoporos Int 2014;25(1):151–8.

68. Lu CW, Chang YK, Chang HH, et al. Fracture risk after bariatric surgery: a 12-year nationwide cohort study. Medicine 2015;94(48):e2087.

69. Maghrabi AH, Wolski K, Abood B, et al. Two-year outcomes on bone density and fracture incidence in patients with T2DM randomized to bariatric surgery versus intensive medical therapy. Obesity (Silver Spring) 2015;23(12):2344–8.

70. Yu EW, Lee MP, Landon JE, et al. Fracture risk after bariatric surgery: Roux-en-Y gastric bypass versus adjustable gastric banding. J Bone Miner Res 2017;32(6):1229–36.

71. Rousseau C, Jean S, Gamache P, et al. Change in fracture risk and fracture pattern after bariatric surgery: nested case-control study. BMJ 2016;354:i3794.

72. Rodríguez-Carmona Y, López-Alavez FJ, González-Garay AG, et al. Bone mineral density after bariatric surgery. A systematic review. Int J Surg 2014;12(9):976–82.

73. Ko BJ, Myung SK, Cho KH, et al. Relationship between bariatric surgery and bone mineral density: a meta-analysis. Obes Surg 2016;26(7):1414–21.

74. Quraishi SA, Bittner EA, Blum L, et al. Association between preoperative 25-hydroxyvitamin D level and hospital-acquired infections following Roux-en-Y gastric bypass surgery. JAMA Surg 2014;149(2):112–8.

75. Schaaf C, Gugenheim J. Impact of preoperative serum vitamin D level on postoperative complications and excess weight loss after gastric bypass. Obes Surg 2017;27(8):1982–5.

76. Carlin AM, Yager KM, Rao DS. Vitamin D depletion impairs hypertension resolution after Roux-en-Y gastric bypass. Am J Surg 2008;195(3):349–52.

77. Zittermann A, Ernst JB, Gummert JF, et al. Vitamin D supplementation, body weight and human serum 25-hydroxyvitamin D response: a systematic review. Eur J Nutr 2014;53(2):367–74.

78. Zittermann A, Frisch S, Berthold HK, et al. Vitamin D supplementation enhances the beneficial effects of weight loss on cardiovascular disease risk markers. Am J Clin Nutr 2009;89(5):1321–7.

79. Mason C, Xiao L, Imayama I, et al. Effects of weight loss on serum vitamin D in postmenopausal women. Am J Clin Nutr 2011;94(1):95–103.

80. Rock CL, Emond JA, Flatt SW, et al. Weight loss is associated with increased serum 25-hydroxyvitamin D in overweight or obese women. Obesity (Silver Spring) 2012;20(11):2296–301.

81. Mason C, Xiao L, Imayama I, et al. Vitamin D3 supplementation during weight loss: a double-blind randomized controlled trial. Am J Clin Nutr 2014;99(5): 1015–25.

82. Aarts E, van Groningen L, Horst R, et al. Vitamin D absorption: consequences of gastric bypass surgery. Eur J Endocrinol 2011;164(5):827–32.

83. Peterson LA, Zeng X, Caufield-Noll CP, et al. Vitamin D status and supplementation before and after bariatric surgery: a comprehensive literature review. Surg Obes Relat Dis 2016;12(3):693–702.

84. Aridi HD, Alami RS, Fouani T, et al. Prevalence of vitamin D deficiency in adults presenting for bariatric surgery in Lebanon. Surg Obes Relat Dis 2016;12(2): 405–11.

85. Chakhtoura MT, Nakhoul NN, Shawwa K, et al. Hypovitaminosis D in bariatric surgery: a systematic review of observational studies. Metabolism 2016;65(4): 574–85.

86. Chan LN, Neilson CH, Kirk EA, et al. Optimization of vitamin D status after Roux-en-Y gastric bypass surgery in obese patients living in northern climate. Obes Surg 2015;25(12):2321–7.

87. Vieth R. Critique of the considerations for establishing the tolerable upper intake level for vitamin D: critical need for revision upwards. J Nutr 2006 Apr;136(4): 1117–22.

88. Gallagher JC, Sai A, Templin T 2nd, et al. Dose response to vitamin D supplementation in postmenopausal women: a randomized trial. Ann Intern Med 2012;156(6):425–37.

89. Ross AC, Taylor CL, Yaktine AL, et al. Dietary reference intakes for calcium and vitamin D. Washington, DC: Institute of Medicine (US) Committee to Review Dietary Reference Intakes for Vitamin D and Calcium. Washington, DC: National Academies Press; 2011.

90. Liu C, Wu D, Zhang JF, et al. Changes in bone metabolism in morbidly obese patients after bariatric surgery: a meta-analysis. Obes Surg 2016; 26(1):91–7.

91. Belfiore A, Cataldi M, Minichini L, et al. Short-term changes in body composition and response to micronutrient supplementation after laparoscopic sleeve gastrectomy. Obes Surg 2015;25(12):2344–51.

92. Lancha A, Moncada R, Valenti V, et al. Comparative effects of gastric bypass and sleeve gastrectomy on plasma osteopontin concentrations in humans. Surg Endosc 2014;28(8):2412–20.

93. Ruiz-Tovar J, Oller I, Priego P, et al. Short- and mid-term changes in bone mineral density after laparoscopic sleeve gastrectomy. Obes Surg 2013;23(7):861–6.

94. Lin E, Armstrong-Moore D, Liang Z, et al. Contribution of adipose tissue to plasma 25-hydroxyvitamin D concentrations during weight loss following gastric bypass surgery. Obesity (Silver Spring) 2011;19(3):588–94.

95. Barake M, Daher RT, Salti I, et al. 25-hydroxyvitamin D assay variations and impact on clinical decision making. J Clin Endocrinol Metab 2012;97(3):835–43.

96. Stein EM, Strain G, Sinha N, et al. Vitamin D insufficiency prior to bariatric surgery: risk factors and a pilot treatment study. Clin Endocrinol (Oxf) 2009; 71(2):176–83.

97. Luger M, Kruschitz R, Kienbacher C, et al. Vitamin D3 loading is superior to conventional supplementation after weight loss surgery in vitamin D-deficient morbidly obese patients: a double-blind randomized placebo-controlled trial. Obes Surg 2017;27(5):1196–207.

98. Wolf E, Utech M, Stehle P, et al. Oral high-dose vitamin D dissolved in oil raised serum 25-hydroxy-vitamin D to physiological levels in obese patients after sleeve gastrectomy–a double-blind, randomized, and placebo-controlled trial. Obes Surg 2016;26(8):1821–9.

99. Sundbom M, Berne B, Hultin H. Short-term UVB treatment or intramuscular cholecalciferol to prevent hypovitaminosis D after gastric bypass–a randomized clinical trial. Obes Surg 2016;26(9):2198–203.

100. Carlin AM, Rao DS, Yager KM, et al. Treatment of vitamin D depletion after Roux-en-Y gastric bypass: a randomized prospective clinical trial. Surg Obes Relat Dis 2009;5(4):444–9.

101. Goldner WS, Stoner JA, Lyden E, et al. Finding the optimal dose of vitamin D following Roux-en-Y gastric bypass: a prospective, randomized pilot clinical trial. Obes Surg 2009;19(2):173–9.

102. Dogan K, Aarts EO, Koehestanie P, et al. Optimization of vitamin suppletion after Roux-en-Y gastric bypass surgery can lower postoperative deficiencies: a randomized controlled trial. Medicine 2014;93(25):e169.

103. Muschitz C, Kocijan R, Haschka J, et al. The impact of vitamin D, calcium, protein supplementation, and physical exercise on bone metabolism after bariatric surgery: the BABS study. J Bone Miner Res 2016;31(3): 672–82.

104. Chouiali A, Mallet PL, Fink G, et al. Comparison of two methods for measuring 25-OH vitamin D in the follow-up of patients after bilio-pancreatic diversion bariatric surgery. Clin Biochem 2017;50(4–5):210–6.

105. King RJ, Chandrajay D, Abbas A, et al. High-dose oral cholecalciferol loading in obesity: impact of body mass index and its utility prior to bariatric surgery to treat vitamin D deficiency. Clin Obes 2017;7(2):92–7.

106. Heaney RP. Vitamin D–baseline status and effective dose. N Engl J Med 2012; 367(1):77–8.

107. Vieth R. Vitamin D. In: Feldman D, Glorieux F, editors. The pharmacology of vitamin D, including fortification strategies. 2nd edition. Chapter 61. Available

at: http://truemedmd.com/wp-content/uploads/2014/01/Pharmacology_Vitamin_D_Fortification_Vieth.pdf. Accessed March, 2017.

108. Sakhaee K, Poindexter J, Aguirre C. The effects of bariatric surgery on bone and nephrolithiasis. Bone 2016;84:1–8.

109. Tarplin S, Ganesan V, Monga M. Stone formation and management after bariatric surgery. Nat Rev Urol 2015;12(5):263–70.

110. Vix M, Liu KH, Diana M, et al. Impact of Roux-en-Y gastric bypass versus sleeve gastrectomy on vitamin D metabolism: short-term results from a prospective randomized clinical trial. Surg Endosc 2014;28(3):821–6.

111. Nogues X, Goday A, Pena MJ, et al. Bone mass loss after sleeve gastrectomy: a prospective comparative study with gastric bypass. Cir Esp 2010; 88(2):103–9.

112. Heber D, Greenway FL, Kaplan LM, et al. Endocrine and nutritional management of the post-bariatric surgery patient: an Endocrine Society Clinical Practice Guideline. J Clin Endocrinol Metab 2010;95(11):4823–43.

113. Mechanick JI, Youdim A, Jones DB, et al. Clinical practice guidelines for the perioperative nutritional, metabolic, and nonsurgical support of the bariatric surgery patient 2013 update: cosponsored by American Association of Clinical Endocrinologists, the Obesity Society, and American Society for Metabolic & Bariatric Surgery. Endocr Pract 2013;19(2):337–72.

114. O'Kane M, Pinkney J, Aasheim E, et al. BOMSS guidelines on perioperative and postoperative biochemical monitoring and micronutrient replacement for patients undergoing bariatric surgery. Adopted by BOMSS Council 2014. Available at: http://www.bomss.org.uk/wp-content/uploads/2014/09/BOMSS-guidelines-Final-version1Oct14.pdf. Accessed August, 2017.

115. Fried M, Yumuk V, Oppert JM, et al. Interdisciplinary European guidelines on metabolic and bariatric surgery. Obes Surg 2014;24(1):42–55.

116. O'Kane M, Parretti HM, Hughes CA, et al. Guidelines for the follow-up of patients undergoing bariatric surgery. Clin Obes 2016;6(3):210–24.

117. Ontario Bariatric Network 2016 Available at: http://www.ontariobariatricnetwork.ca/obn-members/obn-directives-protocols/surgical-program/obn-peri-operative-task-force-recommendations-2016-.pdf Accessed August, 2017.

118. Holick MF, Binkley NC, Bischoff-Ferrari HA, et al. Evaluation, treatment, and prevention of vitamin D deficiency: an Endocrine Society clinical practice guideline. J Clin Endocrinol Metab 2011;96(7):1911–30.

119. Hanley DA, Cranney A, Jones G, et al. Vitamin D in adult health and disease: a review and guideline statement from osteoporosis Canada (summary). CMAJ 2010;182(12):1315–9.

120. Maeda SS, Borba VZ, Camargo MB, et al. Recommendations of the Brazilian Society of Endocrinology and Metabology (SBEM) for the diagnosis and treatment of hypovitaminosis D. Arq Bras Endocrinol Metabol 2014;58(5):411–33.

121. Ziegler O, Sirveaux MA, Brunaud L, et al. Medical follow up after bariatric surgery: nutritional and drug issues. General recommendations for the prevention and treatment of nutritional deficiencies. Diabetes Metab 2009;35(6 Pt 2):544–57.

APPENDIX 1: SUMMARY OF ONGOING/COMPLETED OBSERVATIONAL STUDIES AND RANDOMIZED TRIALS ON VITAMIN D IN BARIATRIC SURGERY

Trial Identifier	Principal Investigator Center Country	Study Design/Surgery Type Intervention/Duration	Sample Size (N) Eligibility Criteria	Outcomes (Primary and Secondary)	Start and Completion Dates
Observational Studies					
NCT00627315 First received: February 28, 2008 Last updated: July 28, 2016 Last verified: July 2016	Judith Korner, MD, Associate Professor of Medicine Columbia University United States	Study design: Observational, prospective cohort Intervention: Gastric bypass or GB Duration: 5 y	N: 240 Inclusion criteria: • >18 y of age • Scheduled for bariatric surgery Exclusion criteria: • Vitamin D deficiency • Primary hyperparathyroidism, osteomalacia • Lithium or thiazide diuretics • Untreated hyperthyroidism, liver disease, renal disease, Cushing syndrome, rheumatoid arthritis, myeloma or Paget disease • Antiobesity medications for >2 wk 90 d before study • Any research study 90 d before study • Malabsorption syndromes such as celiac sprue • Previous bariatric surgery	Primary: Change in bone density Secondary: Change in serum calcium and vitamin D and PTH levels	Start date: March 2015 Study completion date: January 2017 Primary completion date: January 2017

NCT01385098 First received: June 28, 2011 Last updated: Sep. 24, 2015 Last verified: August 2013	Vadim Sherman, MD The Methodist Hospital Research Institute Houston, Texas, United States	Study design: Single arm Surgery type: RYGB SG Intervention: Vitamin D_3 supplementation 2000 IU and calcium 1500 mg Duration: 12 wk	N: 23 Inclusion criteria: • Adult women obese patients undergoing either RYGB or SG • BMI >40 kg/m^2 or BMI >35 kg/m^2 with a comorbidity Exclusion criteria: • Vitamin D deficiency (<20 ng/mL) • Hypercalcemia or hypocalcemia • Renal disease • History of primary hyperparathyroidism • Medications that interfere with vitamin D metabolism • Significant sun exposure or travel to sunny climates during the study	Primary: Serum 25(OH)D level Secondary: The percentage response above baseline comparing RYGB and SG patients	Start date: July 2011 Completion date: September 2015 Primary completion date: May 2013

(continued on next page)

(continued)

Trial Identifier	Principal Investigator Center Country	Study Design/Surgery Type Intervention/Duration	Sample Size (N) Eligibility Criteria	Outcomes (Primary and Secondary)	Start and Completion Dates
NCT01637155 First received: July 10, 2012 Last updated: NA Last verified: July 2012	Violeta Moize, MD Hospital Clinic Provincial de Barcelona Spain	Study design: Single group intervention Surgery type: Gastric bypass SG Intervention: Oral cholecalciferol dose of 50,000 IU to determine pharmacokinetics. After 28 d, patients take a period of 90 d of standardization of cholecalciferol based on baseline levels After this period, patients receive a second oral dose of 50,000 IU Duration: 4 mo	N: 44 Inclusion criteria: • ≥18 y old • Gastric bypass in the last 18 mo (±6 mo) • BMI 25–33 kg/m^2 • 25(OH)D level <20 ng/mL • Clinically stable Exclusion criteria: • Pregnancy, lactation • Menopause • High liver function test • Renal disease or previous renal lithiasis • Digestive disease to suggest malabsorption, granulomatous diseases, diabetic gastroenteropathy • Medication likely to interfere with the absorption of vitamin D, calcium, and bone metabolism, such as corticosteroids and anticonvulsants • Cholecalciferol hypersensitivity	Primary: Comparison of the pharmacokinetic parameters of vitamin D Secondary: • Secondary hyperparathyroidism • Urinary calcium and creatinine • Changes in total protein, albumin, phosphorus, magnesium and calcium, alkaline phosphatase levels • Change in body fat • Change in adherence in both surgeries • Adverse events	NA

NCT01871389 First received: June 4, 2013 Last updated: May 7, 2014 Last verified: May 2014	Lee Mallory Boylan, MD Professor Texas Tech University United States	Study design: Observational Surgery type: Gastric bypass Intervention: Monthly high-dose cholecalciferol (dose NA) Duration: 6 mo	N: 31 Inclusion criteria: • Morbidly obese meeting criteria for gastric bypass • Age >18 y Exclusion criteria: • Medications that affect vitamin D status, increased 25(OH)D or calcium level	Primary: Serum 25(OH)D$_3$	Start date: February 2012 Completion date: August 2013 Primary completion date: August 2013
NCT01910792 First received: June 25, 2012 Last updated: January 11, 2016 Last verified: January 2016	Michael F Holick, PhD, MD Boston University Medical Center United States	Study design: Nonrandomized, open label, parallel assignment Surgery type: Gastric bypass Intervention: Group 1: patients with fat malabsorption syndromes use a UV lamp at home 3 times per week Group 2: patients with gastric bypass use a UV lamp at home 3 times per week Duration: 12 wk	N: 60 Inclusion criteria: • Men and women, age 18 y or older with skin types 2–5 • Fat malabsorption Exclusion criteria: • Treatment with vitamin D • Pregnancy and lactation • History of underlying photosensitivity, or skin type I (develop skin burns after UVB exposure) • History of chronic disease • Medications that cause photosensitivity or influence vitamin D metabolism • History of skin cancer • History of hypocalcemia, hypercalcemia • History of renal, hepatic, hematological, gastrointestinal, endocrine, pulmonary, cardiac, neurologic, or cerebral disease within 3 mo • Travel to sunny climate without sunscreen during 1 mo of the study start	Primary: Vitamin D status Secondary: Erythema	Start date: March 2011 Completion date: February 2014 Primary completion date: February 2014

(continued on next page)

(continued)

Trial Identifier	Principal Investigator Center Country	Study Design/Surgery Type Intervention/Duration	Sample Size (N) Eligibility Criteria	Outcomes (Primary and Secondary)	Start and Completion Dates
Randomized Studies					
NCT01138475 First received: June 4, 2010 Last updated: August 11, 2016 Last verified: August 2016	Kerstyn Zalesin, MD William Beaumont Hospitals Royal Oak, Michigan, United States	Study design: Randomized, double-blind parallel assignment Surgery type: RYGB Intervention: Group 1: paricalcitol 1 μg by mouth daily Group 2: cholecalciferol 5000 IU by mouth daily Group 3: placebo inactive substance, 1 capsule daily Duration: 6 wk	N: 55 Inclusion criteria: • After RYGB (>6 wk and ≤5 y) • >18 y • Negative pregnancy test for women • Normal serum levels of calcium, phosphorous, albumin, iPTH Exclusion criteria: • Vitamin D treatment or allergy to vitamin D • Pregnancy or lactating women • Renal disease or stones • History of hypercalcemia, hyperphosphatemia, or primary hyperparathyroidism • Malignancy within less than 1 year (except nonmelanoma skin cancer) or any history of bone metastasis • Comorbid conditions (malignancy, liver disease) with a life expectancy <1 y • Use of another investigational drug • Poorly controlled hypertension • Drugs affecting the bone or immunosuppressant therapy, steroids, inhibitors or inducers of cytochrome • HIV positive	Primary: Change from baseline in iPTH over 6 wk Secondary: Vitamin and mineral levels and laboratory surveillance	Start date: July 2010 Completion date: August 2015 Primary completion date: August 2015

			Primary/Secondary Outcomes	Dates
NCT02212652 First received: August 6, 2014 Last updated: August 29, 2016 Last verified: August 2016	Kimberley E Steele, MD, PhD Johns Hopkins University United States	Study design: Randomized, double-blind parallel assignment Surgery type: RYGB Vertical SG Intervention: Group 1: vitamin D$_3$ chewable gels 10,000 IU daily Group 2: placebo, gummy button Duration: Intervention duration: 30 d Study duration: 1 y	• History of drug or alcohol abuse, liver or kidney transplant • History of CVA within the last 3 mo N: 70 Inclusion criteria: • RYGBP or vertical SG • 18–64 y of age • BMI of 35–49.9 kg/m² • Serum 25(OH)D concentration <30 ng/mL preoperatively Exclusion criteria: • Dietary restriction for beef gelatin • Expected poor compliance with the medical regimen • Medical conditions that could jeopardize the safety of the subject or the integrity of the study • Pregnancy Primary: Improved postoperative serum 25(OH)D concentration Secondary: • Adverse surgical outcomes[a] • Clinical outcomes[b]	Start date: January 2017 Estimated primary completion date: April 2020
NCT02477956 First received: May 12, 2014 Last updated: June 22, 2015 Last verified: June 2015	David Syn, MD Texas Tech University Health Sciences Center United States	Study design: Randomized, single-blind (investigator), parallel assignment Surgery type: Bariatric surgery (type not specified) Intervention: Dietary supplement: vitamin D$_3$ (Replesta) 2 tablets (100,000 IU/mo) Active comparator: control, standard vitamin D Duration: 6 mo	N: 31 Inclusion criteria: • Morbidly obese and eligible for bariatric surgery Exclusion criteria: • <18 and >60 y of age • Increased serum vitamin D and calcium levels • Pregnant and lactating women Primary: Difference in mean serum 25(OH)D level between groups	Start date: November 2012 Completion date: December 2013 Primary completion date: November 2013

(continued on next page)

(continued)

Trial Identifier	Principal Investigator Center Country	Study Design/Surgery Type Intervention/Duration	Sample Size (N) Eligibility Criteria	Outcomes (Primary and Secondary)	Start and Completion Dates
NCT02483026 First received: April 18, 2015 Last updated: March 6, 2017 Last verified: March 2017	Ram Elazary, MD Head bariatric surgeon Hadassah Ein Cerem Medical Center Israel	Study design: Randomized, double-blind parallel assignment Surgery type: SG Intervention: Supplements care 6 wk presurgery Group 1: multivitamin and vitamin D Group 2: placebo and vitamin D (dose NA) Duration: 1 y	N: 250 Inclusion criteria: • SG • BMI >35 kg/m^2 with comorbidity or >40 kg/m^2 • Vitamin D deficiency before surgery Exclusion criteria: • Previous bariatric surgery • Psychiatric illness • Endocrine problem that affects the weight that is unbalanced • Chronic kidney disease, nephrolithiasis • Metabolic bone disease before surgery, calcium disorders • Pregnancy, breastfeeding • Medications or disease affecting calcium or bone metabolism • Nutritional supplements 2 wk before the study	Primary: Bone density by DXA 1 y after surgery Secondary: • Weight (kg), % excess weight loss • 25(OH)D level (ng/mL) • Vitamin B$_{12}$ level (pg/dL) • Iron level (μg/dL) • PTH level (pg/mL) • Folate level (ng/mL)	Anticipated start date: May 2017 Estimated completion date: October 2019 Estimated primary completion date: October 2018

NCT02817256 First received: June 19, 2016 Last updated: June 26, 2016 Last verified: June 2016	Juma Alkaabi, MD College of Medicine and Health Sciences, United Arab Emirates University United Arab Emirates	Study design: Randomized, double-blind parallel assignment Surgery type: SG Intervention: Group 1: ergocalciferol 300,000 IM every 3 mo; oral, vitamin B_{12} tablets daily (500 µg) calcium/D tables 600–200 mg, iron preparation (47 mg) daily Group 2: ergocalciferol 50,000 IU once every 2 wk, vitamin B_{12} 1000 µg IM every 3 mo, calcium/D tablets 600–200 mg, iron preparation (47 mg) daily Duration: 1 y	N: 105 Inclusion criteria: • 18–60 y • No medical or psychiatric contraindications • BMI>35 kg/m^2 with comorbidities or BMI >40 kg/m^2 before the bariatric surgery Exclusion criteria: • Micronutrient deficiency that requires treatment • Documented poor compliance • Inflammatory bowel disease, malignant or debilitating medical conditions • Hemoglobinopathies or pernicious anemia • Renal stones or history of hypercalcemia • Significant long-standing medical complications that affect micronutrient status • Severe psychiatric illness • Women who are lactating, pregnant, or planning pregnancy	Primary: Change in iron level Secondary: Complications resulting from IM injections Change in level of uric acid, calcium, vitamin A, vitamin D, serum folate, vitamin B_{12}, serum methyl malonate	Start date: October 2016 Estimated completion date: November 2018 Estimated primary completion date: November 2017

(continued on next page)

(continued)

Trial Identifier	Principal Investigator Center Country	Study Design/Surgery Type Intervention/Duration	Sample Size (N) Eligibility Criteria	Outcomes (Primary and Secondary)	Start and Completion Dates
NCT02686905 First received: February 4, 2016 Last updated: September 29, 2016 Last verified: September 2016	Rebecca McDorman, graduate student California State Polytechnic University, Pomona United States	Study design: Randomized, double-blind parallel assignment Surgery type: RYGB Vertical SG Intervention: Group 1: • PatchMD Vitamin D₃/Calcium Patch • PatchMD Multivitamin Patch • PatchMD B12 Energy Plus Patch Group 2: • Chewable Multivitamin with Iron • Chewable calcium • Quick Dissolve B₁₂ (dose NA) Duration: 3 mo	N: 30 Inclusion criteria: • Vertical SG or gastric bypass • Nonpregnant women Exclusion criteria: • Metal objects in the body • Weight >270 kg (600 lb) • Revision surgery	Primary: Glucose (mg/dL) Calcium (mg/dL) Ferritin (ng/mL) B₁₂ (pg/mL) Vitamin D (ng/mL) Hemoglobin A1c (%) Fat mass (kg) Weight (kg); Waist circumference (cm) Hip circumference (cm) Stadiometer measurement (cm) Total body water (kg)	Study date: January 2016 Estimated completion date: June 2017 Estimated primary completion date: June 2017

Abbreviations: CVA, cerebrovascular accident; HIV, human immunodeficiency virus; iPTH, intact PTH; UV, ultraviolet.

A search was conducted on August 11 for all trials completed before 2017, and no results were published.

[a] Surgical site infection, wound separation and dehiscence, anastomotic leak, prolonged length of hospital stay (>3 days), and readmittance to the hospital within 30 days postoperatively.

[b] Wound healing, weight loss, nutritional status, resolution of comorbidities, and other key markers of health, such as vital signs (eg, fever, blood pressure, heart rate, pain) and return of a regular menstrual cycle.

Data from ClinicalTrials.gov and the WHO International Clinical Trials Registry Platform (ICTRP) (March 2017); search strategy: vitamin D AND (bariatric surgery gastric bypass OR sleeve gastrectomy OR gastric banding OR weight loss surgery.)

The Use of Vitamin D Metabolites and Analogues in the Treatment of Chronic Kidney Disease

Ladan Zand, MD[a],*, Rajiv Kumar, MD[a,b],*

KEYWORDS

- Vitamin D analogues • Chronic kidney disease • End-stage renal disease

KEY POINTS

- Secondary hyperparathyroidism and mixed-uremic osteodystrophy are common in chronic kidney disease (CKD) and end-stage renal disease (ESRD).
- Reduced concentrations of 1,25-dihydroxyvitamin D, intestinal malabsorption of calcium, and negative calcium balance contribute to secondary hyperparathyroidism in these conditions.
- A stepwise approach of reducing serum phosphate concentrations with the use of phosphate binders such as sevelamer, calcium salts (eg, calcium acetate, calcium carbonate), lanthanum carbonate, or various iron preparations (ferric citrate, sucroferric oxyhydroxide); correcting negative calcium balance with 1α-hydroxylated vitamin D analogues; and using calcium-sensing receptor agonists such as cinacalcet is generally effective in correcting secondary hyperparathyroidism in CKD and ESRD.
- Treatment with 1-hydroxylated vitamin D metabolites or analogues such as calcitriol, alfacalcidol, doxercalciferol, paricalcitol, maxacalcitol, and falecalcitriol is effective in the treatment of secondary hyperparathyroidism seen in CKD and ESRD.

THE SPECTRUM CHRONIC KIDNEY DISEASE-MINERAL BONE DISORDER
Skeletal Abnormalities in Patients with Chronic Kidney Disease

Alterations in skeletal, cardiovascular, and neurologic function occur in chronic kidney disease (CKD) and end-stage renal disease (ESRD). Abnormalities in bone and mineral metabolism result not only in changes in the skeleton but also alterations in vascular and soft tissue calcification; the entire syndrome is referred to as CKD-mineral bone disorder (MBD).[1] The role of abnormalities in the vitamin D endocrine system is most clearly defined in the pathogenesis of bone disease in CKD-ESRD.[2–4] The salutary

The authors have nothing to disclose.
[a] Division of Nephrology and Hypertension, Department of Medicine, Mayo Clinic, 200 First Street SW, Rochester, MN 55901, USA; [b] Department of Biochemistry and Molecular Biology, Mayo Clinic, 200 First Street SW, Rochester, MN 55901, USA
* Corresponding authors.
E-mail addresses: Zand.ladan@mayo.edu (L.Z.); rkumar@mayo.edu (R.K.)

Endocrinol Metab Clin N Am 46 (2017) 983–1007
http://dx.doi.org/10.1016/j.ecl.2017.07.008
0889-8529/17/© 2017 Elsevier Inc. All rights reserved.

endo.theclinics.com

effects of vitamin D analogues are most apparent in the treatment of disorders of CKD-ESRD–associated bone disease and are of unknown value in the treatment of vascular and soft tissue calcification. When assessed by bone histomorphometry and the rate of bone mineralization, renal osteodystrophy comprises several groups, including secondary hyperparathyroidism of varying severity, mixed uremic osteodystrophy, osteomalacia, and adynamic bone disease.[1,5–11] Hyperparathyroidism is the most frequent type of renal osteodystrophy and is most responsive to therapy with vitamin D analogues. Although hyperparathyroidism is readily detectable by the time the glomerular filtration rate (GFR) reaches 40 to 50 mL/min/1.73 m^2 in both adults[7,11–13] and children,[14,15] histologic changes in bone in the form of abnormal woven osteoid have been described when the GFR has declined to only 80 mL/min/1.73 m^2.[12] Phosphate retention,[7,16–24] a decline in concentrations of the active metabolite of vitamin D, $1\alpha,25$-dihydroxyvitamin D_3 ($1\alpha,25(OH)_2D_3$),[3,4,25–32] with an attendant decrease in intestinal calcium absorption,[33–36] increased fibroblast growth factor (FGF)-23 concentrations,[37–42] and diminished acid excretion by the kidney[43–45] occur when the GFR has decreased to 30 to 50 mL/min/1.73 m^2, and contribute in interrelated ways to the pathogenesis of CKD-MBD. This article briefly reviews some aspects of vitamin D metabolism[46–63] and describes abnormalities that are known to occur in the context of CKD-ESRD. (See J. Wesley Pike and Sylvia Christakos's article "Biology and Mechanisms of Action of the Vitamin D Hormone," in this issue.) The value of various vitamin D analogues in the treatment of CKD-MBD is subsequently discussed.

THE PATHOPHYSIOLOGY OF THE VITAMIN D ENDOCRINE SYSTEM IN CHRONIC KIDNEY DISEASE AND END-STAGE RENAL DISEASE

The major physiologic role of vitamin D, through the action of its active metabolite $1\alpha,25(OH)_2D$, is the maintenance of normal calcium and phosphorus balance.[64–67] Many other biological effects of $1\alpha,25(OH)_2D$ have been described such as the modulation of immune function,[60,68] muscle function,[50,58,69] and cell growth and differentiation[52,54,70] but are not relevant to the pathogenesis of CKD-MBD.

The Generation of Vitamin D in the Skin Is Impaired in Uremia

The endogenous form of vitamin D, vitamin D_3 (cholecalciferol), is formed in the skin as a result of photolysis of the precursor sterol, 7-dehydrocholesterol (DHC)[71–79] (Fig. 1). Ultraviolet light cleaves the B-ring of 7-DHC, giving rise to previtamin D_3, which undergoes equilibration to vitamin D_3.[77–79] Vitamin D_3, bound to vitamin D-binding protein (group-specific component), to which it preferentially binds relative to its precursor, previtamin D_3, exits the skin and enters the circulation.[78] In plants, a precursor sterol, ergosterol, is converted by photolysis to ergocalciferol or vitamin D_2.[72,80,81] In mammals, vitamin D_2 and vitamin D_3 have similar metabolic transformations and equivalent bioactivities. For purposes of this discussion, the term vitamin D refers to both vitamin D_2 and vitamin D_3. The photolytic conversion of 7-DHC to vitamin D_3 is impaired in CKD-ESRD in humans.[82] In uremic white subjects, plasma vitamin D was similar to that seen in normal white subjects but was not detectable in 70% of uremic black subjects studied. Following ultraviolet-B irradiation, the increase in plasma vitamin D was depressed in white subjects on dialysis when compared with healthy white subjects. 7-DHC content was similar in epidermis from site-matched skin of uremic and normal subjects. The precise reason for the impaired production of vitamin D_3 in the skin of uremic subjects is unknown, although one might speculate that the accumulation of various pigments might play a role. Low serum concentrations of vitamin D contribute to a decrease in and circulating concentrations of 25-hydroxyvitamin D, or 25(OH)D.

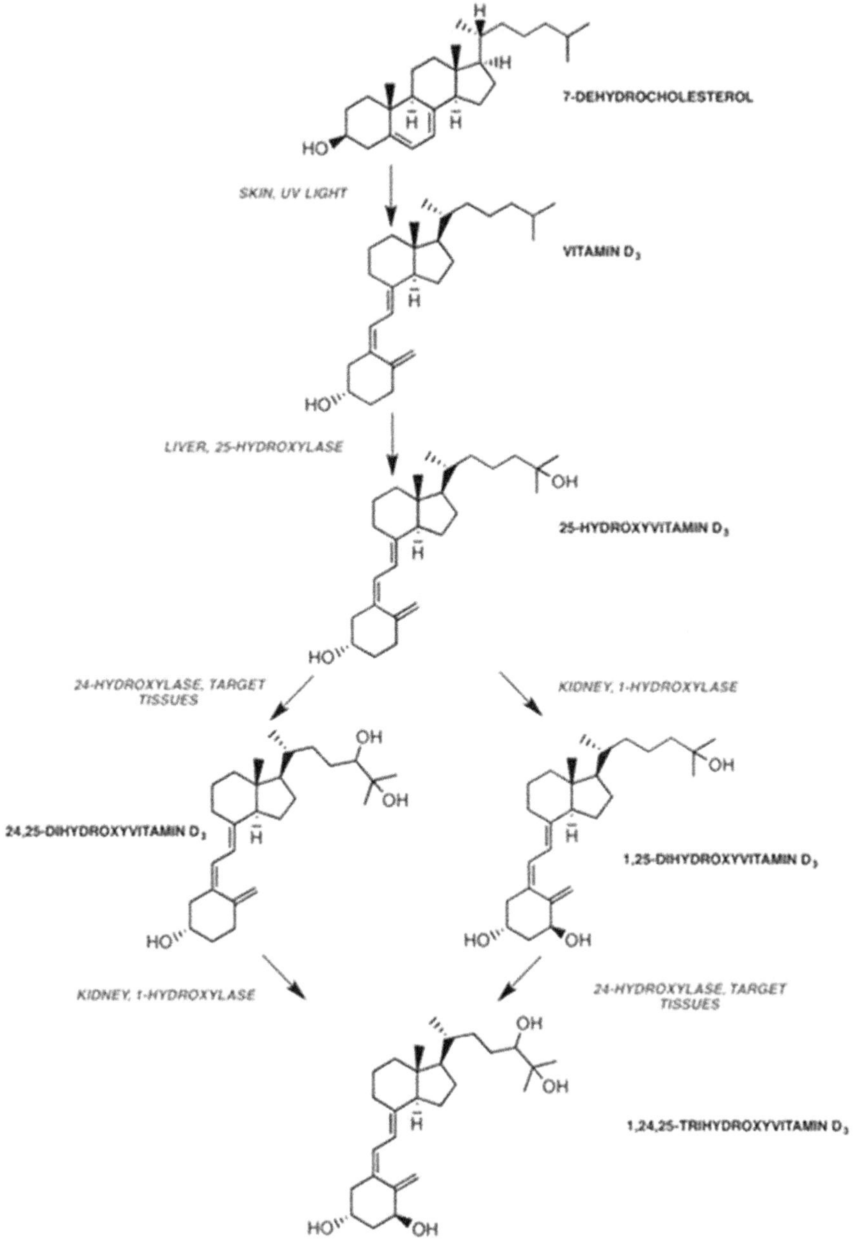

Fig. 1. Metabolism of vitamin D$_3$. UV, ultraviolet.

25-Hydroxyvitamin D Concentrations Are Reduced in Chronic Kidney Disease and End-Stage Renal Disease

Vitamin D is metabolized in the liver microsomes and mitochondria to 25(OH)D$_3$ by the vitamin D$_3$-25-hydroxylase[63,83–93] (see **Fig. 1**). The vitamin D-25-hydroxylase is only partially inhibited by its product, and increasing amounts of administered vitamin D are associated with increases in 25(OH)D. 25(OH)D is the major circulating vitamin

D metabolite,[62–64,75,94,95] and measurements of its concentration are an excellent index of vitamin D nutritional status.[96–99] In CKD, 25(OH)D concentrations are frequently diminished and increase with the administration of vitamin D_3.[100–114] The diminished concentrations of 25(OH)D may be related to a decrease in nutritional intake, a decrease in sun exposure, a reduction in the generation of vitamin D_3 from 7-DHC,[82] or a loss of vitamin D binding protein in proteinuric patients. Lower levels of 25(OH)D have been associated with increased risk of progression of renal disease and mortality.[110,115] 25(OH)D-1α-hydroxylase enzyme activity is present in tissues other than the kidney[116–118] and increased amounts of substrate may result in the generation of 1α,25(OH)$_2$D locally. Therefore, some clinicians have advocated the use of vitamin D supplementation in patients with CKD and ESRD. Before 1α,25(OH)$_2$D$_3$ was available for clinical use, 25(OH)D supplementation was used to suppress parathyroid hormone (PTH) levels in dialysis patients.[119] A meta-analysis of observational and randomized controlled trials has shown that vitamin D supplementation results in a small reduction in PTH level in both CKD and dialysis patients.[107] In a recent randomized controlled trial of 105 dialysis subjects comparing 2 different doses of ergocalciferol with placebo, ergocalciferol did not alter calcium, phosphorous, or PTH levels compared with placebo during a 12-week period.[109] Given these results, the use of vitamin D supplementation in dialysis patients is not recommended. Vitamin D supplementation can be considered in patients with early stages of CKD, in which residual 25(OH)D 1α-hydroxylase enzyme may still be present.

Reduced Intestinal Calcium Absorption and Serum 1α,25-Dihydroxyvitamin-D Is Present in Patients with Chronic Kidney Disease and End-Stage Renal Disease

In CKD and ESRD there is a decrease in the intestinal calcium absorption with concomitant negative calcium balance.[33–36] Reduced serum concentrations of 1α,25(OH)$_2$D[3,4,25–32] are present. The central role of 1α,25(OH)$_2$D in maintaining calcium balance in CKD-ESRD is demonstrated by the observations that not only are 1α,25(OH)$_2$D concentrations reduced in CKD-ESRD but that 1α,25(OH)$_2$D readily increases intestinal calcium transport[121,122] and mobilizes calcium from bone,[123] whereas pharmacologic amounts of precursors, such as vitamin D itself, or intermediary metabolites, such as 25(OH)D, are required to elicit a biological response in anephric animals and patients.[26,123,124] The following sections discuss how 1α,25(OH)$_2$D is synthesized, how the processes are regulated, and what perturbations occur in CKD-ESRD that inhibit the formation of 1α,25(OH)$_2$D.

In states of calcium demand, 25(OH)D is metabolized by the renal 25(OH)D-1α-hydroxylase to the biologically active vitamin D metabolite, 1α,25(OH)$_2$D, in the kidney by PTH-dependent processes[59,64,75,121,122,124–133] (Fig. 2A). Increased concentrations of 1α,25(OH)$_2$D enhance the expression of genes required for the transport of calcium across the enterocyte[134,135] and in the distal convoluted tubule of the kidney. Calcium is absorbed by the intestine by passive paracellular and active transcellular mechanisms.[135–137] Active calcium absorption is 1α,25(OH)$_2$D-dependent, is transcellular, and requires the expenditure of energy.[138,139] Several vitamin D–dependent proteins, each with a specific function, play a role in the movement of calcium across the apical membrane, the enterocyte cytoplasm, and the basal lateral membrane. These include the epithelial calcium or transient receptor potential vanilloid (TRPV) 5 or 6 channels (at the apical membrane), calbindin D_{9K} and D_{28K} (within the cell), and the plasma membrane calcium pump (at the basal lateral membrane).[140] Deletions of TrpV6 and calbindin D_{9K} genes are not associated with alterations in intestinal calcium transport in vivo in the basal state and following the administration of 1α,25(OH)$_2$D,[141,142] although a report suggests that basal calcium transport is normal in TrpV6 knockout mice but

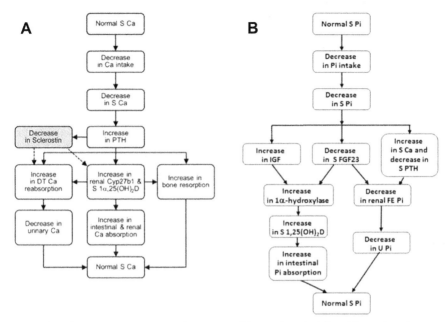

Fig. 2. Physiologic compensation in the setting of hypocalcemia (*A*) and hypophosphatemia (*B*). (*A*) A decrease in serum calcium results in an increase in PTH concentrations that ultimately normalizes serum calcium concentrations by enhancing bone resorption, decreasing urinary calcium excretion, and increasing intestinal calcium absorption through an increase $1\alpha,25(OH)_2D$ concentrations. (*B*) A decrease in serum phosphorous decreases FGF23 and increases in insulin-like growth factor (IGF), which together increase $1\alpha,25(OH)_2D$ concentrations and increase intestinal and renal phosphorous absorption and reabsorption, resulting in a normalization of serum phosphorous. Ca, calcium; FE, fractional excretion; Pi, phosphate.

adaptations to a low calcium diet are impaired.[143] Deletion of the *Pmca1* in the intestine is associated with reduced growth and bone mineralization, and a failure to upregulate calcium absorption in response to $1\alpha,25(OH)_2D_3$, thereby establishing the essential role of the pump in transcellular calcium transport.[144] In states of calcium sufficiency, $1\alpha,25(OH)_2D$ synthesis is reduced, and the synthesis of $24R,25(OH)_2D$,[145–147] a vitamin D metabolite of reduced but uncertain activity, is increased.

Serum phosphate concentrations also regulate the synthesis of $1\alpha,25(OH)_2D$ by PTH-independent mechanisms.[148] Thus, when serum phosphate concentrations are diminished and in states of phosphorous demand, $25(OH)D$ is metabolized to $1\alpha,25(OH)_2D$ and the synthesis of $24R,25(OH)_2D$ is reduced[63,127,148–158] (see **Fig. 2B**). The converse occurs in hyperphosphatemic states. A decrease in serum phosphate concentration is associated with an increase in ionized calcium, a decrease in PTH secretion, and a subsequent decrease in renal phosphate excretion. An increase in renal $25(OH)D$ 1α-hydroxylase activity, increased $1\alpha,25(OH)_2D$ synthesis, and increased phosphorus absorption in the intestine and reabsorption in the kidney occur. In the intestine and kidney, $1\alpha,25(OH)_2D$ regulates the expression of the sodium-phosphate cotransporters IIb, and IIA, and IIc, respectively, thereby regulating the efficiency of phosphate absorption in enterocytes and proximal tubule cells.[140,159–161]

The bioactivity of vitamin D depends on the formation of $1\alpha,25(OH)_2D$. Pharmacologic amounts of precursors, such as vitamin D itself, or intermediary metabolites, such as 25(OH)D, are required to elicit a biological response in anephric animals and patients.[26,123,124] In such individuals, $1\alpha,25(OH)_2D$ readily increases intestinal calcium transport[121,122] and mobilizes calcium from bone.[123] The actions of $1\alpha,25(OH)_2D_3$ require the presence of the vitamin D receptor (VDR), a steroid hormone receptor that binds $1\alpha,25(OH)_2D_3$ with high affinity, and other vitamin D metabolites with lower affinities.[162–165] Following binding of the ligand, $1\alpha,25(OH)_2D_3$ to the VDR, a conformational change in the receptor is associated with the recruitment of other steroid hormone receptors, such as the retinoid x receptor α, and various coactivator (or corepressor) proteins to the transcription start side of $1\alpha,25(OH)_2D_3$-regulated genes.[166–174] (See J. Wesley Pike and Sylvia Christakos's article "Biology and Mechanisms of Action of the Vitamin D Hormone," in this issue.) Several calcium-regulating genes are induced or repressed in vitamin D–responsive target tissues, such as the intestine, kidney, parathyroid gland, and bone.[66,69,175–180]

Retention of Phosphate and Reductions in Renal Mass Are Responsible for Reduced $1\alpha,25$-Dihydroxyvitamin-D Synthesis

As GFR declines (usually less 50 mL/min/SA), hyperphosphatemia develops that is accompanied by hypocalcemia, secondary hyperparathyroidism, a reduction in $1\alpha,25(OH)_2D$ concentrations, and an elevation in FGF 23 (FGF23) levels. The retention of phosphate with decreasing GFR[20,24,181–186] and a reduction in the number of tubular cells[2–4,25,100,187] in which the synthesis of $1\alpha,25(OH)_2D$ occurs are major determinants in evolution of low serum $1\alpha,25(OH)_2D$ concentrations (**Fig. 3**). Decreased phosphate excretion and increased serum phosphate concentrations enhance the production of the phosphaturic factor, FGF23,[42,188] which inhibits the production of $1\alpha,25(OH)_2D$.[189,190] Hyperparathyroidism occurs as a result of reduced concentrations of $1\alpha,25(OH)_2D$ and the attendant negative calcium balance from reduced intestinal calcium absorption, and as a result of loss of inhibition of PTH synthesis

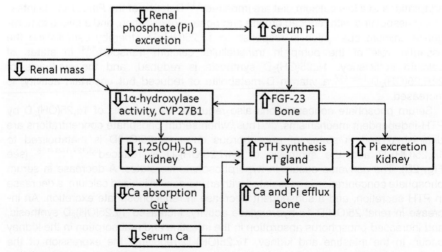

Fig. 3. Reductions in $1\alpha,25(OH)_2D$ concentrations in patients with CKD results from both a reduction in renal mass and an increase in FGF23 levels in response to increases in serum phosphorous concentrations.

associated with the low serum concentrations of $1\alpha,25(OH)_2D$ and decreased parathyroid gland VDR concentrations.[20,191–200]

VITAMIN D ANALOGUES IN THE TREATMENT OF HYPERPARATHYROIDISM IN CHRONIC KIDNEY DISEASE AND END-STAGE RENAL DISEASE

A combined approach aimed at reducing serum phosphate concentrations, improving the negative calcium balance, and inhibiting PTH secretion is required for the effective treatment of hyperparathyroidism in the context of CKD-ESRD. The authors favor a stepwise approach of first reducing serum phosphate concentrations with the use of phosphate binders, such as sevelamer, calcium salts (eg, calcium acetate, calcium carbonate), lanthanum carbonate, or various iron preparations (ferric citrate, sucroferric oxyhydroxide); correcting the negative calcium balance with the use of various 1α-hydroxylated vitamin D analogues; and, finally, using calcium-sensing receptor agonists, such as cinacalcet. The following section describes the use of various vitamin D analogues in the treatment of CKD-MBD in the context of CKD-ESRD. The structures of various compounds used in this regard are shown in **Fig. 4**.

Calcitriol

Calcitriol, or $1\alpha,25(OH)_2D_3$, is the naturally occurring, active form of vitamin D that is available for use in CKD-ESRD patients. Its primary use is to suppress the synthesis of PTH and growth of the PTH gland. An unwanted side effect is increase in calcium and phosphorous levels through its action on the intestine. Both oral and intravenous formulations have been used. Multiple small clinical trials have compared the efficacy of oral versus intravenous calcitriol in patients with ESRD.[201–206] Most studies have shown that oral calcitriol is as effective as intravenous calcitriol in reducing PTH

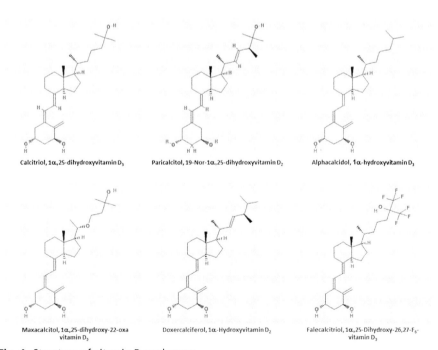

Calcitriol, 1α,25-dihydroxyvitamin D₃   Paricalcitol, 19-Nor-1α,25-dihydroxyvitamin D₂   Alphacalcidol, 1α-hydroxyvitamin D₃

Maxacalcitol, 1α,25-dihydroxy-22-oxa vitamin D₃   Doxercalciferol, 1α-Hydroxyvitamin D₂   Falecalcitriol, 1α,25-Dihydroxy-26,27-F₆-vitamin D₃

Fig. 4. Structure of vitamin D analogues.

concentrations with similar rates of hypercalcemia and hyperphosphatemia. In the most recent meta-analysis of 9 randomized controlled trials, similar findings were noted.[207] Based on the available data, either intravenous or oral formulations are reasonable choices when treating ESRD patients with secondary hyperparathyroidism. The intravenous formulation is more commonly used in the United States, whereas the oral formulation is more frequently used in other countries. The intravenous formulation is more expensive but does ensure adherence. These issues need to be taken into account when deciding on what route to choose.

Paricalcitol

Paricalcitol, or $1,25(OH)_2$-19-nor-D_2, is a vitamin D_2 analogue that lacks the methylene group on the A ring of the sterol. It was the first analogue to be approved for use in patients with CKD. In animal models it is shown to cause equivalent suppression of PTH relative to calcitriol but with less hypercalcemia and hyperphosphatemia.[208] In uremic rat models, paricalcitol has shown to improve the bone histology.[209] In placebo-controlled trials of paricalcitol in dialysis subjects, 68% of subjects treated with paricalcitol achieved 30% reduction in PTH as opposed to 8% of control subjects, and there were few hypercalcemic events recorded in the subjects treated with the drug.[210] Paricalcitol also resulted in a reduction in the bone turnover marker, alkaline phosphatase.[210] In another placebo-controlled trial, paricalcitol resulted in hypercalcemia mainly in subjects who had significant reduction in their PTH concentrations, often with levels less than 100 pg/ml.[211] In a double-blind randomized study comparing calcitriol with paricalcitol in dialysis subjects, those treated with paricalcitol had lower PTH levels at the end of the study and achieved target PTH levels faster with fewer episodes of hypercalcemia and lower calcium x phosphate product compared with those treated with calcitriol.[212] In a large retrospective cohort study of dialysis subjects, those treated with paricalcitol were shown to have a survival advantage compared with those treated with calcitriol.[213] In adjusted models, survival was 16% (95% confidence interval 10%–21%) lower in paricalcitol group compared with calcitriol group. The percentage increase in serum calcium and phosphorous was also lower in those who received paricalcitol compared with calcitriol. This survival advantage, however, has not been evaluated in any randomized controlled trials, and the results of this retrospective study should be interpreted with caution.

Doxercalciferol

Doxercalciferol, or 1α-$(OH)D_2$, is converted to the active form, $1\alpha,25(OH)_2D_2$ through the action of 25-hydroxylase in the liver. Clinical studies of doxercalciferol have shown it to be effective in suppressing PTH levels but have also shown a modest increase in serum calcium and phosphorous levels.[214,215] An intravenous preparation of doxercalciferol is available, and the drug was found to be effective in suppressing PTH with lower rates of hypercalcemia and hyperphosphatemia than 1α-$(OH)D_2$.[216] In a small clinical study comparing the dosing of doxercalciferol with paricalcitol, dosing doxercalciferol at 60% of the dose of paricalcitol resulted in similar reduction in PTH level.[217] In another study comparing doxercalciferol with paricalcitol, doxercalciferol was found to produce a similar reduction in PTH levels and was associated with higher rates of hyperphosphatemia or the calcium X phosphate product.[218]

Alfacalcidol

Alfacalcidol, or 1α-$(OH)D_3$, is converted to the active form, $1\alpha,25(OH)_2D_3$, in the liver. A study comparing alfacalcidol with calcitriol showed that at doses 1.5 to 2 times that of calcitriol, alfacalcidol is equally effective in suppressing PTH with a similar rate of hypercalcemia and hyperphosphatemia.[219] In a randomized crossover trial comparing alfacalcidol with paricalcitol in ESRD patients, alfacalcidol was shown to be as effective in suppressing PTH levels with similar rates of hypercalcemia and hyperphosphatemia as paricalcitol.[220]

Maxacalcitol

The structure of maxacalcitol, or 22-Oxa-1,25(OH)D$_3$, is similar to calcitriol except for the presence of an oxygen between C21 and C23. Maxacalcitol has been shown to result in less hypercalcemia in animal models; however, this has not translated into clinical trials.[221] In humans, maxacalcitol has been shown to be effective in suppressing PTH levels,[222–224] but in a study of 124 dialysis subjects treated with maxacalcitol, 41 experienced hypercalcemia.[223] There is a dose-dependent relationship between the dose of maxacalcitol and risk of hypercalcemia.[222] Intravenous maxacalcitol is not superior to oral calcitriol[225] in as much as decrements in PTH concentrations and the rate of hypercalcemia are similar.[225]

Falecalcitriol

Falecalcitriol, or 1,25(OH)2-26,27-F6-D$_3$, is a newer analogue and is currently only available in Japan. In animal studies, it is suggested to be highly potent in inhibiting PTH.[226] In clinical trials comparing falecalcitriol with alfacalcidol, falecalcitriol has been shown to be more effective than alfacalcidol in reducing PTH with similar rates of hypercalcemia.[227]

A comparison of the various drugs available for the treatment of hyperparathyroidism in CKD-ESRD is shown in **Table 1**.

OTHER EFFECTS OF VITAMIN D AND ITS ANALOGUES
Hypertension and Left Ventricular Hypertrophy

Vitamin D deficiency has been suggested to play a role in both development of cardiac hypertrophy and hypertension. Indeed, VDR knockout mice have been shown to develop both hypertension and left ventricular hypertrophy (LVH), suggesting that vitamin D may directly affect the myocardium.[228] Vitamin D may contribute to development of hypertension and LVH through inhibition of renin. VDR-null mice are shown to have higher expression of renin and angiotensin II associated with both hypertension and LVH.[229] Similarly, hypertensive rats treated with vitamin D analogues have less cardiac hypertrophy than rats treated with vehicle.[230,231] In small clinical trials of dialysis subjects, treatment with calcitriol has been shown to attenuate LVH.[232,233] In a large randomized placebo-controlled trial of 227 subjects with CKD with mild to moderate LVH, treatment with paricalcitol at a dose of 2 μg/d for 48 weeks did not result in any improvement in left ventricular mass index.[234]

Albuminuria

In multiple animal models, vitamin D and its analogues have been shown to reduce albuminuria.[235–239] Similar results have been shown in human clinical trials. Subjects with CKD treated with paricalcitol had lower urinary protein or 24-hour albumin excretion rates compared with placebo.[240,241] In a larger randomized controlled trial involving subjects with type 2 diabetes, those treated with paricalcitol had lower urinary albumin to creatinine ratios compared with placebo-treated subjects, but they also had a lower estimated GFR.[242] Whether the reduction in urinary albumin is a true reduction or reflection of hemodynamic changes remains unclear. Similarly, whether this reduction translates to better renal outcome long-term is also to be

Table 1
Drugs available for the treatment of secondary hyperparathyroidism in chronic kidney disease and end-stage renal disease

Drug	Brand Name	Available in United States	Oral or Intravenous (IV)	Starting Doses	Effect on Calcium[a]	Effect on Phosphorous[a]
Calcitriol	Rocaltrol-Calcijex	Yes	Both	1–2 μg IV thrice weekly	NA	NA
Paricalcitol	Zemplar	Yes	Both	2–4 μg IV thrice weekly	Less hypercalcemia	Less hyperphosphatemia
Alfacalcidol	One-Alpha (Canada)	No	Both		Similar to calcitriol	Similar to calcitriol
Doxercalciferol	Hectorol	Yes	Both	2–4 μg IV thrice weekly	Similar to calcitriol	Similar to calcitriol
Maxacalcitol	Oxarol (Japan)	No	IV		Similar to calcitriol	Similar to calcitriol
Falecalcitriol	Hornel (Japan)	No	Oral		Similar to calcitriol	Similar to calcitriol

[a] Compared with calcitriol.

seen. More recent studies, however, have failed to show a benefit in albuminuria in subjects treated with doxercalciferol.[243]

Mortality

Low 25(OH)D levels have been associated with increased mortality in patients with CKD and ESRD similar to the general population.[110,244–247] Similarly, lower vitamin D levels are associated with an increased rate of progression to ESRD.[110] Many observational studies have suggested that use of active vitamin D in CKD and dialysis subjects improves survival.[248–254] These studies are problematic because subjects who do not receive vitamin D or who had lower vitamin D levels might have been sicker with attendant higher mortality. This type of bias is not accounted for in standard regression models. Tentori and colleagues[255] re-evaluated the data from participants in the Dialysis Outcomes and Practice Patterns Study (DOPPS) study to evaluate the association between vitamin D and mortality. Indeed, subjects who were prescribed vitamin D had fewer comorbidities. When adjusted for confounding variables, vitamin D administration was no longer associated with improved mortality.[255] The lack of mortality benefit with use of vitamin D or its analogues was also shown in a large meta-analysis of 76 trials.[256] Not only did the administration of vitamin D or its analogues not result in mortality benefit, but $1\alpha,25(OH)_2D_3$ administration was associated with higher rate of hypercalcemia and hyperphosphatemia and had a variable effect on reducing PTH levels.[256] It should be noted that in the various trials included in the meta-analysis,[256] the degree of suppression of PTH was variable and there were methodological differences in the measurement of PTH.

SUMMARY

In conclusion, 1-hydroxylated vitamin D analogues are effective in the treatment of secondary hyperparathyroidism in the context of CKD-ESRD. Further studies are required to assess their benefits in the treatment of heart disease and albuminuria.

REFERENCES

1. Moe S, Drueke T, Cunningham J, et al. Definition, evaluation, and classification of renal osteodystrophy: a position statement from kidney disease: improving global outcomes (KDIGO). Kidney Int 2006;69(11):1945–53.
2. McCarthy JT, Kumar R. Behavior of the vitamin D endocrine system in the development of renal osteodystrophy. Semin Nephrol 1986;6(1):21–30.
3. McCarthy JT, Kumar R. Renal osteodystrophy. Endocrinol Metab Clin North Am 1990;19(1):65–93.
4. McCarthy JT, Kumar R. Role of the vitamin D system in the pathogenesis of renal osteodystrophy. In: Kumar R, editor. Vitamin D: basic and clinical aspects. Dortrecht (Netherlands): Martinus Nijhoff Publishers; 1984. p. 611–40.
5. Martin KJ, Olgaard K, Coburn JW, et al. Diagnosis, assessment, and treatment of bone turnover abnormalities in renal osteodystrophy. Am J kidney Dis 2004; 43(3):558–65.
6. Coburn JW, Sherrard DJ, Ott SM, et al. Bone disease in uremia: a reappraisal. In: Norman AW, Schaefer K, Herrath DV, et al, editors. Vitamin D: chemical, biochemical and clinical endocrinology of calcium metabolism. Berlin: Walter de Gruyter; 1982. p. 827–32.
7. Bricker NS, Slatopolsky E, Reiss E, et al. Calcium, phosphorus, and bone in renal disease and transplantation. Arch Intern Med 1969;123(5):543–53.

8. Maung HM, Goldstein DA, Massry SG. Management of renal osteodystrophy with 1,25(OH)$_2$D$_3$. II. Effects on histopathology of bone: evidence for healing of osteomalacia. Mineral Elect Metab 1979;2:48–55.

9. London G, Coyne D, Hruska K, et al. The new kidney disease: improving global outcomes (KDIGO) guidelines - expert clinical focus on bone and vascular calcification. Clin Nephrol 2010;74(6):423–32.

10. Malluche HH. Bone disease in renal failure. Introduction. Miner Electrolyte Metab 1991;17(4):209–10.

11. Malluche HH, Ritz E, Lange HP, et al. Bone histology in incipient and advanced renal failure. Kidney Int 1976;9(4):355–62.

12. Reiss E, Canterbury JM, Kanter A. Circulating parathyroid hormone concentration in chronic renal insufficiency. Arch Intern Med 1969;124(4):417–22.

13. Potts JT, Reita RE, Deftos LJ, et al. Secondary hyperparathyroidism in chronic renal disease. Arch Intern Med 1969;124(4):408–12.

14. Norman ME, Mazur AT, Borden S 4th, et al. Early diagnosis of juvenile renal osteodystrophy. J Pediatr 1980;97(2):226–32.

15. Baron R, Mazur A, Norman M. Histomorphometric classification of juvenile renal osteodystrophy: prevalence of mineralizing defect. In: Norman AW, Schaefer K, Herrath DV, et al, editors. Vitamin D: chemical, biochemical and clinical endocrinology of calcium metabolism. Berlin: Walter de Gruyter; 1982. p. 853–6.

16. Martin DR, Ritter CS, Slatopolsky E, et al. Acute regulation of parathyroid hormone by dietary phosphate. Am J Physiol Endocrinol Metab 2005;289(4): E729–34.

17. Slatopolsky E, Dusso A, Brown AJ. The role of phosphorus in the development of secondary hyperparathyroidism and parathyroid cell proliferation in chronic renal failure. Am J Med Sci 1999;317(6):370–6.

18. Slatopolsky E. The intact nephron hypothesis: the concept and its implications for phosphate management in CKD-related mineral and bone disorder. Kidney Int Suppl 2011;(121):S3–8.

19. Slatopolsky E, Bricker NS. The role of phosphorus restriction in the prevention of secondary hyperparathyroidism in chronic renal disease. Kidney Int 1973;4(2): 141–5.

20. Slatopolsky E, Brown A, Dusso A. Pathogenesis of secondary hyperparathyroidism. Kidney Int Suppl 1999;73:S14–9.

21. Slatopolsky E, Brown A, Dusso A. Role of phosphorus in the pathogenesis of secondary hyperparathyroidism. Am J Kidney Dis 2001;37(1 Suppl 2):S54–7.

22. Slatopolsky E, Brown A, Dusso A. Calcium, phosphorus and vitamin D disorders in uremia. Contrib Nephrol 2005;149:261–71.

23. Slatopolsky E, Caglar S, Gradowska L, et al. On the prevention of secondary hyperparathyroidism in experimental chronic renal disease using "proportional reduction" of dietary phosphorus intake. Kidney Int 1972;2(3):147–51.

24. Slatopolsky E, Delmez JA. Pathogenesis of secondary hyperparathyroidism. Miner Electrolyte Metab 1995;21(1–3):91–6.

25. McCarthy JT, Kumar R. Renal osteodystrophy. In: Jacobson HR, Striker GE, Klahr S, editors. The principles and practice of nephrology. St Louis (MO): Mosby-Year Book, Inc; 1995. p. 1032–45.

26. DeLuca HF. The kidney as an endocrine organ involved in the function of vitamin D. Am J Med 1975;58(1):39–47.

27. Eisman JA, Hamstra AJ, Kream BE, et al. 1,25-Dihydroxyvitamin D in biological fluids: a simplified and sensitive assay. Science 1976;193(4257):1021–3.

28. Hollis BW. Assay of circulating 1,25-dihydroxyvitamin D involving a novel single-cartridge extraction and purification procedure. Clin Chem 1986;32(11):2060–3.

29. Ishimura E, Nishizawa Y, Inaba M, et al. Serum levels of 1,25-dihydroxyvitamin D, 24,25-dihydroxyvitamin D, and 25-hydroxyvitamin D in nondialyzed patients with chronic renal failure. Kidney Int 1999;55(3):1019–27.

30. Mason RS, Lissner D, Wilkinson M, et al. Vitamin D metabolites and their relationship to azotaemic osteodystrophy. Clin Endocrinol (Oxf) 1980;13(4):375–85.

31. Scharla S, Schmidt-Gayk H, Reichel H, et al. A sensitive and simplified radioimmunoassay for 1,25-dihydroxyvitamin D3. Clin Chim Acta 1984;142(3):325–38.

32. Yumita S, Suzuki M, Akiba T, et al. Levels of serum 1,25(OH)2D in patients with pre-dialysis chronic renal failure. Tohoku J Exp Med 1996;180(1):45–56.

33. Coburn JW, Koppel MH, Brickman AS, et al. Study of intestinal absorption of calcium in patients with renal failure. Kidney Int 1973;3(4):264–72.

34. Juttmann JR, Hagenouw-Taal JC, Lameyer LD, et al. Intestinal calcium absorption, serum phosphate, and parathyroid hormone in patients with chronic renal failure and osteodystrophy before and during hemodialysis. Calcif Tissue Res 1978;26(2):119–26.

35. Chanard JM, Drueke T, Zingraff J, et al. Effects of haemodialysis on fractional intestinal absorption of calcium in uraemia. Eur J Clin Invest 1976;6(3):261–4.

36. Recker RR, Saville PD. Calcium absorption in renal failure: its relationship to blood urea nitrogen, dietary calcium intake, time on dialysis, and other variables. J Lab Clin Med 1971;78(3):380–8.

37. Faul C, Amaral AP, Oskouei B, et al. FGF23 induces left ventricular hypertrophy. J Clin Invest 2011;121(11):4393–408.

38. Gutierrez O, Isakova T, Rhee E, et al. Fibroblast growth factor-23 mitigates hyperphosphatemia but accentuates calcitriol deficiency in chronic kidney disease. J Am Soc Nephrol 2005;16(7):2205–15.

39. Gutierrez OM, Januzzi JL, Isakova T, et al. Fibroblast growth factor 23 and left ventricular hypertrophy in chronic kidney disease. Circulation 2009;119(19):2545–52.

40. Gutierrez OM, Mannstadt M, Isakova T, et al. Fibroblast growth factor 23 and mortality among patients undergoing hemodialysis. N Engl J Med 2008;359(6):584–92.

41. Isakova T, Xie H, Yang W, et al. Fibroblast growth factor 23 and risks of mortality and end-stage renal disease in patients with chronic kidney disease. JAMA 2011;305(23):2432–9.

42. Pande S, Ritter CS, Rothstein M, et al. FGF-23 and sFRP-4 in chronic kidney disease and post-renal transplantation. Nephron Physiol 2006;104(1):p23–32.

43. Cunningham J, Fraher LJ, Clemens TL, et al. Chronic acidosis with metabolic bone disease. Effect of alkali on bone morphology and vitamin D metabolism. Am J Med 1982;73(2):199–204.

44. Eiam-ong S, Kurtzman NA. Metabolic acidosis and bone disease. Miner Electrolyte Metab 1994;20(1–2):72–80.

45. Marone CC, Wong NL, Sutton RA, et al. Acidosis and renal calcium excretion in experimental chronic renal failure. Nephron 1981;28(6):294–6.

46. Kumar R. The metabolism of 1,25-dihydroxyvitamin D3. Endocr Rev 1980;1(3):258–67.

47. Gray TK, Lowe W, Lester GE. Vitamin D and pregnancy: the maternal-fetal metabolism of vitamin D. Endocr Rev 1981;2(3):264–74.

48. Norman AW, Roth J, Orci L. The vitamin D endocrine system: steroid metabolism, hormone receptors, and biological response (calcium binding proteins). Endocr Rev 1982;3(4):331–66.
49. Brommage R, DeLuca HF. Evidence that 1,25-dihydroxyvitamin D3 is the physiologically active metabolite of vitamin D3. Endocr Rev 1985;6(4):491–511.
50. Boland R. Role of vitamin D in skeletal muscle function. Endocr Rev 1986;7(4): 434–48.
51. Christakos S, Gabrielides C, Rhoten WB. Vitamin D-dependent calcium binding proteins: chemistry, distribution, functional considerations, and molecular biology. Endocr Rev 1989;10(1):3–26.
52. Bikle DD, Pillai S. Vitamin D, calcium, and epidermal differentiation. Endocr Rev 1993;14(1):3–19.
53. Malloy PJ, Pike JW, Feldman D. The vitamin D receptor and the syndrome of hereditary 1,25-dihydroxyvitamin D-resistant rickets. Endocr Rev 1999;20(2): 156–88.
54. Gurlek A, Pittelkow MR, Kumar R. Modulation of growth factor/cytokine synthesis and signaling by 1alpha,25-dihydroxyvitamin D(3): implications in cell growth and differentiation. Endocr Rev 2002;23(6):763–86.
55. Nagpal S, Na S, Rathnachalam R. Noncalcemic actions of vitamin D receptor ligands. Endocr Rev 2005;26(5):662–87.
56. Bouillon R, Carmeliet G, Verlinden L, et al. Vitamin D and human health: lessons from vitamin D receptor null mice. Endocr Rev 2008;29(6):726–76.
57. Rosen CJ, Adams JS, Bikle DD, et al. The nonskeletal effects of vitamin D: an Endocrine Society scientific statement. Endocr Rev 2012;33(3):456–92.
58. Girgis CM, Clifton-Bligh RJ, Hamrick MW, et al. The roles of vitamin D in skeletal muscle: form, function, and metabolism. Endocr Rev 2013;34(1):33–83.
59. Kumar R. Vitamin D metabolism and mechanisms of calcium transport. J Am Soc Nephrol 1990;1(1):30–42.
60. Griffin MD, Xing N, Kumar R. Vitamin D and its analogs as regulators of immune activation and antigen presentation. Annu Rev Nutr 2003;23:117–45.
61. Christakos S, Dhawan P, Verstuyf A, et al. Vitamin D: metabolism, molecular mechanism of action, and pleiotropic effects. Physiol Rev 2016;96(1):365–408.
62. DeLuca HF, Schnoes HK. Metabolism and mechanism of action of vitamin D. Annu Rev Biochem 1976;45:631–66.
63. DeLuca HF, Schnoes HK. Vitamin D: recent advances. Annu Rev Biochem 1983; 52:411–39.
64. Deluca HF. Historical overview of vitamin D. In: Feldman D, Pke JW, Adams JS, editors. Vitamin D, vol. 1, 3rd edition. Boston: Elsevier; 2011. p. 3–12.
65. DeLuca HF. Evolution of our understanding of vitamin D. Nutr Rev 2008;66(10 Suppl 2):S73–87.
66. Haussler MR, Whitfield GK, Kaneko I, et al. Molecular mechanisms of vitamin D action. Calcif Tissue Int 2013;92(2):77–98.
67. Mizwicki MT, Norman AW. The vitamin D sterol-vitamin D receptor ensemble model offers unique insights into both genomic and rapid-response signaling. Sci Signal 2009;2(75):re4.
68. Griffin MD, Kumar R. Multiple potential clinical benefits for 1alpha,25-dihydroxyvitamin D3 analogs in kidney transplant recipients. J Steroid Biochem Mol Biol 2005;97(1–2):213–8.
69. Ryan ZC, Craig TA, Folmes CD, et al. 1alpha,25-Dihydroxyvitamin D3 regulates mitochondrial oxygen consumption and dynamics in human skeletal muscle cells. J Biol Chem 2016;291(3):1514–28.

70. Gurlek A, Kumar R. Regulation of osteoblast growth by interactions between transforming growth factor-beta and 1alpha,25-dihydroxyvitamin D3. Crit Rev Eukaryot Gene Expr 2001;11(4):299–317.
71. McCollum EV, Simmonds N, Becker JE, et al. Studies on experimental rickets XXI. An experimental demonstration of the existence of a vitamin which promotes calcium deposition. J Biol Chem 1922;53:293–312.
72. Windaus A, Schenck FF, von Weder F. Uber das antirachitisch wirksame bestrahlungs-produkt aus 7-dehydro-cholesterin. Hoppe Seylers Z Physiol Chem 1936;241:100–3.
73. Steenbock H, Black A. Fat-soluble vitamins. XVII. The induction of gross-promoting and calcifying properties in a ration by exposure to ultraviolet light. J Biol Chem 1924;61:405–22.
74. Hess AF, Weinstock M. Anti-rachitic properties imparted to lettuce and to growing wheat by ultraviolet irradiation. Proc Soc Exp Biol Med 1924;22:5–6.
75. DeLuca HF. The metabolism, physiology and function of vitamin D. In: Kumar R, editor. Vitamin D. Boston: Martinus Nijhoff Publishing; 1984. p. 1–68.
76. Esvelt RP, Schnoes HK, DeLuca HF. Vitamin D3 from rat skins irradiated in vitro with ultraviolet light. Arch Biochem Biophys 1978;188(2):282–6.
77. Holick MF, Clark MB. The photobiogenesis and metabolism of vitamin D. Fed Proc 1978;37(12):2567–74.
78. Holick MF, MacLaughlin JA, Clark MB, et al. Photosynthesis of previtamin D3 in human skin and the physiologic consequences. Science 1980;210(4466): 203–5.
79. Holick MF, Richtand NM, McNeill SC, et al. Isolation and identification of previtamin D3 from the skin of rats exposed to ultraviolet irradiation. Biochemistry 1979;18(6):1003–8.
80. Windaus A, Linsert O, Luttringhaus A, et al. Crystalline-vitamin D 2. Annalen de Chem 1932;492:226–41.
81. Steenbock H, Kletzien SWF, Halpin JG. The reaction of the chicken to irradiated ergosterol and irradiated yeast as contrasted with the natural vitamin of fish liver oils. J Biol Chem 1932;97:249–64.
82. Jacob AI, Sallman A, Santiz Z, et al. Defective photoproduction of cholecalciferol in normal and uremic humans. J Nutr 1984;114(7):1313–9.
83. Blunt JW, DeLuca HF, Schnoes HK. 25-hydroxycholecalciferol. A biologically active metabolite of vitamin D3. Biochemistry 1968;7(10):3317–22.
84. Suda T, DeLuca HF, Schnoes H, et al. 25-hydroxyergocalciferol: a biologically active metabolite of vitamin D2. Biochem Biophys Res Commun 1969;35(2): 182–5.
85. Suda T, DeLuca HF, Schnoes HK, et al. The isolation and identification of 25-hydroxyergocalciferol. Biochemistry 1969;8(9):3515–20.
86. Ponchon G, DeLuca HF. The role of the liver in the metabolism of vitamin D. J Clin Invest 1969;48(7):1273–9.
87. Ponchon G, Kennan AL, DeLuca HF. "Activation" of vitamin D by the liver. J Clin Invest 1969;48(11):2032–7.
88. Bhattacharyya MH, DeLuca HF. The regulation of rat liver calciferol-25-hydroxylase. J Biol Chem 1973;248(9):2969–73.
89. Bhattacharyya MH, DeLuca HF. Subcellular location of rat liver calciferol-25-hydroxylase. Arch Biochem Biophys 1974;160(1):58–62.
90. Madhok TC, DeLuca HF. Characteristics of the rat liver microsomal enzyme system converting cholecalciferol into 25-hydroxycholecalciferol. Evidence for the participation of cytochrome p-450. Biochem J 1979;184(3):491–9.

91. Cheng JB, Levine MA, Bell NH, et al. Genetic evidence that the human CYP2R1 enzyme is a key vitamin D 25-hydroxylase. Proc Natl Acad Sci U S A 2004; 101(20):7711–5.

92. Zhu J, DeLuca HF. Vitamin D 25-hydroxylase - Four decades of searching, are we there yet? Arch Biochem Biophys 2012;523(1):30–6.

93. Zhu JG, Ochalek JT, Kaufmann M, et al. CYP2R1 is a major, but not exclusive, contributor to 25-hydroxyvitamin D production in vivo. Proc Natl Acad Sci U S A 2013;110(39):15650–5.

94. Haddad JG Jr. Transport of vitamin D metabolites. Clin Orthop Relat Res 1979;(142):249–61.

95. Schwartz JB, Lai J, Lizaola B, et al. Variability in free 25(OH) vitamin D levels in clinical populations. J Steroid Biochem Mol Biol 2014;144(Pt A):156–8.

96. Chung M, Balk EM, Brendel M, et al. Vitamin D and calcium: a systematic review of health outcomes. Evid Rep Technol Assess (Full Rep) 2009;(183):1–420.

97. Rosen CJ, Gallagher JC. The 2011 IOM report on vitamin D and calcium requirements for North America: clinical implications for providers treating patients with low bone mineral density. J Clin Densitom 2011;14(2):79–84.

98. Holick MF, Binkley NC, Bischoff-Ferrari HA, et al. Evaluation, treatment, and prevention of vitamin D deficiency: an Endocrine Society clinical practice guideline. J Clin Endocrinol Metab 2011;96(7):1911–30.

99. Institute of Medicine (US) Committee. Dietary reference intakes for calcium and vitamin D. In: Ross AC, Taylor CL, Yaktine AL, et al, editors. The National Academies Collection: Reports funded by National Institutes of Health. Washington (DC): National Academies Press (US); 2011.

100. Al-Badr W, Martin KJ. Vitamin D and kidney disease. Clin J Am Soc Nephrol 2008;3(5):1555–60.

101. Dusso A, Gonzalez EA, Martin KJ. Vitamin D in chronic kidney disease. Best Pract Res Clin Endocrinol Metab 2011;25(4):647–55.

102. Echida Y, Mochizuki T, Uchida K, et al. Risk factors for vitamin D deficiency in patients with chronic kidney disease. Intern Med 2012;51(8):845–50.

103. Elder GJ, Mackun K. 25-Hydroxyvitamin D deficiency and diabetes predict reduced BMD in patients with chronic kidney disease. J Bone Miner Res 2006;21(11):1778–84.

104. Gonzalez EA, Sachdeva A, Oliver DA, et al. Vitamin D insufficiency and deficiency in chronic kidney disease. A single center observational study. Am J Nephrol 2004;24(5):503–10.

105. Hari P, Gupta N, Hari S, et al. Vitamin D insufficiency and effect of cholecalciferol in children with chronic kidney disease. Pediatr Nephrol 2010;25(12):2483–8.

106. Helvig CF, Cuerrier D, Hosfield CM, et al. Dysregulation of renal vitamin D metabolism in the uremic rat. Kidney Int 2010;78(5):463–72.

107. Kandula P, Dobre M, Schold JD, et al. Vitamin D supplementation in chronic kidney disease: a systematic review and meta-analysis of observational studies and randomized controlled trials. Clin J Am Soc Nephrol 2011;6(1):50–62.

108. LaClair RE, Hellman RN, Karp SL, et al. Prevalence of calcidiol deficiency in CKD: a cross-sectional study across latitudes in the United States. Am J Kidney Dis 2005;45(6):1026–33.

109. Mehrotra R, Kermah D, Budoff M, et al. Hypovitaminosis D in chronic kidney disease. Clin J Am Soc Nephrol 2008;3(4):1144–51.

110. Ravani P, Malberti F, Tripepi G, et al. Vitamin D levels and patient outcome in chronic kidney disease. Kidney Int 2009;75(1):88–95.

111. Rucker D, Tonelli M, Coles MG, et al. Vitamin D insufficiency and treatment with oral vitamin D3 in northern-dwelling patients with chronic kidney disease. J Nephrol 2009;22(1):75–82.
112. Satirapoj B, Limwannata P, Chaiprasert A, et al. Vitamin D insufficiency and deficiency with stages of chronic kidney disease in an Asian population. BMC Nephrol 2013;14:206.
113. Zehnder D, Landray MJ, Wheeler DC, et al. Cross-sectional analysis of abnormalities of mineral homeostasis, vitamin D and parathyroid hormone in a cohort of pre-dialysis patients. The chronic renal impairment in Birmingham (CRIB) study. Nephron Clin Pract 2007;107(3):c109–16.
114. Cheng S, Coyne D. Vitamin D and outcomes in chronic kidney disease. Curr Opin Nephrol Hypertens 2007;16(2):77–82.
115. Mehrotra R, Kermah DA, Salusky IB, et al. Chronic kidney disease, hypovitaminosis D, and mortality in the United States. Kidney Int 2009;76(9):977–83.
116. Hewison M, Burke F, Evans KN, et al. Extra-renal 25-hydroxyvitamin D3-1alpha-hydroxylase in human health and disease. J Steroid Biochem Mol Biol 2007; 103(3–5):316–21.
117. Zehnder D, Bland R, Chana RS, et al. Synthesis of 1,25-dihydroxyvitamin D(3) by human endothelial cells is regulated by inflammatory cytokines: a novel autocrine determinant of vascular cell adhesion. J Am Soc Nephrol 2002;13(3): 621–9.
118. Zehnder D, Bland R, Williams MC, et al. Extrarenal expression of 25-hydroxyvitamin d(3)-1 alpha-hydroxylase. J Clin Endocrinol Metab 2001;86(2):888–94.
119. Recker R, Schoenfeld P, Letteri J, et al. The efficacy of calcifediol in renal osteodystrophy. Arch Intern Med 1978;138(Spec No):857–63.
120. Bhan I, Dobens D, Tamez H, et al. Nutritional vitamin D supplementation in dialysis: a randomized trial. Clin J Am Soc Nephrol 2015;10(4):611–9.
121. Holick MF, Schnoes HK, DeLuca HF. Identification of 1,25-dihydroxycholecalciferol, a form of vitamin D3 metabolically active in the intestine. Proc Natl Acad Sci U S A 1971;68(4):803–4.
122. Holick MF, Schnoes HK, DeLuca HF, et al. Isolation and identification of 1,25-dihydroxycholecalciferol. A metabolite of vitamin D active in intestine. Biochemistry 1971;10(14):2799–804.
123. Holick MF, Garabedian M, DeLuca HF. 1,25-dihydroxycholecalciferol: metabolite of vitamin D3 active on bone in anephric rats. Science 1972;176(4039):1146–7.
124. Reeve L, Tanaka Y, DeLuca HF. Studies on the site of 1,25-dihydroxyvitamin D3 synthesis in vivo. J Biol Chem 1983;258(6):3615–7.
125. Bilezikian JP, Canfield RE, Jacobs TP, et al. Response of 1alpha,25-dihydroxyvitamin D3 to hypocalcemia in human subjects. N Engl J Med 1978;299(9): 437–41.
126. Boyle IT, Gray RW, DeLuca HF. Regulation by calcium of in vivo synthesis of 1,25-dihydroxycholecalciferol and 21,25-dihydroxycholecalciferol. Proc Natl Acad Sci U S A 1971;68(9):2131–4.
127. DeLuca HF. Regulation of vitamin D metabolism in the kidney. Adv Exp Med Biol 1977;81:195–209.
128. Kumar R. Metabolism of 1,25-dihydroxyvitamin D3. Physiol Rev 1984;64(2): 478–504.
129. Fraser DR, Kodicek E. Unique biosynthesis by kidney of a biological active vitamin D metabolite. Nature 1970;228(5273):764–6.

130. Garabedian M, Holick MF, Deluca HF, et al. Control of 25-hydroxycholecalciferol metabolism by parathyroid glands. Proc Natl Acad Sci U S A 1972;69(7): 1673–6.
131. Shultz TD, Fox J, Heath H 3rd, et al. Do tissues other than the kidney produce 1,25-dihydroxyvitamin D3 in vivo? A reexamination. Proc Natl Acad Sci U S A 1983;80(6):1746–50.
132. Ryan ZC, Ketha H, McNulty MS, et al. Sclerostin alters serum vitamin D metabolite and fibroblast growth factor 23 concentrations and the urinary excretion of calcium. Proc Natl Acad Sci U S A 2013;110(15):6199–204.
133. Kumar R, Vallon V. Reduced renal calcium excretion in the absence of sclerostin expression: evidence for a novel calcium-regulating bone kidney axis. J Am Soc Nephrol 2014;25(10):2159–68.
134. DeLuca HF. Overview of general physiologic features and functions of vitamin D. Am J Clin Nutr 2004;80(6 Suppl):1689S–96S.
135. Tebben PJ, Kumar R. The hormonal regulation of calcium metabolism. In: Alpern RJ, Moe OW, Caplan M, editors. Seldin and Giebisch's the kidney, physiology and pathophysiology, vol. 2. New York: Academic Press; 2013. p. 2273–330.
136. Wasserman RH, Corradino RA, Fullmer CS, et al. Some aspects of vitamin D action; calcium absorption and the vitamin D-dependent calcium-binding protein. Vitam Horm 1974;32:299–324.
137. Wasserman RH, Fullmer CS. Vitamin D and intestinal calcium transport: facts, speculations and hypotheses. J Nutr 1995;125(7 Suppl):1971S–9S.
138. Wasserman RH, Smith CA, Brindak ME, et al. Vitamin D and mineral deficiencies increase the plasma membrane calcium pump of chicken intestine. Gastroenterology 1992;102(3):886–94.
139. Wasserman RH, Chandler JS, Meyer SA, et al. Intestinal calcium transport and calcium extrusion processes at the basolateral membrane. J Nutr 1992;122(3 Suppl):662–71.
140. Berndt T, Thompson JR, Kumar R. The regulation of calcium, magnesium, and phosphate excretion by the kidney. In: Skorecki K, Chertow G, Marsden P, et al, editors. Brenner and Rector's the kidney, vol. 1, 10th edition. Philadelphia: Elsevier; 2015. p. 185–203.
141. Benn BS, Ajibade D, Porta A, et al. Active intestinal calcium transport in the absence of transient receptor potential vanilloid type 6 and calbindin-D9k. Endocrinology 2008;149(6):3196–205.
142. Kutuzova GD, Sundersingh F, Vaughan J, et al. TRPV6 is not required for 1alpha,25-dihydroxyvitamin D3-induced intestinal calcium absorption in vivo. Proc Natl Acad Sci U S A 2008;105(50):19655–9.
143. Lieben L, Benn BS, Ajibade D, et al. Trpv6 mediates intestinal calcium absorption during calcium restriction and contributes to bone homeostasis. Bone 2010; 47(2):301–8.
144. Ryan ZC, Craig TA, Filoteo AG, et al. Deletion of the intestinal plasma membrane calcium pump, isoform 1, Atp2b1, in mice is associated with decreased bone mineral density and impaired responsiveness to 1, 25-dihydroxyvitamin D3. Biochem Biophys Res Commun 2015;467(1):152–6.
145. Holick MF, Schnoes HK, DeLuca HF, et al. Isolation and identification of 24,25-dihydroxycholecalciferol, a metabolite of vitamin D made in the kidney. Biochemistry 1972;11(23):4251–5.
146. Lam HY, Schnoes HK, DeLuca HF, et al. 24,25-Dihydroxyvitamin D3. Synthesis and biological activity. Biochemistry 1973;12(24):4851–5.

147. Tanaka Y, DeLuca HF, Ikekawa N, et al. Determination of stereochemical configuration of the 24-hydroxyl group of 24,25-dihydroxyvitamin D3 and its biological importance. Arch Biochem Biophys 1975;170(2):620–6.

148. Tanaka Y, Deluca HF. The control of 25-hydroxyvitamin D metabolism by inorganic phosphorus. Arch Biochem Biophys 1973;154(2):566–74.

149. Baxter LA, DeLuca HF. Stimulation of 25-hydroxyvitamin D3-1alpha-hydroxylase by phosphate depletion. J Biol Chem 1976;251(10):3158–61.

150. Ribovich ML, DeLuca HF. 1,25-Dihydroxyvitamin D3 metabolism. The effect of dietary calcium and phosphorus. Arch Biochem Biophys 1978;188(1):164–71.

151. Dominguez JH, Gray RW, Lemann J Jr. Dietary phosphate deprivation in women and men: effects on mineral and acid balances, parathyroid hormone and the metabolism of 25-OH-vitamin D. J Clin Endocrinol Metab 1976;43(5):1056–68.

152. Gray RW, Wilz DR, Caldas AE, et al. The importance of phosphate in regulating plasma 1,25-(OH)2-vitamin D levels in humans: studies in healthy subjects in calcium-stone formers and in patients with primary hyperparathyroidism. J Clin Endocrinol Metab 1977;45(2):299–306.

153. Steele TH, Engle JE, Tanaka Y, et al. Phosphatemic action of 1,25-dihydroxyvitamin D3. Am J Physiol 1975;229(2):489–95.

154. Gray RW. Control of plasma 1,25-(OH)2-vitamin D concentrations by calcium and phosphorus in the rat: effects of hypophysectomy. Calcif Tissue Int 1981; 33(5):485–8.

155. Gray RW. Effects of age and sex on the regulation of plasma 1,25-(OH)2-D by phosphorus in the rat. Calcif Tissue Int 1981;33(5):477–84.

156. Gray RW, Garthwaite TL. Activation of renal 1,25-dihydroxyvitamin D3 synthesis by phosphate deprivation: evidence for a role for growth hormone. Endocrinology 1985;116(1):189–93.

157. Gray RW, Garthwaite TL, Phillips LS. Growth hormone and triiodothyronine permit an increase in plasma 1,25(OH)2D concentrations in response to dietary phosphate deprivation in hypophysectomized rats. Calcif Tissue Int 1983;35(1): 100–6.

158. Gray RW, Haasch ML, Brown CE. Regulation of plasma 1,25-(OH)2-D3 by phosphate: evidence against a role for total or acid-soluble renal phosphate content. Calcif Tissue Int 1983;35(6):773–7.

159. Kido S, Kaneko I, Tatsumi S, et al. Vitamin D and type II sodium-dependent phosphate cotransporters. Contrib Nephrol 2013;180:86–97.

160. Taketani Y, Segawa H, Chikamori M, et al. Regulation of type II renal Na+-dependent inorganic phosphate transporters by 1,25-dihydroxyvitamin D3. Identification of a vitamin D-responsive element in the human NAPi-3 gene. J Biol Chem 1998;273(23):14575–81.

161. Wagner CA, Hernando N, Forster IC, et al. The SLC34 family of sodium-dependent phosphate transporters. Pflugers Arch 2014;466(1):139–53.

162. Baker AR, McDonnell DP, Hughes M, et al. Cloning and expression of full-length cDNA encoding human vitamin D receptor. Proc Natl Acad Sci U S A 1988; 85(10):3294–8.

163. Jehan F, DeLuca HF. Cloning and characterization of the mouse vitamin D receptor promoter. Proc Natl Acad Sci U S A 1997;94(19):10138–43.

164. Lu Z, Hanson K, DeLuca HF. Cloning and origin of the two forms of chicken vitamin D receptor. Arch Biochem Biophys 1997;339(1):99–106.

165. Brumbaugh PF, Haussler MR. 1Alpha,25-dihydroxyvitamin D3 receptor: competitive binding of vitamin D analogs. Life Sci 1973;13(12):1737–46.

166. Rachez C, Lemon BD, Suldan Z, et al. Ligand-dependent transcription activation by nuclear receptors requires the DRIP complex. Nature 1999;398(6730): 824–8.

167. Ciesielski F, Rochel N, Moras D. Adaptability of the Vitamin D nuclear receptor to the synthetic ligand Gemini: remodelling the LBP with one side chain rotation. J Steroid Biochem Mol Biol 2007;103(3–5):235–42.

168. Hourai S, Rodrigues LC, Antony P, et al. Structure-based design of a superagonist ligand for the vitamin D nuclear receptor. Chem Biol 2008;15(4):383–92.

169. Rochel N, Hourai S, Perez-Garcia X, et al. Crystal structure of the vitamin D nuclear receptor ligand binding domain in complex with a locked side chain analog of calcitriol. Arch Biochem Biophys 2007;460(2):172–6.

170. Rochel N, Wurtz JM, Mitschler A, et al. The crystal structure of the nuclear receptor for vitamin D bound to its natural ligand. Mol Cell 2000;5(1):173–9.

171. Molnar F, Perakyla M, Carlberg C. Vitamin D receptor agonists specifically modulate the volume of the ligand-binding pocket. J Biol Chem 2006;281(15): 10516–26.

172. Vaisanen S, Ryhanen S, Saarela JT, et al. Structurally and functionally important amino acids of the agonistic conformation of the human vitamin D receptor. Mol Pharmacol 2002;62(4):788–94.

173. Yamada S, Shimizu M, Yamamoto K. Structure-function relationships of vitamin D including ligand recognition by the vitamin D receptor. Med Res Rev 2003; 23(1):89–115.

174. Yamamoto K, Masuno H, Choi M, et al. Three-dimensional modeling of and ligand docking to vitamin D receptor ligand binding domain. Proc Natl Acad Sci U S A 2000;97(4):1467–72.

175. Darwish H, DeLuca HF. Vitamin D-regulated gene expression. Crit Rev Eukaryot Gene Expr 1993;3(2):89–116.

176. Haussler MR, Jurutka PW, Mizwicki M, et al. Vitamin D receptor (VDR)-mediated actions of 1alpha,25(OH)(2)vitamin D(3): genomic and non-genomic mechanisms. Best Pract Res Clin Endocrinol Metab 2011;25(4):543–59.

177. Jurutka PW, Whitfield GK, Hsieh JC, et al. Molecular nature of the vitamin D receptor and its role in regulation of gene expression. Rev Endocr Metab Disord 2001;2(2):203–16.

178. Lowe KE, Maiyar AC, Norman AW. Vitamin D-mediated gene expression. Crit Rev Eukaryot Gene Expr 1992;2(1):65–109.

179. Craig TA, Zhang Y, Magis AT, et al. Detection of 1alpha,25-dihydroxyvitamin D-regulated miRNAs in zebrafish by whole transcriptome sequencing. Zebrafish 2014;11(3):207–18.

180. Craig TA, Zhang Y, McNulty MS, et al. Research resource: whole transcriptome RNA sequencing detects multiple 1alpha,25-dihydroxyvitamin D(3)-sensitive metabolic pathways in developing zebrafish. Mol Endocrinol 2012;26(9): 1630–42.

181. Dusso AS, Arcidiacono MV, Sato T, et al. Molecular basis of parathyroid hyperplasia. J Ren Nutr 2007;17(1):45–7.

182. Dusso AS, Sato T, Arcidiacono MV, et al. Pathogenic mechanisms for parathyroid hyperplasia. Kidney Int Suppl 2006;(102):S8–11.

183. Slatopolsky E, Gradowska L, Kashemsant C, et al. The control of phosphate excretion in uremia. J Clin Invest 1966;45(5):672–7.

184. Slatopolsky E, Robson AM, Elkan I, et al. Control of phosphate excretion in uremic man. J Clin Invest 1968;47(8):1865–74.

185. Slatopolsky E, Rutherford WE, Hruska K, et al. How important is phosphate in the pathogenesis of renal osteodystrophy? Arch Intern Med 1978;138(Spec No):848–52.

186. Slatopolsky E, Rutherford WE, Martin K, et al. The role of phosphate and other factors on the pathogenesis of renal osteodystrophy. Adv Exp Med Biol 1977; 81:467–75.

187. Nigwekar SU, Tamez H, Thadhani RI. Vitamin D and chronic kidney disease-mineral bone disease (CKD-MBD). Bonekey Rep 2014;3:498.

188. Larsson T, Nisbeth U, Ljunggren O, et al. Circulating concentration of FGF-23 increases as renal function declines in patients with chronic kidney disease, but does not change in response to variation in phosphate intake in healthy volunteers. Kidney Int 2003;64(6):2272–9.

189. Quarles LD. Endocrine functions of bone in mineral metabolism regulation. J Clin Invest 2008;118(12):3820–8.

190. Shimada T, Kakitani M, Yamazaki Y, et al. Targeted ablation of Fgf23 demonstrates an essential physiological role of FGF23 in phosphate and vitamin D metabolism. J Clin Invest 2004;113(4):561–8.

191. Naveh-Many T, Marx R, Keshet E, et al. Regulation of 1,25-dihydroxyvitamin D3 receptor gene expression by 1,25-dihydroxyvitamin D3 in the parathyroid in vivo. J Clin Invest 1990;86(6):1968–75.

192. Naveh-Many T, Rahamimov R, Livni N, et al. Parathyroid cell proliferation in normal and chronic renal failure rats. The effects of calcium, phosphate, and vitamin D. J Clin Invest 1995;96(4):1786–93.

193. Naveh-Many T, Silver J. Regulation of parathyroid hormone gene expression by hypocalcemia, hypercalcemia, and vitamin D in the rat. J Clin Invest 1990;86(4): 1313–9.

194. Silver J, Naveh-Many T, Mayer H, et al. Regulation by vitamin D metabolites of parathyroid hormone gene transcription in vivo in the rat. J Clin Invest 1986; 78(5):1296–301.

195. Silver J, Russell J, Sherwood LM. Regulation by vitamin D metabolites of messenger ribonucleic acid for preproparathyroid hormone in isolated bovine parathyroid cells. Proc Natl Acad Sci U S A 1985;82(12):4270–3.

196. Brown AJ, Zhong M, Finch J, et al. The roles of calcium and 1,25-dihydroxyvitamin D3 in the regulation of vitamin D receptor expression by rat parathyroid glands. Endocrinology 1995;136(4):1419–25.

197. Denda M, Finch J, Brown AJ, et al. 1,25-dihydroxyvitamin D3 and 22-oxacalcitriol prevent the decrease in vitamin D receptor content in the parathyroid glands of uremic rats. Kidney Int 1996;50(1):34–9.

198. Dusso AS, Thadhani R, Slatopolsky E. Vitamin D receptor and analogs. Semin Nephrol 2004;24(1):10–6.

199. Slatopolsky E, Finch J, Ritter C, et al. Effects of 19-nor-1,25(OH)2D2, a new analogue of calcitriol, on secondary hyperparathyroidism in uremic rats. Am J Kidney Dis 1998;32(2 Suppl 2):S40–7.

200. Takahashi F, Finch JL, Denda M, et al. A new analog of 1,25-(OH)2D3, 19-NOR-1,25-(OH)2D2, suppresses serum PTH and parathyroid gland growth in uremic rats without elevation of intestinal vitamin D receptor content. Am J Kidney Dis 1997;30(1):105–12.

201. Bacchini G, Fabrizi F, Pontoriero G, et al. 'Pulse oral' versus intravenous calcitriol therapy in chronic hemodialysis patients. A prospective and randomized study. Nephron 1997;77(3):267–72.

202. Fischer ER, Harris DC. Comparison of intermittent oral and intravenous calcitriol in hemodialysis patients with secondary hyperparathyroidism. Clin Nephrol 1993;40(4):216–20.

203. Indridason OS, Quarles LD. Comparison of treatments for mild secondary hyperparathyroidism in hemodialysis patients. Durham Renal Osteodystrophy Study Group. Kidney Int 2000;57(1):282–92.

204. Liou HH, Chiang SS, Huang TP, et al. Comparative effect of oral or intravenous calcitriol on secondary hyperparathyroidism in chronic hemodialysis patients. Miner Electrolyte Metab 1994;20(3):97–102.

205. Mazzaferro S, Pasquali M, Ballanti P, et al. Intravenous versus oral calcitriol therapy in renal osteodystrophy: results of a prospective, pulsed and dose-comparable study. Miner Electrolyte Metab 1994;20(3):122–9.

206. Quarles LD, Yohay DA, Carroll BA, et al. Prospective trial of pulse oral versus intravenous calcitriol treatment of hyperparathyroidism in ESRD. Kidney Int 1994;45(6):1710–21.

207. Haiyang Z, Chenggang X. Comparison of intermittent intravenous and oral calcitriol in the treatment of secondary hyperparathyroidism in chronic hemodialysis patients: a meta-analysis of randomized controlled trials. Clin Nephrol 2009; 71(3):276–85.

208. Slatopolsky E, Finch J, Ritter C, et al. A new analog of calcitriol, 19-nor-1,25-(OH)2D2, suppresses parathyroid hormone secretion in uremic rats in the absence of hypercalcemia. Am J Kidney Dis 1995;26(5):852–60.

209. Slatopolsky E, Cozzolino M, Lu Y, et al. Efficacy of 19-Nor-1,25-(OH)2D2 in the prevention and treatment of hyperparathyroid bone disease in experimental uremia. Kidney Int 2003;63(6):2020–7.

210. Martin KJ, Gonzalez EA, Gellens M, et al. 19-Nor-1-alpha-25-dihydroxyvitamin D2 (Paricalcitol) safely and effectively reduces the levels of intact parathyroid hormone in patients on hemodialysis. J Am Soc Nephrol 1998;9(8):1427–32.

211. Martin KJ, Gonzalez EA, Gellens ME, et al. Therapy of secondary hyperparathyroidism with 19-nor-1alpha,25-dihydroxyvitamin D2. Am J Kidney Dis 1998;32(2 Suppl 2):S61–6.

212. Sprague SM, Llach F, Amdahl M, et al. Paricalcitol versus calcitriol in the treatment of secondary hyperparathyroidism. Kidney Int 2003;63(4):1483–90.

213. Teng M, Wolf M, Lowrie E, et al. Survival of patients undergoing hemodialysis with paricalcitol or calcitriol therapy. N Engl J Med 2003;349(5):446–56.

214. Frazao JM, Chesney RW, Coburn JW. Intermittent oral 1alpha-hydroxyvitamin D2 is effective and safe for the suppression of secondary hyperparathyroidism in haemodialysis patients. 1alphad2 Study Group. Nephrol Dial Transplant 1998; 13(Suppl 3):68–72.

215. Tan AU Jr, Levine BS, Mazess RB, et al. Effective suppression of parathyroid hormone by 1 alpha-hydroxy-vitamin D2 in hemodialysis patients with moderate to severe secondary hyperparathyroidism. Kidney Int 1997;51(1):317–23.

216. Maung HM, Elangovan L, Frazao JM, et al. Efficacy and side effects of intermittent intravenous and oral doxercalciferol (1alpha-hydroxyvitamin D(2)) in dialysis patients with secondary hyperparathyroidism: a sequential comparison. Am J Kidney Dis 2001;37(3):532–43.

217. Zisman AL, Ghantous W, Schinleber P, et al. Inhibition of parathyroid hormone: a dose equivalency study of paricalcitol and doxercalciferol. Am J Nephrol 2005; 25(6):591–5.

218. Joist HE, Ahya SN, Giles K, et al. Differential effects of very high doses of doxercalciferol and paricalcitol on serum phosphorus in hemodialysis patients. Clin Nephrol 2006;65(5):335–41.
219. Kiattisunthorn K, Wutyam K, Indranoi A, et al. Randomized trial comparing pulse calcitriol and alfacalcidol for the treatment of secondary hyperparathyroidism in haemodialysis patients. Nephrology (Carlton) 2011;16(3):277–84.
220. Hansen D, Rasmussen K, Danielsen H, et al. No difference between alfacalcidol and paricalcitol in the treatment of secondary hyperparathyroidism in hemodialysis patients: a randomized crossover trial. Kidney Int 2011;80(8):841–50.
221. Murayama E, Miyamoto K, Kubodera N, et al. Synthetic studies of vitamin D3 analogues. VIII. Synthesis of 22-oxavitamin D3 analogues. Chem Pharm Bull (Tokyo) 1986;34(10):4410–3.
222. Akizawa T, Ohashi Y, Akiba T, et al. Dose-response study of 22-oxacalcitriol in patients with secondary hyperparathyroidism. Ther Apher Dial 2004;8(6):480–91.
223. Akizawa T, Suzuki M, Akiba T, et al. Long-term effect of 1,25-dihydroxy-22-oxavitamin D(3) on secondary hyperparathyroidism in haemodialysis patients. One-year administration study. Nephrol Dial Transplant 2002;17(Suppl 10):28–36.
224. Yasuda M, Akiba T, Nihei H. Multicenter clinical trial of 22-oxa-1,25-dihydroxyvitamin D3 for chronic dialysis patients. Am J Kidney Dis 2003;41(3 Suppl 1):S108–11.
225. Tamura S, Ueki K, Mashimo K, et al. Comparison of the efficacy of an oral calcitriol pulse or intravenous 22-oxacalcitriol therapies in chronic hemodialysis patients. Clin Exp Nephrol 2005;9(3):238–43.
226. Nishizawa Y, Morii H, Ogura Y, et al. Clinical trial of 26,26,26,27,27,27-hexafluoro-1,25-dihydroxyvitamin D3 in uremic patients on hemodialysis: preliminary report. Contrib Nephrol 1991;90:196–203.
227. Ito H, Ogata H, Yamamoto M, et al. Comparison of oral falecalcitriol and intravenous calcitriol in hemodialysis patients with secondary hyperparathyroidism: a randomized, crossover trial. Clin Nephrol 2009;71(6):660–8.
228. Xiang W, Kong J, Chen S, et al. Cardiac hypertrophy in vitamin D receptor knockout mice: role of the systemic and cardiac renin-angiotensin systems. Am J Physiol Endocrinol Metab 2005;288(1):E125–32.
229. Li YC, Kong J, Wei M, et al. 1,25-Dihydroxyvitamin D(3) is a negative endocrine regulator of the renin-angiotensin system. J Clin Invest 2002;110(2):229–38.
230. Kong J, Kim GH, Wei M, et al. Therapeutic effects of vitamin D analogs on cardiac hypertrophy in spontaneously hypertensive rats. Am J Pathol 2010;177(2):622–31.
231. Bodyak N, Ayus JC, Achinger S, et al. Activated vitamin D attenuates left ventricular abnormalities induced by dietary sodium in Dahl salt-sensitive animals. Proc Natl Acad Sci U S A 2007;104(43):16810–5.
232. Kim HW, Park CW, Shin YS, et al. Calcitriol regresses cardiac hypertrophy and QT dispersion in secondary hyperparathyroidism on hemodialysis. Nephron Clin Pract 2006;102(1):c21–9.
233. Park CW, Oh YS, Shin YS, et al. Intravenous calcitriol regresses myocardial hypertrophy in hemodialysis patients with secondary hyperparathyroidism. Am J Kidney Dis 1999;33(1):73–81.
234. Thadhani R, Appelbaum E, Pritchett Y, et al. Vitamin D therapy and cardiac structure and function in patients with chronic kidney disease: the PRIMO randomized controlled trial. JAMA 2012;307(7):674–84.

235. Lillevang ST, Rosenkvist J, Andersen CB, et al. Single and combined effects of the vitamin D analogue KH1060 and cyclosporin A on mercuric-chloride-induced autoimmune disease in the BN rat. Clin Exp Immunol 1992;88(2):301–6.

236. Branisteanu DD, Leenaerts P, van Damme B, et al. Partial prevention of active Heymann nephritis by 1 alpha, 25 dihydroxyvitamin D3. Clin Exp Immunol 1993;94(3):412–7.

237. Schwarz U, Amann K, Orth SR, et al. Effect of 1,25 (OH)2 vitamin D3 on glomerulosclerosis in subtotally nephrectomized rats. Kidney Int 1998;53(6):1696–705.

238. Migliori M, Giovannini L, Panichi V, et al. Treatment with 1,25-dihydroxyvitamin D3 preserves glomerular slit diaphragm-associated protein expression in experimental glomerulonephritis. Int J Immunopathol Pharmacol 2005;18(4):779–90.

239. Zhang Z, Zhang Y, Ning G, et al. Combination therapy with AT1 blocker and vitamin D analog markedly ameliorates diabetic nephropathy: blockade of compensatory renin increase. Proc Natl Acad Sci U S A 2008;105(41):15896–901.

240. Alborzi P, Patel NA, Peterson C, et al. Paricalcitol reduces albuminuria and inflammation in chronic kidney disease: a randomized double-blind pilot trial. Hypertension 2008;52(2):249–55.

241. Fishbane S, Chittineni H, Packman M, et al. Oral paricalcitol in the treatment of patients with CKD and proteinuria: a randomized trial. Am J Kidney Dis 2009; 54(4):647–52.

242. de Zeeuw D, Agarwal R, Amdahl M, et al. Selective vitamin D receptor activation with paricalcitol for reduction of albuminuria in patients with type 2 diabetes (VITAL study): a randomised controlled trial. Lancet 2010;376(9752):1543–51.

243. Moe SM, Saifullah A, LaClair RE, et al. A randomized trial of cholecalciferol versus doxercalciferol for lowering parathyroid hormone in chronic kidney disease. Clin J Am Soc Nephrol 2010;5(2):299–306.

244. Drechsler C, Pilz S, Obermayer-Pietsch B, et al. Vitamin D deficiency is associated with sudden cardiac death, combined cardiovascular events, and mortality in haemodialysis patients. Eur Heart J 2010;31(18):2253–61.

245. Drechsler C, Verduijn M, Pilz S, et al. Vitamin D status and clinical outcomes in incident dialysis patients: results from the NECOSAD study. Nephrol Dial Transplant 2011;26(3):1024–32.

246. Wolf M, Shah A, Gutierrez O, et al. Vitamin D levels and early mortality among incident hemodialysis patients. Kidney Int 2007;72(8):1004–13.

247. Dobnig H, Pilz S, Scharnagl H, et al. Independent association of low serum 25-hydroxyvitamin d and 1,25-dihydroxyvitamin d levels with all-cause and cardiovascular mortality. Arch Intern Med 2008;168(12):1340–9.

248. Kalantar-Zadeh K, Kuwae N, Regidor DL, et al. Survival predictability of time-varying indicators of bone disease in maintenance hemodialysis patients. Kidney Int 2006;70(4):771–80.

249. Kovesdy CP, Ahmadzadeh S, Anderson JE, et al. Association of activated vitamin D treatment and mortality in chronic kidney disease. Arch Intern Med 2008;168(4):397–403.

250. Melamed ML, Eustace JA, Plantinga L, et al. Changes in serum calcium, phosphate, and PTH and the risk of death in incident dialysis patients: a longitudinal study. Kidney Int 2006;70(2):351–7.

251. Shoben AB, Rudser KD, de Boer IH, et al. Association of oral calcitriol with improved survival in nondialyzed CKD. J Am Soc Nephrol 2008;19(8):1613–9.

252. Shoji T, Shinohara K, Kimoto E, et al. Lower risk for cardiovascular mortality in oral 1alpha-hydroxy vitamin D3 users in a haemodialysis population. Nephrol Dial Transplant 2004;19(1):179–84.
253. Teng M, Wolf M, Ofsthun MN, et al. Activated injectable vitamin D and hemodialysis survival: a historical cohort study. J Am Soc Nephrol 2005;16(4):1115–25.
254. Wolf M, Betancourt J, Chang Y, et al. Impact of activated vitamin D and race on survival among hemodialysis patients. J Am Soc Nephrol 2008;19(7):1379–88.
255. Tentori F, Albert JM, Young EW, et al. The survival advantage for haemodialysis patients taking vitamin D is questioned: findings from the Dialysis Outcomes and Practice Patterns Study. Nephrol Dial Transplant 2009;24(3):963–72.
256. Palmer SC, McGregor DO, Macaskill P, et al. Meta-analysis: vitamin D compounds in chronic kidney disease. Ann Intern Med 2007;147(12):840–53.

Vitamin D Receptor Signaling and Cancer

Moray J. Campbell, MS, PhD[a],*, Donald L. Trump, MD[b]

KEYWORDS

- Vitamin D • Chemoprevention • Chemotherapy • TCGA • Genomics

KEY POINTS

- Preclinical and epidemiologic data justify the concept that vitamin D compounds could be exploited as a differentiation therapy for a wide range of malignancies.
- Clinical evaluation of vitamin D compounds has been more equivocal and, although biological responses can be measured in vivo, clinical responses have not justified further evaluation.
- Dissecting mechanisms of cellular resistance is one route to defining patient groups with greater precision who may respond more fully to clinical targeting.
- Large genomic and population datasets are available that can be mined to define patient responses more completely and identify which tumor types may be most effectively targeted.

A PRIMER ON VITAMIN D BIOLOGY AND MEDICINE

The primary biological action of the secosteroid hormone vitamin D ($1,25(OH)_2D_3$) is to bind to the vitamin D receptor (NR1I1/VDR) and to regulate serum calcium levels. As a downstream consequence, the actions of the receptor control bone formation and maintenance. The first clinical manifestation of insufficient VDR endocrine signaling, rickets, was discovered by Daniel Whistler in the Netherlands in the 17th century; 300 years later, the VDR gene was cloned by Bert O'Malley and coworkers.[1] Between these dates, research into vitamin D was at the forefront of areas of public health, chemistry and biochemistry including the light catalyzed synthesis of vitamin D_3 by Adolf Windaus. For this work, he received the Nobel Prize in Chemistry (1928). Work in the 1960s and 1970s led to analyses of vitamin D endocrine metabolism and led to remarkable strides describing biochemical synthesis of $1,25(OH)_2D_3$ and the diverse biology in which VDR participates.

[a] Division of Pharmaceutics and Pharmaceutical Chemistry, College of Pharmacy, The Ohio State University, 536 Parks Hall, Columbus, OH 43210, USA; [b] Department of Medicine, Inova Schar Cancer Institute, Virginia Commonwealth University, 3221 Gallows Road, Fairfax, VA 22031, USA
* Corresponding author.
E-mail address: Campbell.1933@osu.edu

Endocrinol Metab Clin N Am 46 (2017) 1009–1038
http://dx.doi.org/10.1016/j.ecl.2017.07.007   endo.theclinics.com
0889-8529/17/© 2017 The Author(s). Published by Elsevier Inc. This is an open access article under the CC BY-NC-ND license (http://creativecommons.org/licenses/by-nc-nd/4.0/).

The precursor of 1,25$(OH)_2D_3$, cholecalciferol or vitamin D_3, is produced in the skin and converted in the liver to 25-hydroxyvitamin D_3, (25$(OH)D_3$); circulating levels of 25$(OH)D_3$ serve as a useful index of vitamin D total body stores. A further hydroxylation occurs in the principally in the kidney at the carbon 1 position by 25-hydroxyvitamin D-1α-hydroxylase (encoded by *CYP27B1*) to produce the biologically active hormone, 1,25$(OH)_2D_3$. A second mitochondrial cytochrome P450 enzyme, the 24-hydroxylase (encoded by *CYP24A1*), can use both 25$(OH)D$ and 1,25$(OH)_2D_3$ as substrates, and is the first step in the inactivation pathway for these metabolites. Because of the direct role 1,25$(OH)_2D_3$ plays in control of serum calcium levels, elevated levels of 1,25$(OH)_2D_3$ block its synthesis and induce inactivation and accelerate catabolism[2] via induction of CYP24A1, in a classical negative feedback loop.

In parallel to these VDR-centered discoveries a greater awareness emerged of the 48 members of the nuclear hormone receptor (NR) superfamily, of which the VDR is a member. As a result, the VDR and other NRs represent some of the most well-studied human transcription factors and have yielded significant insight into the mechanisms of transcriptional control.

It is worth stressing the fundamental importance of the precise monitoring and regulation of serum calcium levels to human health; hence, the endocrine role of the VDR in the regulation of calcium homeostasis is critical. The levels of vitamin D depend on cutaneous synthesis initiated by solar radiation and on dietary intake; a decrease of either one or both sources leads to insufficiency. The contribution from the ultraviolet light (UV)-initiated cutaneous conversion of 7-dehydrocholesterol to vitamin D_3 is the greater, contributing more than 90% toward final 1,25$(OH)_2D_3$ synthesis in a vitamin D–sufficient individual.

The importance of the relationships between solar exposure and the ability to capture UV-mediated energy is underscored by the inverse correlation between human skin pigmentation and latitude and associated 25$(OH)D$ levels. That is, skin pigmentation was lost as humans migrated out of Africa to adjust to life with reduced solar UV exposure. As a result, individual capacity to generate vitamin D_3 in response to solar UV exposure is intimately associated with forebear environmental adaptation. The correct and sufficient level of solar exposure and serum vitamin D_3 are matters of considerable debate, and an Institute of Medicine report[3] in 2010 recommended daily vitamin D_3 intake at the levels of 600 IU/d for most groups in the population (800 IU/d for those >70 years of age). However, this recommendation is not without controversy; parallel reassessment of the vitamin D impact on the prevention of osteoporosis has suggested that the correct level may be as high as 2 to 3000 IU/d, which may reflect more accurately ancestral serum levels.[4] Another challenge is determining how a given intake relates to serum levels among individuals[5,6] and what are the appropriate biochemical readouts for measuring systemic response.

However, given that there has been a concerted research focus on VDR signaling, there now exists a fairly sophisticated appreciation of this process, and it has been extensively reviewed.[7–13]

WHY CONSIDER TREATING CANCER WITH VITAMIN D COMPOUNDS?

The first report that VDR actions could control cancer cell growth were discovered partly through serendipity, and partly through logical extension of other studies. Reports in the 1970s identified purified cell fractions that bound 1,25$(OH)_2D_3$ with high affinity,[14] and encouraged investigators to begin to consider what were the molecular actions of the VDR in the classic tissues involved in calcium homeostasis, for example, skin, bone, intestine, and kidney.[15] In 1981, Kay Colston and coworkers[16] were first to demonstrate that $1\alpha,25(OH)_2D_3$ at nanomolar concentrations inhibited human melanoma cell proliferation in vitro. That the workers used a cancer cell model was serendipitous; cancer cell models are more readily available to study in cell culture experiments than nonmalignant counterparts, and in this case[16] the cells chosen were available in an adjacent laboratory.

In parallel, it was also known that retinoids, which are also small lipophilic molecules that target NRs, could drive cell differentiation, for example, in HL60 leukemia cells lines cells.[17] In turn these studies led to the pharmacologic exploitation of all-*trans* retinoic acid in acute promyelocytic leukemia (APL). The molecular cause of APL are translocations of the RARγ receptor forming chimeric proteins such as PML-RARγ. These chimeric proteins disrupt the control of differentiation and give rise to APL.[18–20] Pharmacologic doses of all-*trans* retinoic acid are able to trigger differentiation and, therefore, this therapy in APL is a dramatic example of targeted cancer therapies; in addition, these findings contributed significantly to the rise of the concept of differentiation therapy.[21–29] All-*trans* retinoic acid remains the mainstay of therapy for APL[30,31] and this is a major catalyst for studying RARs across cancers.[29,32,33] As a result, workers began to consider exploiting the antiproliferative actions of $1,25(OH)_2D_3$ as a differentiation therapy in cancers. In the first instance, the ability of $1,25(OH)_2D_3$ to induce differentiation in cultured mouse and human myeloid leukemia cells was examined.[34,35] From the early 1980s onwards the antiproliferative effects of $1,25(OH)_2D_3$ have been explored in a wide variety of cancer cell lines, which include all major solid tumors and leukemia.[36–43]

WHAT HAS BEEN LEARNED FROM PRECLINICAL STUDIES?

One of the most highly cited papers in the last 20 years of cancer research is the *Hallmarks of Cancer* paper by Douglas Hanahan and Robert Weinberg.[44] This landmark paper defined 6 stages necessary for cancer to develop and be sustained. Although this work has been expanded to include additional steps, this original thesis provides a highly significant backdrop against which to examine anticancer VDR functions.

Insensitivity to Antigrowth Signals and Evasion of Apoptosis

Cancer cells sustain their own proliferative signals and silence cues for programmed cell death. Signaling via $1,25(OH)_2D_3$ drives antiproliferative events, and counters the insensitivity to antigrowth signals and the evasion of apoptosis in cancer cells. Multiple investigators have examined the mechanistic basis for cell sensitivity to VDR antiproliferative responses. For example, early studies focused on understanding antiproliferative pathways, be they mediating cell cycle arrest[37,45–47] or programmed cell death.[48–50] However, other studies supported a role for $1,25(OH)_2D_3$ to block or impede programmed cell death.[51,52] Historically, hematologic malignancies combined an ease of interrogation with robust classification of cellular differentiation capacity that were envied by investigators of solid tumors. It is, therefore, no coincidence that these cell systems led to the identification of VDR control of genes that control cell cycle progression, including p21$^{(waf1/cip1)}$ and p27$^{(kip1)}$, as well as the direct binding sites on the gene *CDKN1A* (encodes p21$^{(waf1/cip1)}$).[53,54] The regulation of p27$^{(kip1)}$ seems to be mechanistically enigmatic and exemplifies the broad effects of VDR signaling in that both transcriptional and translational regulation, such as enhanced mRNA translation, and attenuating degradative mechanisms are described?[55–58]

The upregulation of p21$^{(waf1/cip1)}$ and p27$^{(kip1)}$ principally mediate G_1 cell cycle arrest, but $1\alpha,25(OH)_2D_3$ has been shown to mediate a G_2/M cell cycle arrest in a number of cancer cell lines via direct induction of GADD45α.[59–61] Concomitant with these events is a downregulation of cyclins such as cyclin A, a decrease in kinase activities associated with activated complexes, and ultimately the dephosphorylation of the retinoblastoma protein and sequestration of E2F family members in a repressive complex.[62] Concomitant with changes in the cell cycle, $1,25(OH)_2D_3$ induces differentiation, most clearly evident in myeloid cell lines, but also supported by other cell types and most likely reflects the intimate links that exist between the regulation of the G_1 transition and the induction of cellular differentiation.[63-72]

Programmed cell death has been reported in breast cancer models and leukemia models,[73-76] with evidence that the levels of BCL-2 family of proteins are tightly regulated.[77] Treatment with $1\alpha,25(OH)_2D_3$ upregulates vitamin D upregulated protein 1, which binds to the disulfide reducing protein thioredoxin and inhibits its ability to neutralize reactive oxygen species, which in turn can lead to stress-induced apoptosis.[78-80]

Tissue Invasion and Metastasis

VDR signaling enhances adhesion and suppresses the invasive capacity of cells; many of these effects are associated with a more differentiated phenotype. In an elegant series of studies, Munoz and coworkers have dissected the relationships between VDR signaling and invasion in colon cancer cell lines and primary tumors.[81-86] These workers established the delicate interplay between VDR, E-cadherin, and the Wnt signaling pathway in cell lines and clinical samples. Others have examined adhesion protein expression in other cancer models, suggesting that these mechanisms may be generalizable beyond colon cancer cells.[38,87-89]

Limitless Replicative Potential

An essential component of cancer is the ability to replicate without limits that often requires silencing of mechanisms of genomic surveillance. The VDR seems to play roles in maintaining genomic integrity and facilitating DNA repair. There is close cooperation between VDR actions and the p53 tumor suppressor pathway. Correlative data suggest that, generally, cells that respond to $1,25(OH)_2D_3$ most profoundly have wild-type p53, and at the molecular level several target genes are shared by both signaling pathways, such as *CDKN1A* and *GADD45A*.[53,54,59,90-95] Notably in the skin, VDR signaling is combined with surveillance of genomic damage to regulate mitosis negatively.[96,97] In other epithelial tissues, close cooperation between VDR regulates *BRCA1* mRNA and protein via transcriptional activation, again supporting a role in genomic surveillance.[98-100]

IDENTIFYING VITAMIN D RECEPTOR–MEDIATED TRANSCRIPTOMES

To identify critical target genes that mediate these actions, comprehensive genome-wide transcriptomic screens have revealed broad consensus on certain targets, but have also highlighted variability.[36,60,101,102] There is a significant history of VDR-centric transcriptomic studies that support the cell phenotypes observed.[36,60,61,101-111] For example, the study of isogenic cell pairs with differing sensitivities to $1,25(OH)_2D_3$ signaling has identified networks that mediate antiproliferative sensitivity. In this manner, a significant role of cross-talk between VDR and transforming growth factor (TGF)-β signaling has been revealed.[112,113] In addition, similar studies have shown that VDR transcriptional targets can distinguish leukemia aggressiveness.[114] The list of gene targets that is common across cell models seems to be short; the most clearly shared target is CYP24A1. Beyond that, commonly enriched gene networks often focus on cell cycle control and signal transduction. However, substantial variations in experimental design (eg, dose, exposure time, and use of $1,25(OH)_2D_3$ or an analog) limit strict comparisons. Thus, although a formal metaanalysis to reveal common themes has not been applied,[115,116] it seems clear that there is little overlap between the transcriptomic studies. It is also noteworthy that datasets have been developed that are aimed at noncoding RNA species.[117,118] Therefore, the diversity of the VDR regulated transcriptome is likely to increase.

More recently, these transcriptomic studies have been complemented by VDR ChIP-Seq studies in which the VDR genomic binding patterns have been captured. VDR ChIP-seq studies have been performed in several human cell types,[119–123] in the presence and/or absence of ligand, and revealed the impact of ligand binding on VDR genomic targeting. Arguably, VDR ChIP-seq studies are more important than transcriptomic studies because they reveal direct VDR genomic interactions, whereas transcriptomic analyses inevitably include direct and indirect VDR-mediated effects. Each VDR ChIP-Seq analysis revealed approximately 2000 to 6000 genomic loci normally distributed around transcription start sites, reflecting the binomial distributions found for other transcription factors,[123,124] but many loci are found at considerable distance from the transcription start sites. Another important finding from these studies is that the dual hexameric DNA motif spaced by 3 bp, a so-called DR3 motif,[125,126] is found in the majority but not all of the most prominent genomic VDR binding sites. Other binding motifs have also been suggested, for example, an inverted palindrome spaced by 9 bp, a so-called IP-9.[127,128] The application of ChIP-Seq approaches to NRs in general has revealed greater binding site diversity than previously expected; in addition the importance of flanking regions for cofactors to be biologically important to determine function.[129] These aspects of transcriptional regulation are described in greater depth in J. Wesley Pike and Sylvia Christakos' article, "Biology and Mechanisms of Action of the Vitamin D Hormone," in this issue.

The precise frequency of DR3 type elements in part remains ambiguous, because it depends on a number of variables that include the depth of the sequence read, the precise discovery motif algorithm applied, and the statistical thresholds used. Regardless of the actual percentage of VDR binding sites that contain DR3 motifs, it is clear that the VDR binds in significant levels to genomic regions that do not contain a canonical DR3. This may be explained by the VDR interacting with the genome in both direct (VDR–DNA) and indirect (VDR–protein–DNA) modes (reviewed in reference[8]).

There is a compelling case to be made for the reanalysis of the VDR ChIP-Seq data, from genomic alignment to differential peak calling. The rationale for reanalyses is two-part. Analyses of ChIP-Seq is not trivial in terms of statistical assumptions, and the existing studies have all been analyzed in a different manner. Therefore, there is the possibility that thresholds and cutoffs differ between studies. Second, the methodologies for ChIP-Seq processing are an area of active development and advancement, and the most recent approaches display a number of benefits over earlier analytical workflows.[130]

IN VIVO VITAMIN D RECEPTOR ANTICANCER ACTIONS

Given this wealth of understanding of the broad anticancer actions of the VDR, and the aim to exploit this understanding in cancer settings, the use of rodent models is a major intermediary step before clinical exploitation of VDR signaling in either chemoprevention or chemotherapy settings.

A clear difficulty in investigating the efficacy of targeting VDR with either $1,25(OH)_2D_3$ or analogues that have more attractive pharmacologic propterits[33,126,131–140] is that mice are not humans. Their spectra of age-associated malignancies are different from humans and other key metabolic differences exist. Recapitulating these lifetime effects are further compounded by the need to establish the window in which chemoprevention effects may play a role in either tumor initiation or progression.

Notwithstanding these caveats, the $Vdr^{-/-}$ animals are extremely useful tools to elucidate more clearly the role for the VDR to act in a cancer preventive manner.[2,141,142] A series of animals have been generated in which the VDR-ablated background has been crossed into animals with tumor disposition phenotypes. In the first instance, there is evidence that deleting or reducing VDR levels alters the morphology in the colon[143,144] and breast.[145] Furthermore, crossing the Vdr-deficient and heterozygote mice with mouse mammary tumor virus–neu transgenic mice has generated animals that show a degree of Vdr haplosufficiency.[145] The mammary tumor burden in the crossed mice is reduced with the presence of one wild-type Vdr allele and further with 2 wild-type Vdr alleles. Alternatively, the $Vdr^{-/-}$ animals demonstrate greater susceptibility to carcinogen challenge. For example, challenging $Vdr^{-/-}$ mice with DMBA induced more preneoplastic lesions in the mammary glands than in wild-type mice.[146]

Previously, other workers have established that deletion of the Adenomatous polyposis coli (Apc) gene in a mouse can faithfully recapitulate human colon cancer. In turn, these mice have been exploited to examine the impact of Vdr deletion on the progression of colon cancer[147]; similar studies support an antitumorogenic role for the VDR in the skin.[148] Numerous studies have examined the ability of dietary or pharmacologic addition of vitamin D compounds to either prevent tumor formation or inhibit the growth of xenograft tumors.[82,149–159]

One area of investigation is the impact of experimental dietary variations and their impact on tumor predisposition. Long-term studies of mice fed with a Western-style diet (eg, high fat and phosphate and low vitamin D and calcium content) have been exploited to examine the impact of vitamin D on colon cancer proliferation.[160] Similarly, vitamin D and calcium dietary interventions and can modulate colon crypt hyperplasia[161] and provide a rationale for how diet, inflammation, and premalignant cells could all interact and modulate cancer progression.[143,162–165]

HUMAN EPIDEMIOLOGIC FINDINGS AND CLINICAL TRIALS

Epidemiologic studies by Cedric Garland and coworkers were the first to investigate relationships between intensity of sunlight exposure and cancer incidence and revealed an inverse correlation with risk of colon cancer, and subsequently extended these findings to implicate a relationship with other cancers.[166–170] For example, levels of 25OH-D, the major circulating metabolite of vitamin D, are significantly lower in breast cancer patients than in age-matched controls.[171–173] However, these relationships are clearly complex and reflect lifetime exposures, and indeed controlling for lifestyle factors can significantly impact the strength of the relationships.[174] Although these are all association studies, and therefore function cannot be readily inferred, there are some suggestive findings that low serum levels of 25OH-D are an unfavorable prognostic indicator[175–178] or may trigger worse chemotherapy responses.[179] In other cancers, prostate for example, the relationships are more equivocal, with some positive findings,[180,181] although more generally the results are not able to support a cancer-preventative impact of vitamin D levels.[182–185] To address these ambiguities, investigators are now in the first stages of randomized supplementation trials,[186] one of which, VITAL (VITamin D and omega-3 TriaL), has now accrued 25,000 people and is examining the impact of supplementing vitamin D and omega

3 fatty acid on a range of pathologies, principally cancer and heart disease incidence[187]

Collectively, these preclinical studies and aspects of the epidemiologic findings encouraged academic and pharmaceutical partnerships in the design of vitamin D analogues that may have an optimal balance of in vivo properties to be used as a chemoprevention or chemotherapy agent. Optimizing vitamin D compounds for in vivo anticancer efficacy is aimed at ensuring a favorable balance between calcium mobilizing actions, which result in hypercalcemia, and enhancing the anticancer actions of targeting the VDR. Several medicinal chemistry groups undertook this goal, led in many ways by the group of Milan Uskokovic at Hoffman la Roche,[64,188-200] alongside Lisa Binderup at Leo Pharmaceuticals,[201-204] as well as other groups in academic settings, including Gary Posner.[205-208] Together, these and other investigators have synthesized a blizzard of vitamin D analogues that have many promising properties, being resistant to metabolism and yet have tolerable impact on serum calcium levels.

Several of these analogues have served as the lead compounds in the search for disease settings where the anticancer actions of vitamin D compounds can be exploited. For example, phase I trials have been undertaken in a range of advanced cancers[209,210] and led to more targeted phase II trials in pancreatic,[211] liver,[212] prostate,[213-216] and breast cancers.[186,217] In all cases, the regimens were well-tolerated but clinical responses were at times modest. However, this in part may reflect that the doses chosen were too conservative and the correct endpoints for these trials would be measuring cellular differentiation (or reduced proliferation or enhanced apoptosis), and this is not readily undertaken in the context of clinical trials.

These challenges are illustrated by considering prostate cancer in more detail. A number of investigators have considered the option of treating men with localized disease before surgery and then studying the prostate tumor after surgery for characterization of known VDR target genes. In a trial of nearly 40 patients with localized prostate cancer, Beer and colleagues[218] administered either $1,25(OH)_2D_3$ or placebo for 4 weeks before radical prostatectomy. Expression changes in the VDR or known candidate VDR target genes of markers of cell proliferation were examined. Interestingly VDR was downregulated in the treatment group, whereas the other genes chosen (eg, *TGFBR2*) were unchanged. Others replicated this approach but with doxercalciferol and revealed significant modulation of *TGFBR2*. Interestingly, microarray studies of $1,25(OH)_2D_3$ sensitivity in isogenic breast cancer cell lines established that *TGFBR2* was a critical mediator and marker of sensitivity toward $1,25(OH)_2D_3$.[112] Other investigators have examined the question of efficacy by escalating dose to assess how well higher levels of $1,25(OH)_2D_3$ can be tolerated.[219] Together these studies suggest that $1,25(OH)_2D_3$ can be given to prostate cancer patients at quite high doses and changes in expression of VDR-dependent genes can be observed.

This finding has also led others to consider how chemotherapy with $1,25(OH)_2D_3$ could be potentiated by combinations with other cytotoxic agents for added clinical benefit. Such combination studies are intrinsically challenging; in the vitamin D arena, Novocea undertook such an approach in their development of DN-101 (a new formulation of $1,25(OH)_2D_3$) as a cancer therapy in combination with docetaxel for men with advanced prostate cancer that had failed hormonal therapy, so-called castration resistant prostate cancer. Based on numerous preclinical studies and a single institution clinical study, Novocea conducted a randomized phase III study (ASCENT I [AIPC Study of Calcitriol ENhancing Taxotere]) to determine whether the prostate-specific antigen response rate (defined as a >50% decline in prostate-specific antigen for >1 month) was different for the standard therapy for castration resistant prostate cancer at the time (docetaxel 36 mg/m^2 weekly intravenously for 4 weeks every 6 weeks) compared with the same dose and schedule of docetaxel plus DN-101, 45 μg weekly.[220] Although this study did not meet the prostate-specific antigen response criteria, it did alter the overall survival and therefore justified a large randomized trial to assess survival. This new trial (ASCENT II) was halted before full recruitment because survival in the DN-101 arm was reduced compared with standard of care. However, the ASCENT II trial design was seriously flawed: the chemotherapy in each arm was not equal in efficacy. The design of the trial was docetaxel A + DN-101 versus docetaxel B + placebo. Substantial data existed at the time that the trial was initiated that docetaxel A was clearly inferior to docetaxel B in terms of survival in men with castration resistant prostate cancer. Therefore, the trial was actually designed to ask the question, can DN-101 overcome the inferiority of docetaxel regimen A.

A more fundamental flaw of both trials was that the dose of 1,25(OH)$_2$D$_3$ chosen was neither the biologically optimal nor the maximum tolerated dose. Other studies have clearly shown that a 2 to 3 times higher doses of calcitriol can be given safely to such patients. However, the result of ASCENT II has been interpreted as "calcitriol does not potentiate docetaxel (and hence any chemotherapy) in a large clinical trial." This is a conclusion based on no adequate data. As a result, the application of vitamin D formulations have probably been left in a challenging development point.[221]

Given these tantalizing preclinical and epidemiologic findings, the question then is why have the clinical trials not been successful? It is clear that clinical exploitation of any drug is hard, and there is a very high attrition rate of drugs passing from preclinical development to clinical implementation.[222] There are many therapies that struggle to balance preclinical promise with clinical realities, and the clinical development pipeline is often challenged by ensuring optimal clinical trial design, as illustrated by PARP inhibitors and antiangiogenesis therapies[223–227] that, although approved by the US Food and Drug Administration, have required further reanalyses to define optimal efficacy.[228,229] Therefore, it is possible that vitamin D–centered chemotherapies will fall to a similar fate. It may well be that, to date, an incomplete understanding of what are the desirable anticancer actions and inappropriate clinical trial design have impeded clinical success with vitamin D compounds.

CELLULAR MECHANISMS OF RESISTANCE

A major focus emerged on dissecting how cancer cells vary in their response to 1,25(OH)$_2$D$_3$. One initial focus was on genetic variation in the 3′ and 5′ regions of the VDR gene itself.[230–233] For example, a start codon polymorphism in exon II at the 5′ end of the gene, determined using the *fok*-I restriction enzyme, result in a truncated protein.[234] These findings were initially suggestive of a functional relationship between VDR gene genetic variation and cancer risk, but in larger studies these associations seem to be equivocal, or more nuanced.[235–242] Indeed, this is also reflected by the fact that the National Human Genome Research Institute genome-wide association studies (GWAS) catalog does not list any genome-wide significant genetic variation that is annotated to the VDR and related to cancer phenotypes; rather the genetic variation of the VDR seems to associate with immune, diabetic, and reproduction phenotypes.[243–245]

Also at the genetic level, various investigators have considered how cell responsiveness to 1,25(OH)$_2$D$_3$ may be determined by the expression of the activating (CYP27B1) and metabolizing (CYP24A1) enzymes. For example, comparative genome hybridization studies found that *CYP24A1* is amplified in human breast cancer in relation to paired normal tissue.[246,247] Others have revealed reduced *CYP27B1* mRNA and protein levels in a wide variety of cancer cell lines and primary tumors.[248–254] Together these findings suggest that cancer cell sensitivity toward 1,25(OH)$_2$D$_3$ may primarily depend on autocrine metabolism in target cells rather than the endocrine synthesis and uptake in target cells. This raises the possibility that local control of these enzymes could be exploited in targeted VDR-centric therapies.

Finally, others have considered how epigenetic mechanisms may disrupt VDR signaling. Evidence for this approach arises from the observation that 1,25(OH)$_2$D$_3$-reclacitrant cells still often respond transcriptionally, but lack transcriptional responsiveness to antiproliferative target genes such as *CDKN1A*, but sustain or even enhance induction of *CYP24A1* gene.[61,100,112,118,255] These data suggest that the VDR transcriptome is skewed in cancer cells to disfavor antiproliferative target genes, and that lack of functional VDR alone cannot explain resistance. The interactions of transcriptional corepressors such as NCOR1 and NCOR2/SMRT have been examined to investigate this possibility.[61,256–261] In turn, altered VDR–corepressor interactions may form a molecular lesion that could be targeted by cotreatment of 1,25(OH)$_2$D$_3$ plus the HDAC inhibitors.[262–267]

LESSONS FOR BIG DATA TO OPTIMIZE VITAMIN D RECEPTOR–CENTERED THERAPIES

Biology is very clearly in the genomic era, in which the sum total of genes, transcripts, proteins and metabolites in cells are captured and analyzed. Arguably, the achievements of the Human Genome Project[268] served as a major catalyst for this approach, and other research consortia have applied similar technologies and approaches to tackle other fundamental challenges in biology. Powerful examples are illustrated by Encyclopedia of DNA coding elements (ENCODE),[269,270] RoadMap Epigenome,[271] Functional and Taxonomic Analysis of Metagenomes,[272] International Human Epigenome Consortium,[273,274] the Cancer Genome Atlas (TCGA),[275] and the Genotype-Tissue Expression (GTEx) project.[276] The volume of data generated by these projects is unprecedented and truly transformative in terms of the questions that can be addressed, the manner in which they are tackled, and the how the findings are interpreted and widely translated.

Bioinformatic analyses are central to both the generation of these complex datasets and their investigation. Unbiased bioinformatics analyses can reveal organizational insight that is neither obvious nor intuitive. Unbiased and agnostic analyses are achieved by applying algorithmic approaches that depend on discrete mathematics and information theory, combined with graph theory, data mining, and computer science generally, with a central role for the statistical sciences. In this manner, bioinformatic approaches offer the promise to reveal underlying mechanisms of biology in health and disease.

For example, -omic technologies can be applied to capture genomic structural variants and mutations, gene and protein expression patterns, protein posttranslational modifications, and metabolites across cell states. Bioinformatics analyses is applied to all steps from data capture, to data processing (eg, filtering and normalization), to establishing reproducible changes between states A and B, and to more complex integrative analyses from combining different -omic datasets. The statistical sciences are central to all these steps. The ultimate goal from these workflows is to identify network changes between states, and finally to identify nodes that exert control. Such nodes would then form attractive targets for interventionist wet laboratory-based experiments.

Several points are worth stressing from this theoretic workflow. First, study design and phenotype definition are critical. Second, all analyses include a denominator (eg, the genome, the detectable transcriptome, etc) so that any change is considered against the appropriate backdrop of all events occurring in the cell. Third, all data processing includes normalization across samples, including replicates and states, and subsequent filtering to remove the large component of the signal that is unchanging to, therefore, control the penalties of false discovery. Finally, the integrative steps have very high potential for creativity and novelty. That is, as the volume of publicly available data grows, the statistical approaches and types of data integration that can occur are varied and represent where many of the key biological questions of the future will be framed.

The mechanics of VDR signaling and disruption in cancer can, therefore, be analyzed in the paradigm of mining and analyzing large biological datasets. Therefore, there are several bioinformatics approaches that are applicable to the VDR. In the first instance, applying the genome as the denominator allows the question to be addressed of where VDR biology is significant. For example, in what cancer does a significant role for the VDR emerge when considering all genetic variations or gene expression?

At the simplest, GTEx project[277] and the TCGA data can be investigated to identify in which normal tissue is the VDR most highly expressed, or in what cancer is it most commonly altered. The GTEx data reveal that the VDR is most abundant in tissues of the colon and small intestine, and least abundant in basal ganglia and brain tissues. The TCGA data reveal that the VDR is most commonly altered by deletion in 2 cohorts of adenoid cystic carcinoma of the breast.[278,279] Interestingly, the GTEx data clearly reflect the focus at the preclinical and epidemiologic level of investigated VDR in colon cancer. However, no studies to date have examined VDR in the context of adenoid cystic carcinoma of breast cancer.

The TCGA[280,281] data are derived from more than 33 different cancer types that were collected from approximately 11,000 patients. The analyses of these data have been the subject of more than 350 papers to date and it is striking that none of these papers identified a genome-wide significant role for disruption or association of the VDR with tumor phenotypes. By comparison, more than 100 TCGA papers report a significant relationship with TP53.

Often, biological signals are extremely contextual. Analyses of myeloid[282] and megakaryocyte[283] cells illustrate that there is a significant role for the VDR to act in distinct transcriptional units that control specific points of cell differentiation. These findings reveal the intricate mechanistic basis to some of the earliest cancer studies on VDR signaling in leukemia,[284,285] which revealed that exogenous vitamin D compounds can trigger cell differentiation. Therefore, reflecting on the role VDR seems to be playing in myeloid systems, it is worth stressing the apparent importance of VDR in immune phenotypes. That is, GWAS identify significant roles for VDR genetic variation in immune phenotypes.[244,286,287]

Perhaps reflecting the reproduction-related functions of the VDR in murine systems,[288] the Vdr$^{-/-}$ mice display a mammary gland phenotype, and this genotype can modulate cancer incidence in murine cancer models.[145,289,290] However, transcriptional and epigenomic control of breast epithelial systems in human cells does not reveal a genome-wide significant role for the VDR,[291] and the major breast cancer papers from TCGA have not identified a genome-wide significant role for the VDR to act as a cancer driver.[292–295]

Putting these findings together from leukemia and common cancers suggests that the VDR itself does not act as a direct cancer driver, either through loss or gain of function. This finding may limit the likelihood of therapeutic exploitation in the cancer context.

Other approaches can be applied to leverage public data by changing the denominator. It is possible to address questions centered around the VDR and related genes, and thereby limit the penalties of false discovery. For example, previously we analyzed 13 transcription factor families implicated in cancer, including the NR superfamily, across 3000 tumors from 6 different tumor types.[296–300] Bootstrapping approaches[301] established that, across cancers, only the NR family was significantly downregulated, but was neither significantly mutated nor altered by copy number variation.[302] Within the NRs, we found that several NRs were uniquely suppressed in only one tumor site, including VDR in the colon cancer (COAD) cohort; this finding may reflect the strong expression of VDR in the normal colon. VDR downregulation was not found to be driven by copy number variation or mutation and thus epigenetic mechanisms may be primarily responsible for altered expression.[301,302] There is a very well-established literature supporting links between corrupted VDR signaling and colon cancer.[85,147,303–308] Our pan-cancer analyses add to these findings, suggesting that loss of VDR-induced growth restraint may be more apparent in colon cancer than in other cancers where alterations are not apparent.

The VDR ChIP-seq data also lend themselves to be combined with other types of publicly available data to ask further questions concerning VDR function. For example, an attractive integration approach is to examine how significant genetic variation in transcription factor binding site can relate to phenotypes and disease susceptibility. Testing the possibility that genetic variation impacts transcription factor function underpins trait differences and disease phenotypes is analytically challenging, given the size of the datasets and the potential for false discovery. Various groups have addressed this challenge; notably, both the ENCODE and Roadmap Epigenome consortia leveraged the remarkable volume of ChIP-seq data they generated and merged the binding sites with GWAS data to reveal and rank sites where single nucleotide polymorphisms (SNPs) seem to have a significant impact on the activity of multiple transcription factors.[124,271,309]

However, given that VDR has not been considered in any of these consortia, we have recently integrated VDR ChIP-Seq[119–123] with National Human Genome Research Institute GWAS SNPs, and SNPs in linkage disequilibrium, to provide novel insight into the interaction between disease- and phenotype-associated SNPs and VDR binding. From these analyses, we applied transcription factor motif searching and exploited other ChIP-Seq data to identify significant interactions between the VDR and other transcription factors and disease traits. In this manner, we identified genetic variation that was significant at the genome-wide level enriched in VDR binding sites that were shared with nuclear factor-κB binding regions related to immune phenotypes, including self-reported allergy.[310] However, none of the GWAS SNPs identified in VDR binding sites were neither in a DR3 type motif, again underscoring the diversity of VDR binding sites, nor related to cancer phenotypes.

However, there does seem to be a significant relationship between VDR and colon cancer, given that the VDR is highly expressed in the normal colon, associated with the control of local immunity,[82,308,311–315] and that, of all the NRs, the VDR is commonly and significantly downregulated in colon cancer. To test this possibility, we leveraged VDR ChIP-Seq data derived in LS180 colon cancer cells[121] with the expression of VDR target genes in the TCGA–COAD cohort.[298] Clustering the tumors by expression patterns then allowed testing the relationships between expression of VDR target genes and clinical outcome. Expression of VDR target genes were either significantly repressed or activated in the COAD cohort, suggesting that VDR functions in both activating and repressing complexes at the basal (or physiologically activated) state.[316] For instance, *LGALS4* is a VDR target gene that is specific to colonic cells and is downregulated in colon cancer, acting as a tumor suppressor,[303,317,318] and *LGALS4* quartile expression patterns significantly associated with disease-free survival in specific patient subgroups.

A further opportunity available for meaningful data integration of ChIP-Seq studies is in the judicious choice of the cell line of study. For example, there are 3 tier 1 cell lines in the ENCODE project including K562 cells, which has approximately 600 publicly available genome-wide datasets. Therefore, there is an exciting opportunity once VDR ChIP-Seq is undertaken in one of these models in terms of integrative analyses[319] that could leverage ENCODE or RoadMap Epigenome data.

FUTURE CONSIDERATIONS AND SUMMARY

Enthusiasm remains for exploiting vitamin D signaling in cancer systems. This partly reflects that the biology is now very well-understood, that the toxicities associated with vitamin D compounds are easily monitored and managed and that in an era of high dimensional biological data it is possible to measure and dissect the actions of VDR signaling in very great detail. It seems likely that efforts will continue to exploit vitamin D compounds in the clinical setting, and it may well be that by exploiting tools to very accurately measure tumor type and burden will allow vitamin D-centered therapies to be applied with great precision. It seems likely that among the actions of VDR, the immunomodulatory capacity may ultimately be the ones that are most advantageous in cancer therapies.

ACKNOWLEDGMENTS

M.J. Campbell acknowledges support in part from the Prostate program of the Department of Defense Congressionally Directed Medical Research Programs [W81XWH-14-1-0608, W81XWH-11-2-0033]. D.L. Trump acknowledges the support of the Inova Schar Cancer Institute and the generosity of the Schar Family.

REFERENCES

1. Baker AR, McDonnell DP, Hughes M, et al. Cloning and expression of full-length cDNA encoding human vitamin D receptor. Proc Natl Acad Sci U S A 1988;85: 3294–8.
2. Takeyama K, Kitanaka S, Sato T, et al. 25-Hydroxyvitamin D3 1alpha-hydroxylase and vitamin D synthesis. Science 1997;277:1827–30.
3. Ross AC, Manson JE, Abrams SA, et al. The 2011 report on dietary reference intakes for calcium and vitamin D from the institute of medicine: what clinicians need to know. J Clin Endocrinol Metab 2011;96:53–8.
4. Dawson-Hughes B, Heaney RP, Holick MF, et al. Estimates of optimal vitamin D status. Osteoporos Int 2005;16:713–6.
5. King L, Dear K, Harrison SL, et al. Investigating the patterns and determinants of seasonal variation in vitamin D status in Australian adults: the Seasonal D Cohort Study. BMC Public Health 2016;16:892.
6. Diffey BL. Modelling the seasonal variation of vitamin D due to sun exposure. Br J Dermatol 2010;162:1342–8.
7. Campbell MJ. Vitamin D and the RNA transcriptome: more than mRNA regulation. Front Physiol 2014;5:181.

8. Carlberg C, Campbell MJ. Vitamin D receptor signaling mechanisms: integrated actions of a well-defined transcription factor. Steroids 2013;78:127–36.
9. Carlberg C. Molecular approaches for optimizing vitamin D supplementation. Vitam Horm 2016;100:255–71.
10. Narvaez CJ, Matthews D, LaPorta E, et al. The impact of vitamin D in breast cancer: genomics, pathways, metabolism. Front Physiol 2014;5:213.
11. White JH. Vitamin D metabolism and signaling in the immune system. Rev Endocr Metab Disord 2012;13:21–9.
12. Bikle DD. Extraskeletal actions of vitamin D. Ann N Y Acad Sci 2016;1376:29–52.
13. Jeffery LE, Raza K, Hewison M. Vitamin D in rheumatoid arthritis-towards clinical application. Nat Rev Rheumatol 2016;12:201–10.
14. Brumbaugh PF, Hughes MR, Haussler MR. Cytoplasmic and nuclear binding components for 1alpha25-dihydroxyvitamin D3 in chick parathyroid glands. Proc Natl Acad Sci U S A 1975;72:4871–5.
15. Jones PG, Haussler MR. Scintillation autoradiographic localization of 1,25-dihydroxyvitamin D3 in chick intestine. Endocrinology 1979;104:313–21.
16. Colston K, Colston MJ, Feldman D. 1,25-dihydroxyvitamin D3 and malignant melanoma: the presence of receptors and inhibition of cell growth in culture. Endocrinology 1981;108:1083–6.
17. Strickland S, Mahdavi V. The induction of differentiation in teratocarcinoma stem cells by retinoic acid. Cell 1978;15:393–403.
18. Raelson JV, Nervi C, Rosenauer A, et al. The PML/RAR alpha oncoprotein is a direct molecular target of retinoic acid in acute promyelocytic leukemia cells. Blood 1996;88:2826–32.
19. Grignani F, Ferrucci PF, Testa U, et al. The acute promyelocytic leukemia-specific PML-RAR alpha fusion protein inhibits differentiation and promotes survival of myeloid precursor cells. Cell 1993;74:423–31.
20. de The H, Lavau C, Marchio A, et al. The PML-RAR alpha fusion mRNA generated by the t(15;17) translocation in acute promyelocytic leukemia encodes a functionally altered RAR. Cell 1991;66:675–84.
21. Chen SJ, Zhu YJ, Tong JH, et al. Rearrangements in the second intron of the RARA gene are present in a large majority of patients with acute promyelocytic leukemia and are used as molecular marker for retinoic acid-induced leukemic cell differentiation. Blood 1991;78:2696–701.
22. Douer D, Koeffler HP. Retinoic acid. Inhibition of the clonal growth of human myeloid leukemia cells. J Clin Invest 1982;69:277–83.
23. Breitman TR, Selonick SE, Collins SJ. Induction of differentiation of the human promyelocytic leukemia cell line (HL-60) by retinoic acid. Proc Natl Acad Sci U S A 1980;77:2936–40.
24. Castaigne S, Chomienne C, Daniel MT, et al. Retinoic acids in the treatment of acute promyelocytic leukemia. Nouv Rev Fr Hematol 1990;32:36–8.
25. Huang ME, Ye YC, Chen SR, et al. Use of all-trans retinoic acid in the treatment of acute promyelocytic leukemia. Haematol Blood Transfus 1989;32:88–96.
26. Grignani F, De Matteis S, Nervi C, et al. Fusion proteins of the retinoic acid receptor-alpha recruit histone deacetylase in promyelocytic leukaemia. Nature 1998;391:815–8.
27. Lin RJ, Nagy L, Inoue S, et al. Role of the histone deacetylase complex in acute promyelocytic leukaemia. Nature 1998;391:811–4.
28. Spira AI, Carducci MA. Differentiation therapy. Curr Opin Pharmacol 2003;3: 338–43.

29. Ferrari AC, Waxman S. Differentiation agents in cancer therapy. Cancer Chemother Biol Response Modif 1994;15:337–66.

30. Lo-Coco F, Di Donato L, GIMEMA, et al, German-Austrian Acute Myeloid Leukemia Study Group and Study Alliance Leukemia. Targeted therapy alone for acute promyelocytic leukemia. N Engl J Med 2016;374:1197–8.

31. Uray IP, Dmitrovsky E, Brown PH. Retinoids and rexinoids in cancer prevention: from laboratory to clinic. Semin Oncol 2016;43:49–64.

32. Bhutani T, Koo J. A review of the chemopreventative effects of oral retinoids for internal neoplasms. J Drugs Dermatol 2011;10:1292–8.

33. Campbell MJ, Park S, Uskokovic MR, et al. Expression of retinoic acid receptor-beta sensitizes prostate cancer cells to growth inhibition mediated by combinations of retinoids and a 19-nor hexafluoride vitamin D3 analog. Endocrinology 1998;139:1972–80.

34. Miyaura C, Abe E, Kuribayashi T, et al. 1 alpha,25-dihydroxyvitamin D3 induces differentiation of human myeloid leukemia cells. Biochem Biophys Res Commun 1981;102:937–43.

35. Abe E, Miyaura C, Sakagami H, et al. Differentiation of mouse myeloid leukemia cells induced by 1 alpha,25-dihydroxyvitamin D3. Proc Natl Acad Sci U S A 1981;78:4990–4.

36. Palmer HG, Sanchez-Carbayo M, Ordonez-Moran P, et al. Genetic signatures of differentiation induced by 1alpha,25-dihydroxyvitamin D3 in human colon cancer cells. Cancer Res 2003;63:7799–806.

37. Koike M, Elstner E, Campbell MJ, et al. 19-nor-hexafluoride analogue of vitamin D3: a novel class of potent inhibitors of proliferation of human breast cell lines. Cancer Res 1997;57:4545–50.

38. Campbell MJ, Elstner E, Holden S, et al. Inhibition of proliferation of prostate cancer cells by a 19-nor-hexafluoride vitamin D3 analogue involves the induction of p21waf1, p27kip1 and E-cadherin. J Mol Endocrinol 1997;19:15–27.

39. Elstner E, Campbell MJ, Munker R, et al. Novel 20-epi-vitamin D3 analog combined with 9-cis-retinoic acid markedly inhibits colony growth of prostate cancer cells. Prostate 1999;40:141–9.

40. Peehl DM, Skowronski RJ, Leung GK, et al. Antiproliferative effects of 1,25-dihydroxyvitamin D3 on primary cultures of human prostatic cells. Cancer Res 1994; 54:805–10.

41. Welsh J, Wietzke JA, Zinser GM, et al. Impact of the vitamin D3 receptor on growth-regulatory pathways in mammary gland and breast cancer. J Steroid Biochem Mol Biol 2002;83:85–92.

42. Colston KW, Berger U, Coombes RC. Possible role for vitamin D in controlling breast cancer cell proliferation. Lancet 1989;1:188–91.

43. Colston K, Colston MJ, Fieldsteel AH, et al. 1,25-dihydroxyvitamin D3 receptors in human epithelial cancer cell lines. Cancer Res 1982;42:856–9.

44. Hanahan D, Weinberg RA. The hallmarks of cancer. Cell 2000;100:57–70.

45. Yen A, Varvayanis S. RB phosphorylation in sodium butyrate-resistant HL-60 cells: cross-resistance to retinoic acid but not vitamin D3. J Cell Physiol 1995; 163:502–9.

46. Hager G, Formanek M, Gedlicka C, et al. 1,25(OH)2 vitamin D3 induces elevated expression of the cell cycle-regulating genes P21 and P27 in squamous carcinoma cell lines of the head and neck. Acta Otolaryngol 2001;121:103–9.

47. Kumagai T, O'Kelly J, Said JW, et al. Vitamin D2 analog 19-nor-1,25-dihydroxy-vitamin D2: antitumor activity against leukemia, myeloma, and colon cancer cells. J Natl Cancer Inst 2003;95:896–905.

48. Davoust N, Wion D, Chevalier G, et al. Vitamin D receptor stable transfection restores the susceptibility to 1,25-dihydroxyvitamin D3 cytotoxicity in a rat glioma resistant clone. J Neurosci Res 1998;52:210–9.

49. Fife RS, Sledge GW Jr, Proctor C. Effects of vitamin D3 on proliferation of cancer cells in vitro. Cancer Lett 1997;120:65–9.

50. Naveilhan P, Berger F, Haddad K, et al. Induction of glioma cell death by 1,25(OH)2 vitamin D3: towards an endocrine therapy of brain tumors? J Neurosci Res 1994;37:271–7.

51. Wang X, Studzinski GP. Antiapoptotic action of 1,25-dihydroxyvitamin D3 is associated with increased mitochondrial MCL-1 and RAF-1 proteins and reduced release of cytochrome c. Exp Cell Res 1997;235:210–7.

52. Xu HM, Tepper CG, Jones JB, et al. 1,25-Dihydroxyvitamin D3 protects HL60 cells against apoptosis but down-regulates the expression of the bcl-2 gene. Exp Cell Res 1993;209:367–74.

53. Liu M, Lee MH, Cohen M, et al. Transcriptional activation of the Cdk inhibitor p21 by vitamin D3 leads to the induced differentiation of the myelomonocytic cell line U937. Genes Dev 1996;10:142–53.

54. Saramaki A, Banwell CM, Campbell MJ, et al. Regulation of the human p21(waf1/cip1) gene promoter via multiple binding sites for p53 and the vitamin D3 receptor. Nucleic Acids Res 2006;34:543–54.

55. Wang QM, Jones JB, Studzinski GP. Cyclin-dependent kinase inhibitor p27 as a mediator of the G1-S phase block induced by 1,25-dihydroxyvitamin D3 in HL60 cells. Cancer Res 1996;56:264–7.

56. Li P, Li C, Zhao X, et al. p27(Kip1) stabilization and G(1) arrest by 1,25-dihydroxyvitamin D(3) in ovarian cancer cells mediated through down-regulation of cyclin E/cyclin-dependent kinase 2 and Skp1-Cullin-F-box protein/Skp2 ubiquitin ligase. J Biol Chem 2004;279:25260–7.

57. Huang YC, Chen JY, Hung WC. Vitamin D(3) receptor/Sp1 complex is required for the induction of p27(Kip1) expression by vitamin D(3). Oncogene 2004; 23(28):4856–61.

58. Hengst L, Reed SI. Translational control of p27Kip1 accumulation during the cell cycle. Science 1996;271:1861–4.

59. Jiang F, Li P, Fornace AJ Jr, et al. G2/M arrest by 1,25-dihydroxyvitamin D3 in ovarian cancer cells mediated through the induction of GADD45 via an exonic enhancer. J Biol Chem 2003;278:48030–40.

60. Akutsu N, Lin R, Bastien Y, et al. Regulation of gene Expression by 1alpha,25-dihydroxyvitamin D3 and Its analog EB1089 under growth-inhibitory conditions in squamous carcinoma Cells. Mol Endocrinol 2001;15:1127–39.

61. Khanim FL, Gommersall LM, Wood VH, et al. Altered SMRT levels disrupt vitamin D3 receptor signalling in prostate cancer cells. Oncogene 2004;23: 6712–25.

62. Wu G, Fan RS, Li W, et al. Modulation of cell cycle control by vitamin D3 and its analogue, EB1089, in human breast cancer cells. Oncogene 1997;15:1555–63.

63. Lubbert M, Salser W, Prokocimer M, et al. Stable methylation patterns of MYC and other genes regulated during terminal myeloid differentiation. Leukemia 1991;5:533–9.

64. Zhou JY, Norman AW, Lubbert M, et al. Novel vitamin D analogs that modulate leukemic cell growth and differentiation with little effect on either intestinal calcium absorption or bone mobilization. Blood 1989;74:82–93.

65. Zile MH, Cullum ME, Simpson RU, et al. Induction of differentiation of human promyelocytic leukemia cell line HL-60 by retinoyl glucuronide, a biologically active metabolite of vitamin A. Proc Natl Acad Sci U S A 1987;84:2208–12.

66. Wang JK, Johnson MD, Morgan JI, et al. Vitamin D3 derivatives inhibit the differentiation of Friend erythroleukemia cells. Mol Pharmacol 1986;30:639–42.

67. Brelvi ZS, Studzinski GP. Inhibition of DNA synthesis by an inducer of differentiation of leukemic cells, 1 alpha, 25 dihydroxy vitamin D3, precedes down regulation of the c-myc gene. J Cell Physiol 1986;128:171–9.

68. Munker R, Norman A, Koeffler HP. Vitamin D compounds. Effect on clonal proliferation and differentiation of human myeloid cells. J Clin Invest 1986;78:424–30.

69. Palmer HG, Gonzalez-Sancho JM, Espada J, et al. Vitamin D(3) promotes the differentiation of colon carcinoma cells by the induction of E-cadherin and the inhibition of beta-catenin signaling. J Cell Biol 2001;154.369–87.

70. Lazzaro G, Agadir A, Qing W, et al. Induction of differentiation by 1alpha-hydroxyvitamin D(5) in T47D human breast cancer cells and its interaction with vitamin D receptors. Eur J Cancer 2000;36:780–6.

71. Konety BR, Schwartz GG, Acierno JS Jr, et al. The role of vitamin D in normal prostate growth and differentiation. Cell Growth Differ 1996;7:1563–70.

72. Kim YR, Abraham NG, Lutton JD. Mechanisms of differentiation of U937 leukemic cells induced by GM-CSF and 1,25(OH)2 vitamin D3. Leuk Res 1991;15:409–18.

73. Narvaez CJ, Byrne BM, Romu S, et al. Induction of apoptosis by 1,25-dihydroxyvitamin D3 in MCF-7 vitamin D3-resistant variant can be sensitized by TPA. J Steroid Biochem Mol Biol 2003;84:199–209.

74. Diaz GD, Paraskeva C, Thomas MG, et al. Apoptosis is induced by the active metabolite of vitamin D3 and its analogue EB1089 in colorectal adenoma and carcinoma cells: possible implications for prevention and therapy. Cancer Res 2000;60:2304–12.

75. Elstner E, Linker-Israeli M, Le J, et al. Synergistic decrease of clonal proliferation, induction of differentiation, and apoptosis of acute promyelocytic leukemia cells after combined treatment with novel 20-epi vitamin D3 analogs and 9-cis retinoic acid. J Clin Invest 1997;99:349–60.

76. Elstner E, Linker-Israeli M, Said J, et al. 20-epi-vitamin D3 analogues: a novel class of potent inhibitors of proliferation and inducers of differentiation of human breast cancer cell lines. Cancer Res 1995;55:2822–30.

77. Narvaez CJ, Vanweelden K, Byrne I, et al. Characterization of a vitamin D3-resistant MCF-7 cell line. Endocrinology 1996;137:400–9.

78. Byrne BM, Welsh J. Altered thioredoxin subcellular localization and redox status in MCF-7 cells following 1,25-dihydroxyvitamin D3 treatment. J Steroid Biochem Mol Biol 2005;97:57–64.

79. Jeon JH, Lee KN, Hwang CY, et al. Tumor suppressor VDUP1 increases p27(kip1) stability by inhibiting JAB1. Cancer Res 2005;65:4485–9.

80. Junn E, Han SH, Im JY, et al. Vitamin D3 up-regulated protein 1 mediates oxidative stress via suppressing the thioredoxin function. J Immunol 2000;164:6287–95.

81. Ferrer-Mayorga G, Gomez-Lopez G, Barbachano A, et al. Vitamin D receptor expression and associated gene signature in tumour stromal fibroblasts predict clinical outcome in colorectal cancer. Gut 2017;66(8):1449–62.

82. Alvarez-Diaz S, Valle N, Garcia JM, et al. Cystatin D is a candidate tumor suppressor gene induced by vitamin D in human colon cancer cells. J Clin Invest 2009;119:2343–58.

83. Pendas-Franco N, Garcia JM, Pena C, et al. DICKKOPF-4 is induced by TCF/beta-catenin and upregulated in human colon cancer, promotes tumour cell invasion and angiogenesis and is repressed by 1alpha,25-dihydroxyvitamin D3. Oncogene 2008;27:4467–77.

84. Larriba MJ, Valle N, Palmer HG, et al. The inhibition of Wnt/beta-catenin signalling by 1alpha,25-dihydroxyvitamin D3 is abrogated by Snail1 in human colon cancer cells. Endocr Relat Cancer 2007;14:141–51.

85. Palmer HG, Larriba MJ, Garcia JM, et al. The transcription factor SNAIL represses vitamin D receptor expression and responsiveness in human colon cancer. Nat Med 2004;10:917–9.

86. Tenbaum SP, Ordonez-Moran P, Puig I, et al. Beta-catenin confers resistance to PI3K and AKT inhibitors and subverts FOXO3a to promote metastasis in colon cancer. Nat Med 2012;18:892–901.

87. Chiang KC, Yeh CN, Hsu JT, et al. The vitamin D analog, MART-10, represses metastasis potential via downregulation of epithelial-mesenchymal transition in pancreatic cancer cells. Cancer Lett 2014;354:235–44.

88. Upadhyay SK, Verone A, Shoemaker S, et al. 1,25-dihydroxyvitamin D3 (1,25(OH)2D3) signaling capacity and the epithelial-mesenchymal transition in non-small cell lung cancer (NSCLC): implications for use of 1,25(OH)2D3 in NSCLC treatment. Cancers (Basel) 2013;5:1504–21.

89. Gniadecki R, Gajkowska B, Hansen M. 1,25-dihydroxyvitamin D3 stimulates the assembly of adherens junctions in keratinocytes: involvement of protein kinase C. Endocrinology 1997;138:2241–8.

90. Prudencio J, Akutsu N, Benlimame N, et al. Action of low calcemic 1alpha,25-dihydroxyvitamin D3 analogue EB1089 in head and neck squamous cell carcinoma. J Natl Cancer Inst 2001;93:745–53.

91. Baudet C, Chevalier G, Chassevent A, et al. 1,25-dihydroxyvitamin D3 induces programmed cell death in a rat glioma cell line. J Neurosci Res 1996;46:540–50.

92. Asada M, Yamada T, Fukumuro K, et al. p21Cip1/WAF1 is important for differentiation and survival of U937 cells. Leukemia 1998;12:1944–50.

93. Munker R, Kobayashi T, Elstner E, et al. A new series of vitamin D analogs is highly active for clonal inhibition, differentiation, and induction of WAF1 in myeloid leukemia. Blood 1996;88:2201–9.

94. Schwaller J, Koeffler HP, Niklaus G, et al. Posttranscriptional stabilization underlies p53-independent induction of p21WAF1/CIP1/SDI1 in differentiating human leukemic cells. J Clin Invest 1995;95:973–9.

95. Stambolsky P, Tabach Y, Fontemaggi G, et al. Modulation of the vitamin D3 response by cancer-associated mutant p53. Cancer Cell 2010;17:273–85.

96. Reichrath J, Reichrath S, Heyne K, et al. Tumor suppression in skin and other tissues via cross-talk between vitamin D- and p53-signaling. Front Physiol 2014;5:166.

97. Ellison TI, Smith MK, Gilliam AC, et al. Inactivation of the vitamin D receptor enhances susceptibility of murine skin to UV-induced tumorigenesis. J Invest Dermatol 2008;128:2508–17.

98. Graziano S, Johnston R, Deng O, et al. Vitamin D/vitamin D receptor axis regulates DNA repair during oncogene-induced senescence. Oncogene 2016;35: 5362–76.

99. Pickholtz I, Saadyan S, Keshet GI, et al. Cooperation between BRCA1 and vitamin D is critical for histone acetylation of the p21waf1 promoter and growth inhibition of breast cancer cells and cancer stem-like cells. Oncotarget 2014;5: 11827–46.

100. Campbell MJ, Gombart AF, Kwok SH, et al. The anti-proliferative effects of 1alpha,25(OH)2D3 on breast and prostate cancer cells are associated with induction of BRCA1 gene expression. Oncogene 2000;19:5091–7.

101. Eelen G, Verlinden L, Van Camp M, et al. Microarray analysis of 1alpha,25-dihydroxyvitamin D3-treated MC3T3-E1 cells. J Steroid Biochem Mol Biol 2004; 89-90:405–7.

102. Wang TT, Tavera-Mendoza LE, Laperriere D, et al. Large-scale in silico and microarray-based identification of direct 1,25-dihydroxyvitamin D3 target genes. Mol Endocrinol 2005;19(11):2685–95.

103. Savli H, Aalto Y, Nagy B, et al. Gene expression analysis of 1,25(OH)2D3-dependent differentiation of HL-60 cells: a cDNA array study. Br J Haematol 2002;118:1065–70.

104. Lin R, Nagai Y, Sladek R, et al. Expression profiling in squamous carcinoma cells reveals pleiotropic effects of vitamin D3 analog EB1089 signaling on cell proliferation, differentiation, and immune system regulation. Mol Endocrinol 2002;16: 1243–56.

105. Ferreira GB, Vanherwegen AS, Eelen G, et al. Vitamin D3 induces tolerance in human dendritic cells by activation of intracellular metabolic pathways. Cell Rep 2015. [Epub ahead of print].

106. Bosse Y, Maghni K, Hudson TJ. 1alpha,25-dihydroxy-vitamin D3 stimulation of bronchial smooth muscle cells induces autocrine, contractility, and remodeling processes. Physiol Genomics 2007;29:161–8.

107. Kawata H, Kamiakito T, Takayashiki N, et al. Vitamin D3 suppresses the androgen-stimulated growth of mouse mammary carcinoma SC-3 cells by transcriptional repression of fibroblast growth factor 8. J Cell Physiol 2006;207: 793–9.

108. Guzey M, Luo J, Getzenberg RH. Vitamin D3 modulated gene expression patterns in human primary normal and cancer prostate cells. J Cell Biochem 2004;93:271–85.

109. Kobayashi T, Uehara S, Ikeda T, et al. Vitamin D3 up-regulated protein-1 regulates collagen expression in mesangial cells. Kidney Int 2003;64:1632–42.

110. Hilpert J, Wogensen L, Thykjaer T, et al. Expression profiling confirms the role of endocytic receptor megalin in renal vitamin D3 metabolism. Kidney Int 2002;62: 1672–81.

111. Takahashi Y, Nagata T, Ishii Y, et al. Up-regulation of vitamin D3 up-regulated protein 1 gene in response to 5-fluorouracil in colon carcinoma SW620. Oncol Rep 2002;9:75–9.

112. Towsend K, Trevino V, Falciani F, et al. Identification of VDR-responsive gene signatures in breast cancer cells. Oncology 2006;71:111–23.

113. Larsen JE, Nathan V, Osborne JK, et al. ZEB1 drives epithelial-to-mesenchymal transition in lung cancer. J Clin Invest 2016;126:3219–35.

114. Tagliafico E, Tenedini E, Manfredini R, et al. Identification of a molecular signature predictive of sensitivity to differentiation induction in acute myeloid leukemia. Leukemia 2006;20:1751–8.

115. Engreitz JM, Chen R, Morgan AA, et al. ProfileChaser: searching microarray repositories based on genome-wide patterns of differential expression. Bioinformatics 2011;27:3317–8.

116. Shah NH, Jonquet C, Chiang AP, et al. Ontology-driven indexing of public datasets for translational bioinformatics. BMC Bioinformatics 2009;10(Suppl 2):S1.

117. Jiang YJ, Bikle DD. LncRNA: a new player in 1alpha, 25(OH)2 vitamin D3/VDR protection against skin cancer formation. Exp Dermatol 2014;23:147–50.

118. Singh PK, Long MD, Battaglia S, et al. VDR regulation of microRNA differs across prostate cell models suggesting extremely flexible control of transcription. Epigenetics 2015;10:40–9.

119. Ding N, Yu RT, Subramaniam N, et al. A vitamin D receptor/SMAD genomic circuit gates hepatic fibrotic response. Cell 2013;153:601–13.

120. Heikkinen S, Vaisanen S, Pehkonen P, et al. Nuclear hormone 1alpha,25-dihydroxyvitamin D3 elicits a genome-wide shift in the locations of VDR chromatin occupancy. Nucleic Acids Res 2011;39:9181–93.

121. Meyer MB, Goetsch PD, Pike JW. VDR/RXR and TCF4/beta-catenin cistromes in colonic cells of colorectal tumor origin: impact on c-FOS and c-MYC gene expression. Mol Endocrinol 2012;26:37–51.

122. Ramagopalan SV, Heger A, Berlanga AJ, et al. A ChIP-seq defined genome-wide map of vitamin D receptor binding: associations with disease and evolution. Genome Res 2010;20:1352–60.

123. Tuoresmaki P, Vaisanen S, Neme A, et al. Patterns of genome-wide VDR locations. PLoS One 2014;9:e96105.

124. Djebali S, Davis CA, Merkel A, et al. Landscape of transcription in human cells. Nature 2012;489:101–8.

125. Shaffer PL, Gewirth DT. Structural analysis of RXR-VDR interactions on DR3 DNA. J Steroid Biochem Mol Biol 2004;89-90:215–9.

126. Sasaki H, Harada H, Handa Y, et al. Transcriptional activity of a fluorinated vitamin D analog on VDR-RXR-mediated gene expression. Biochemistry 1995; 34:370–7.

127. Nayeri S, Danielsson C, Kahlen JP, et al. The anti-proliferative effect of vitamin D3 analogues is not mediated by inhibition of the AP-1 pathway, but may be related to promoter selectivity. Oncogene 1995;11:1853–8.

128. Quack M, Carlberg C. Selective recognition of vitamin D receptor conformations mediates promoter selectivity of vitamin D analogs. Mol Pharmacol 1999;55: 1077–87.

129. Phan TQ, Jow MM, Privalsky ML. DNA recognition by thyroid hormone and retinoic acid receptors: 3,4,5 rule modified. Mol Cell Endocrinol 2010;319:88–98.

130. Lun AT, Smyth GK. From reads to regions: a bioconductor workflow to detect differential binding in ChIP-seq data. F1000Res 2015;4:1080.

131. Yoon JS, Kim JY, Park HK, et al. Antileukemic effect of a synthetic vitamin D3 analog, HY-11, with low potential to cause hypercalcemia. Int J Oncol 2008; 32:387–96.

132. Vaisanen S, Perakyla M, Karkkainen JI, et al. Structural evaluation of the agonistic action of a vitamin D analog with two side chains binding to the nuclear vitamin D receptor. Mol Pharmacol 2003;63:1230–7.

133. Peleg S, Ismail A, Uskokovic MR, et al. Evidence for tissue- and cell-type selective activation of the vitamin D receptor by Ro-26-9228, a noncalcemic analog of vitamin D3. J Cell Biochem 2003;88:267–73.

134. Evans SR, Soldatenkov V, Shchepotin EB, et al. Novel 19-nor-hexafluoride vitamin D3 analog (Ro 25-6760) inhibits human colon cancer in vitro via apoptosis. Int J Oncol 1999;14:979–85.

135. Takahashi F, Finch JL, Denda M, et al. A new analog of 1,25-(OH)2D3, 19-NOR-1,25-(OH)2D2, suppresses serum PTH and parathyroid gland growth in uremic rats without elevation of intestinal vitamin D receptor content. Am J Kidney Dis 1997;30:105–12.

136. O'Kelly J, Uskokovic M, Lemp N, et al. Novel Gemini-vitamin D3 analog inhibits tumor cell growth and modulates the Akt/mTOR signaling pathway. J Steroid Biochem Mol Biol 2006;100:107–16.

137. Zhou JY, Norman AW, Akashi M, et al. Development of a novel 1,25(OH)2-vitamin D3 analog with potent ability to induce HL-60 cell differentiation without modulating calcium metabolism. Blood 1991;78:75–82.

138. Belorusova AY, Rochel N. Structural studies of vitamin D nuclear receptor ligand-binding properties. Vitam Horm 2016;100:83–116.

139. Eelen G, Valle N, Sato Y, et al. Superagonistic fluorinated vitamin D3 analogs stabilize helix 12 of the vitamin D receptor. Chem Biol 2008;15:1029–34.

140. Eelen G, Verlinden L, Rochel N, et al. Superagonistic action of 14-epi-analogs of 1,25-dihydroxyvitamin D explained by vitamin D receptor-coactivator interaction. Mol Pharmacol 2005;67:1566–73.

141. Amling M, Priemel M, Holzmann T, et al. Rescue of the skeletal phenotype of vitamin D receptor-ablated mice in the setting of normal mineral ion homeostasis: formal histomorphometric and biomechanical analyses. Endocrinology 1999;140:4982–7.

142. Van Cromphaut SJ, Dewerchin M, Hoenderop JG, et al. Duodenal calcium absorption in vitamin D receptor-knockout mice: functional and molecular aspects. Proc Natl Acad Sci U S A 2001;98:13324–9.

143. Kallay E, Pietschmann P, Toyokuni S, et al. Characterization of a vitamin D receptor knockout mouse as a model of colorectal hyperproliferation and DNA damage. Carcinogenesis 2001;22:1429–35.

144. Jin D, Wu S, Zhang YG, et al. Lack of vitamin D receptor causes dysbiosis and changes the functions of the murine intestinal microbiome. Clin Ther 2015;37:996–1009.e7.

145. Zinser GM, Welsh J. Vitamin D receptor status alters mammary gland morphology and tumorigenesis in MMTV-neu mice. Carcinogenesis 2004;25:2361–72.

146. Zinser GM, Sundberg JP, Welsh J. Vitamin D(3) receptor ablation sensitizes skin to chemically induced tumorigenesis. Carcinogenesis 2002;23:2103–9.

147. Larriba MJ, Ordonez-Moran P, Chicote I, et al. Vitamin D receptor deficiency enhances Wnt/beta-catenin signaling and tumor burden in colon cancer. PLoS One 2011;6:e23524.

148. Teichert AE, Elalieh H, Elias PM, et al. Overexpression of hedgehog signaling is associated with epidermal tumor formation in vitamin D receptor-null mice. J Invest Dermatol 2011;131:2289–97.

149. Colston KW, Chander SK, Mackay AG, et al. Effects of synthetic vitamin D analogues on breast cancer cell proliferation in vivo and in vitro. Biochem Pharmacol 1992;44:693–702.

150. Oades GM, Dredge K, Kirby RS, et al. Vitamin D receptor-dependent antitumour effects of 1,25-dihydroxyvitamin D3 and two synthetic analogues in three in vivo models of prostate cancer. BJU Int 2002;90:607–16.

151. Zugmaier G, Jager R, Grage B, et al. Growth-inhibitory effects of vitamin D analogues and retinoids on human pancreatic cancer cells. Br J Cancer 1996;73: 1341–6.
152. El Abdaimi K, Dion N, Papavasiliou V, et al. The vitamin D analogue EB 1089 prevents skeletal metastasis and prolongs survival time in nude mice transplanted with human breast cancer cells. Cancer Res 2000;60:4412–8.
153. Li Z, Jia Z, Gao Y, et al. Activation of vitamin D receptor signaling downregulates the expression of nuclear FOXM1 protein and suppresses pancreatic cancer cell stemness. Clin Cancer Res 2015;21:844–53.
154. Zhang X, Jiang F, Li P, et al. Growth suppression of ovarian cancer xenografts in nude mice by vitamin D analogue EB1089. Clin Cancer Res 2005;11:323–8.
155. Dackiw AP, Ezzat S, Huang P, et al. Vitamin D3 administration induces nuclear p27 accumulation, restores differentiation, and reduces tumor burden in a mouse model of metastatic follicular thyroid cancer. Endocrinology 2004;145: 5840–6.
156. Kim JS, Roberts JM, Bingman WE 3rd, et al. The prostate cancer TMPRSS2:ERG fusion synergizes with the vitamin D receptor (VDR) to induce CYP24A1 expression-limiting VDR signaling. Endocrinology 2014;155:3262–73.
157. Tangpricha V, Spina C, Yao M, et al. Vitamin D deficiency enhances the growth of MC-26 colon cancer xenografts in Balb/c mice. J Nutr 2005;135:2350–4.
158. Peleg S, Khan F, Navone NM, et al. Inhibition of prostate cancer-mediated osteoblastic bone lesions by the low-calcemic analog 1alpha-hydroxymethyl-16-ene-26,27-bishomo-25-hydroxy vitamin D3. J Steroid Biochem Mol Biol 2005; 97:203–11.
159. Verone-Boyle AR, Shoemaker S, Attwood K, et al. Diet-derived 25-hydroxyvitamin D3 activates vitamin D receptor target gene expression and suppresses EGFR mutant non-small cell lung cancer growth in vitro and in vivo. Oncotarget 2016;7:995–1013.
160. Newmark HL, Yang K, Kurihara N, et al. Western-style diet-induced colonic tumors and their modulation by calcium and vitamin D in C57Bl/6 mice: a preclinical model for human sporadic colon cancer. Carcinogenesis 2009;30:88–92.
161. Thomas MG, Tebbutt S, Williamson RC. Vitamin D and its metabolites inhibit cell proliferation in human rectal mucosa and a colon cancer cell line. Gut 1992;33: 1660–3.
162. Cross HS, Nittke T, Kallay E. Colonic vitamin D metabolism: implications for the pathogenesis of inflammatory bowel disease and colorectal cancer. Mol Cell Endocrinol 2011;347:70–9.
163. Kallay E, Bises G, Bajna E, et al. Colon-specific regulation of vitamin D hydroxylases–a possible approach for tumor prevention. Carcinogenesis 2005;26: 1581–9.
164. Cross HS, Kallay E, Lechner D, et al. Phytoestrogens and vitamin D metabolism: a new concept for the prevention and therapy of colorectal, prostate, and mammary carcinomas. J Nutr 2004;134:1207S–12S.
165. Aggarwal A, Kallay E. Cross talk between the calcium-sensing receptor and the vitamin D system in prevention of cancer. Front Physiol 2016;7:451.
166. Garland CF, Gorham ED, Mohr SB, et al. Vitamin D for cancer prevention: global perspective. Ann Epidemiol 2009;19:468–83.
167. Garland CF, Gorham ED, Mohr SB, et al. Vitamin D and prevention of breast cancer: pooled analysis. J Steroid Biochem Mol Biol 2007;103:708–11.
168. Gorham ED, Garland CF, Garland FC, et al. Vitamin D and prevention of colorectal cancer. J Steroid Biochem Mol Biol 2005;97:179–94.

169. Garland C, Shekelle RB, Barrett-Connor E, et al. Dietary vitamin D and calcium and risk of colorectal cancer: a 19-year prospective study in men. Lancet 1985; 1:307–9.

170. Garland CF, Garland FC. Do sunlight and vitamin D reduce the likelihood of colon cancer? Int J Epidemiol 1980;9:227–31.

171. Engel P, Fagherazzi G, Boutten A, et al. Serum 25(OH) vitamin D and risk of breast cancer: a nested case-control study from the French E3N cohort. Cancer Epidemiol Biomarkers Prev 2010;19:2341–50.

172. Chen P, Hu P, Xie D, et al. Meta-analysis of vitamin D, calcium and the prevention of breast cancer. Breast Cancer Res Treat 2010;121:469–77.

173. Abbas S, Linseisen J, Slanger T, et al. Serum 25-hydroxyvitamin D and risk of post-menopausal breast cancer–results of a large case-control study. Carcinogenesis 2008;29:93–9.

174. Vrieling A, Seibold P, Johnson TS, et al. Circulating 25-hydroxyvitamin D and postmenopausal breast cancer survival: influence of tumor characteristics and lifestyle factors? Int J Cancer 2014;134:2972–83.

175. Meeker S, Seamons A, Maggio-Price L, et al. Protective links between vitamin D, inflammatory bowel disease and colon cancer. World J Gastroenterol 2016;22: 933–48.

176. Shirazi L, Almquist M, Borgquist S, et al. Serum vitamin D (25OHD3) levels and the risk of different subtypes of breast cancer: a nested case-control study. Breast 2016;28:184–90.

177. Yao S, Kwan ML, Ergas IJ, et al. Association of serum level of vitamin D at diagnosis with breast cancer survival: a case-cohort analysis in the pathways study. JAMA Oncol 2017;3:351–7.

178. Yuan C, Qian ZR, Babic A, et al. Prediagnostic plasma 25-hydroxyvitamin D and pancreatic cancer survival. J Clin Oncol 2016;34:2899–905.

179. Bittenbring JT, Neumann F, Altmann B, et al. Vitamin D deficiency impairs rituximab-mediated cellular cytotoxicity and outcome of patients with diffuse large B-cell lymphoma treated with but not without rituximab. J Clin Oncol 2014;32:3242–8.

180. Choo CS, Mamedov A, Chung M, et al. Vitamin D insufficiency is common in patients with nonmetastatic prostate cancer. Nutr Res 2011;31:21–6.

181. Bonjour JP, Chevalley T, Fardellone P. Calcium intake and vitamin D metabolism and action, in healthy conditions and in prostate cancer. Br J Nutr 2007;97: 611–6.

182. Shui IM, Mondul AM, Lindstrom S, et al, Breast and Prostate Cancer Cohort Consortium Group. Circulating vitamin D, vitamin D-related genetic variation, and risk of fatal prostate cancer in the National Cancer Institute Breast and Prostate Cancer Cohort Consortium. Cancer 2015;121:1949–56.

183. Holt SK, Kolb S, Fu R, et al. Circulating levels of 25-hydroxyvitamin D and prostate cancer prognosis. Cancer Epidemiol 2013;37:666–70.

184. Albanes D, Mondul AM, Yu K, et al. Serum 25-hydroxy vitamin D and prostate cancer risk in a large nested case-control study. Cancer Epidemiol Biomarkers Prev 2011;20:1850–60.

185. Park SY, Cooney RV, Wilkens LR, et al. Plasma 25-hydroxyvitamin D and prostate cancer risk: the multiethnic cohort. Eur J Cancer 2010;46:932–6.

186. Jacot W, Firmin N, Roca L, et al. Impact of a tailored oral vitamin D supplementation regimen on serum 25-hydroxyvitamin D levels in early breast cancer patients: a randomized phase III study. Ann Oncol 2016;27:1235–41.

187. Bassuk SS, Manson JE, Lee IM, et al. Baseline characteristics of participants in the VITamin D and omega-3 TriaL (VITAL). Contemp Clin Trials 2016;47:235–43.
188. Flarakos CC, Weiskopf A, Robinson M, et al. Metabolism of selective 20-epi-vitamin D3 analogs in rat osteosarcoma UMR-106 cells: isolation and identification of four novel C-1 fatty acid esters of 1alpha,25-dihydroxy-16-ene-20-epi-vitamin D3. Steroids 2017;119:18–30.
189. Okamoto R, Gery S, Kuwayama Y, et al. Novel Gemini vitamin D3 analogs: large structure/function analysis and ability to induce antimicrobial peptide. Int J Cancer 2014;134:207–17.
190. Huet T, Maehr H, Lee HJ, et al. Structure-function study of gemini derivatives with two different side chains at C-20, Gemini-0072 and Gemini-0097. Medchemcomm 2011;2:424–9.
191. Reddy GS, Omdahl JL, Robinson M, et al. 23-carboxy-24,25,26,27-tetranorvitamin D3 (calcioic acid) and 24-carboxy-25,26,27-trinorvitamin D3 (cholacalcioic acid): end products of 25-hydroxyvitamin D3 metabolism in rat kidney through C-24 oxidation pathway. Arch Biochem Biophys 2006;455:18–30.
192. Uskokovic MR, Manchand P, Marczak S, et al. C-20 cyclopropyl vitamin D3 analogs. Curr Top Med Chem 2006;6:1289–96.
193. Weinstein EA, Rao DS, Siu-Caldera ML, et al. Isolation and identification of 1alpha-hydroxy-24-oxovitamin D3 and 1alpha,23-dihydroxy-24-oxovitamin D3: metabolites of 1alpha,24(R)-dihydroxyvitamin D3 produced in rat kidney. Biochem Pharmacol 1999;58:1965–73.
194. Sekimoto H, Siu-Caldera ML, Weiskopf A, et al. 1alpha,25-dihydroxy-3-epi-vitamin D3: in vivo metabolite of 1alpha,25-dihydroxyvitamin D3 in rats. FEBS Lett 1999;448:278–82.
195. Gardner JP, Zhang F, Uskokovic MR, et al. Vitamin D analog 25-(OH)-16,23E-Diene-26,27-hexafluoro-vitamin D3 induces differentiation of HL60 cells with minimal effects on cellular calcium homeostasis. J Cell Biochem 1996;63:500–12.
196. Rao LG, Sutherland MK, Reddy GS, et al. Effects of 1alpha,25-dihydroxy-16ene, 23yne-vitamin D3 on osteoblastic function in human osteosarcoma SaOS-2 cells: differentiation-stage dependence and modulation by 17-beta estradiol. Bone 1996;19:621–7.
197. Napoli JL, Sommerfeld JL, Pramanik BC, et al. 19-nor-10-ketovitamin D derivatives: unique metabolites of vitamin D3, vitamin D2, and 25-hydroxyvitamin D3. Biochemistry 1983;22:3636–40.
198. Reinhardt TA, Napoli JL, Praminik B, et al. 1 Alpha-25,26-trihydroxyvitamin D3: an in vivo and in vitro metabolite of vitamin D3. Biochemistry 1981;20:6230–5.
199. Narwid TA, Blount JF, Iacobelli JA, et al. Vitamin D3 metabolites. 3. Synthesis and X-ray analysis of 1 alpha,25-dihydroxycholesterol. Helv Chim Acta 1974; 57:781–9.
200. Asou H, Koike M, Elstner E, et al. 19-nor vitamin-D analogs: a new class of potent inhibitors of proliferation and inducers of differentiation of human myeloid leukemia cell lines. Blood 1998;92:2441–9.
201. Maenpaa PH, Vaisanen S, Jaaskelainen T, et al. Vitamin D(3) analogs (MC 1288, KH 1060, EB 1089, GS 1558, and CB 1093): studies on their mechanism of action. Steroids 2001;66:223–5.
202. Wang X, Chen X, Akhter J, et al. The in vitro effect of vitamin D3 analogue EB-1089 on a human prostate cancer cell line (PC-3). Br J Urol 1997;80:260–2.
203. Akhter J, Goerdel M, Morris DL. Vitamin D3 analogue (EB 1089) inhibits in vitro cellular proliferation of human colon cancer cells. Br J Surg 1996;83:229–30.

204. Mathiasen IS, Colston KW, Binderup L. EB 1089, a novel vitamin D analogue, has strong antiproliferative and differentiation inducing effects on cancer cells. J Steroid Biochem Mol Biol 1993;46:365–71.

205. Sundaram S, Beckman MJ, Bajwa A, et al. QW-1624F2-2, a synthetic analogue of 1,25-dihydroxyvitamin D3, enhances the response to other deltanoids and suppresses the invasiveness of human metastatic breast tumor cells. Mol Cancer Ther 2006;5:2806–14.

206. Kahraman M, Sinishtaj S, Dolan PM, et al. Potent, selective and low-calcemic inhibitors of CYP24 hydroxylase: 24-sulfoximine analogues of the hormone 1alpha,25-dihydroxyvitamin D(3). J Med Chem 2004;47:6854–63.

207. Somjen D, Waisman A, Lee JK, et al. A non-calcemic analog of 1 alpha,25 dihydroxy vitamin D(3) (JKF) upregulates the induction of creatine kinase B by 17 beta estradiol in osteoblast-like ROS 17/2.8 cells and in rat diaphysis. J Steroid Biochem Mol Biol 2001;77:205–12.

208. Posner GH. New vitamin D analogues. Nephrol Dial Transplant 1996;11(Suppl 3):32–6.

209. Gulliford T, English J, Colston KW, et al. A phase I study of the vitamin D analogue EB 1089 in patients with advanced breast and colorectal cancer. Br J Cancer 1998;78:6–13.

210. Jain RK, Trump DL, Egorin MJ, et al. A phase I study of the vitamin D3 analogue ILX23-7553 administered orally to patients with advanced solid tumors. Invest New Drugs 2011;29:1420–5.

211. Evans TR, Colston KW, Lofts FJ, et al. A phase II trial of the vitamin D analogue Seocalcitol (EB1089) in patients with inoperable pancreatic cancer. Br J Cancer 2002;86:680–5.

212. Dalhoff K, Dancey J, Astrup L, et al. A phase II study of the vitamin D analogue Seocalcitol in patients with inoperable hepatocellular carcinoma. Br J Cancer 2003;89:252–7.

213. Flaig TW, Barqawi A, Miller G, et al. A phase II trial of dexamethasone, vitamin D, and carboplatin in patients with hormone-refractory prostate cancer. Cancer 2006;107:266–74.

214. Jarrard D, Konety B, Huang W, et al. Phase IIa, randomized placebo-controlled trial of single high dose cholecalciferol (vitamin D3) and daily Genistein (G-2535) versus double placebo in men with early stage prostate cancer undergoing prostatectomy. Am J Clin Exp Urol 2016;4:17–27.

215. Chadha MK, Tian L, Mashtare T, et al. Phase 2 trial of weekly intravenous 1,25 dihydroxy cholecalciferol (calcitriol) in combination with dexamethasone for castration-resistant prostate cancer. Cancer 2010;116:2132–9.

216. Osborn JL, Schwartz GG, Smith DC, et al. Phase II trial of oral 1,25-dihydroxy-vitamin D (calcitriol) in hormone refractory prostate cancer. Urol Oncol 1995;1:195–8.

217. Amir E, Simmons CE, Freedman OC, et al. A phase 2 trial exploring the effects of high-dose (10,000 IU/day) vitamin D(3) in breast cancer patients with bone metastases. Cancer 2010;116:284–91.

218. Beer TM, Myrthue A, Garzotto M, et al. Randomized study of high-dose pulse calcitriol or placebo prior to radical prostatectomy. Cancer Epidemiol Biomarkers Prev 2004;13:2225–32.

219. Wagner D, Trudel D, Van der Kwast T, et al. Randomized clinical trial of vitamin D3 doses on prostatic vitamin D metabolite levels and ki67 labeling in prostate cancer patients. J Clin Endocrinol Metab 2013;98:1498–507.

220. Beer TM, Ryan CW, Venner PM, et al, ASCENT (AIPC Study of Calcitriol ENhancing Taxotere) Investigators. Intermittent chemotherapy in patients with metastatic androgen-independent prostate cancer: results from ASCENT, a double-blinded, randomized comparison of high-dose calcitriol plus docetaxel with placebo plus docetaxel. Cancer 2008;112:326–30.
221. Scher HI, Jia X, Chi K, et al. Randomized, open-label phase III trial of docetaxel plus high-dose calcitriol versus docetaxel plus prednisone for patients with castration-resistant prostate cancer. J Clin Oncol 2011;29:2191–8.
222. Stahel R, Bogaerts J, Ciardiello F, et al. Optimising translational oncology in clinical practice: strategies to accelerate progress in drug development. Cancer Treat Rev 2015;41:129–35.
223. Leichman L, Groshen S, O'Neil BH, et al. Phase II study of olaparib (AZD-2281) after standard systemic therapies for disseminated colorectal cancer. Oncologist 2016;21:172–7.
224. Ledermann JA, Harter P, Gourley C, et al. Overall survival in patients with platinum-sensitive recurrent serous ovarian cancer receiving olaparib maintenance monotherapy: an updated analysis from a randomised, placebo-controlled, double-blind, phase 2 trial. Lancet Oncol 2016;17:1579–89.
225. Guha M. PARP inhibitors stumble in breast cancer. Nat Biotechnol 2011;29: 373–4.
226. Martin M, Loibl S, von Minckwitz G, et al. Phase III trial evaluating the addition of bevacizumab to endocrine therapy as first-line treatment for advanced breast cancer: the letrozole/fulvestrant and avastin (LEA) study. J Clin Oncol 2015; 33:1045–52.
227. Sharma SP. Avastin saga reveals debate over clinical trial endpoints. J Natl Cancer Inst 2012;104:800–1.
228. Azvolinsky A. PARP inhibitors: targeting the right patients. J Natl Cancer Inst 2012;104:1851–2.
229. Bang YJ, Im SA, Lee KW, et al. Double-blind phase II trial with prospective classification by ATM protein level to evaluate the efficacy and tolerability of olaparib plus paclitaxel in patients with recurrent or metastatic gastric cancer. J Clin Oncol 2015;33:3858–65.
230. Tworoger SS, Gates MA, Lee IM, et al. Polymorphisms in the vitamin D receptor and risk of ovarian cancer in four studies. Cancer Res 2009;69:1885–91.
231. Murtaugh MA, Sweeney C, Ma KN, et al. Vitamin D receptor gene polymorphisms, dietary promotion of insulin resistance, and colon and rectal cancer. Nutr Cancer 2006;55:35–43.
232. Buyru N, Tezol A, Yosunkaya-Fenerci E, et al. Vitamin D receptor gene polymorphisms in breast cancer. Exp Mol Med 2003;35:550–5.
233. Ingles SA, Ross RK, Yu MC, et al. Association of prostate cancer risk with genetic polymorphisms in vitamin D receptor and androgen receptor. J Natl Cancer Inst 1997;89:166–70.
234. Bretherton-Watt D, Given-Wilson R, Mansi JL, et al. Vitamin D receptor gene polymorphisms are associated with breast cancer risk in a UK Caucasian population. Br J Cancer 2001;85:171–5.
235. Gu H, Wang X, Zheng L, et al. Vitamin D receptor gene polymorphisms and esophageal cancer risk in a Chinese population: a negative study. Med Oncol 2014;31:827.
236. Kang S, Zhao Y, Liu J, et al. Association of vitamin D receptor Fok I polymorphism with the risk of prostate cancer: a meta-analysis. Oncotarget 2016;7: 77878–89.

237. Lu D, Jing L, Zhang S. Vitamin D receptor polymorphism and breast cancer risk: a meta-analysis. Medicine (Baltimore) 2016;95:e3535.

238. Clendenen TV, Ge W, Koenig KL, et al. Genetic polymorphisms in vitamin D metabolism and signaling genes and risk of breast cancer: a nested case-control study. PLoS One 2015;10:e0140478.

239. Ashmore JH, Gallagher CJ, Lesko SM, et al. No association between vitamin D intake, VDR polymorphisms, and colorectal cancer in a population-based case-control study. Cancer Epidemiol Biomarkers Prev 2015;24:1635–7.

240. Yang B, Liu S, Yang X, et al. Current evidence on the four polymorphisms of VDR and breast cancer risk in Caucasian women. Meta Gene 2014;2:41–9.

241. Zhang Q, Shan Y. Genetic polymorphisms of vitamin D receptor and the risk of prostate cancer: a meta-analysis. J BUON 2013;18:961–9.

242. Luo S, Guo L, Li Y, et al. Vitamin D receptor gene ApaI polymorphism and breast cancer susceptibility: a meta-analysis. Tumour Biol 2014;35:785–90.

243. Perry JR, Day F, Elks CE, et al. Parent-of-origin-specific allelic associations among 106 genomic loci for age at menarche. Nature 2014;514:92–7.

244. Jostins L, Ripke S, Weersma RK, et al. Host-microbe interactions have shaped the genetic architecture of inflammatory bowel disease. Nature 2012;491:119–24.

245. Lai HM, Chen CJ, Su BY, et al. Gout and type 2 diabetes have a mutual interdependent effect on genetic risk factors and higher incidences. Rheumatology (Oxford) 2012;51:715–20.

246. Rennstam K, Jonsson G, Tanner M, et al. Cytogenetic characterization and gene expression profiling of the trastuzumab-resistant breast cancer cell line JIMT-1. Cancer Genet Cytogenet 2007;172:95–106.

247. Albertson DG, Ylstra B, Segraves R, et al. Quantitative mapping of amplicon structure by array CGH identifies CYP24 as a candidate oncogene. Nat Genet 2000;25:144–6.

248. Lopes N, Sousa B, Martins D, et al. Alterations in vitamin D signalling and metabolic pathways in breast cancer progression: a study of VDR, CYP27B1 and CYP24A1 expression in benign and malignant breast lesions. BMC Cancer 2010;10:483.

249. Holick CN, Stanford JL, Kwon EM, et al. Comprehensive association analysis of the vitamin D pathway genes, VDR, CYP27B1, and CYP24A1, in prostate cancer. Cancer Epidemiol Biomarkers Prev 2007;16:1990–9.

250. Brozek W, Manhardt T, Kallay E, et al. Relative expression of vitamin D hydroxylases, CYP27B1 and CYP24A1, and of cyclooxygenase-2 and heterogeneity of human colorectal cancer in relation to age, gender, tumor location, and malignancy: results from factor and cluster analysis. Cancers (Basel) 2012;4:763–76.

251. Cross HS, Kallay E, Farhan H, et al. Regulation of extrarenal vitamin D metabolism as a tool for colon and prostate cancer prevention. Recent Results Cancer Res 2003;164:413–25.

252. Singh R, Yadav V, Kumar S, et al. MicroRNA-195 inhibits proliferation, invasion and metastasis in breast cancer cells by targeting FASN, HMGCR, ACACA and CYP27B1. Sci Rep 2015;5:17454.

253. Ma JF, Nonn L, Campbell MJ, et al. Mechanisms of decreased Vitamin D 1alpha-hydroxylase activity in prostate cancer cells. Mol Cell Endocrinol 2004;221:67–74.

254. Townsend K, Banwell CM, Guy M, et al. Autocrine metabolism of vitamin D in normal and malignant breast tissue. Clin Cancer Res 2005;11:3579–86.

255. Peng X, Tiwari N, Roy S, et al. Regulation of CYP24 splicing by 1,25-dihydroxyvitamin D(3) in human colon cancer cells. J Endocrinol 2012;212:207–15.
256. Doig CL, Singh PK, Dhiman VK, et al. Recruitment of NCOR1 to VDR target genes is enhanced in prostate cancer cells and associates with altered DNA methylation patterns. Carcinogenesis 2013;34:248–56.
257. Meyer MB, Pike JW. Corepressors (NCoR and SMRT) as well as coactivators are recruited to positively regulated 1alpha,25-dihydroxyvitamin D3-responsive genes. J Steroid Biochem Mol Biol 2013;136:120–4.
258. Abedin SA, Thorne JL, Battaglia S, et al. Elevated NCOR1 disrupts a network of dietary-sensing nuclear receptors in bladder cancer cells. Carcinogenesis 2009;30:449–56.
259. Saramaki A, Diermeier S, Kellner R, et al. Cyclical chromatin looping and transcription factor association on the regulatory regions of the p21 (CDKN1A) gene in response to 1alpha,25-dihydroxyvitamin D3. J Biol Chem 2009;284:8073–82.
260. Peng X, Jhaveri P, Hussain-Hakimjee EA, et al. Overexpression of ER and VDR is not sufficient to make ER-negative MDA-MB231 breast cancer cells responsive to 1alpha-hydroxyvitamin D5. Carcinogenesis 2007;28:1000–7.
261. Tse AK, Zhu GY, Wan CK, et al. 1alpha,25-Dihydroxyvitamin D3 inhibits transcriptional potential of nuclear factor kappa B in breast cancer cells. Mol Immunol 2010;47:1728–38.
262. Tavera-Mendoza LE, Quach TD, Dabbas B, et al. Incorporation of histone deacetylase inhibition into the structure of a nuclear receptor agonist. Proc Natl Acad Sci U S A 2008;105:8250–5.
263. Rashid SF, Moore JS, Walker E, et al. Synergistic growth inhibition of prostate cancer cells by 1 alpha,25 Dihydroxyvitamin D(3) and its 19-nor-hexafluoride analogs in combination with either sodium butyrate or trichostatin A. Oncogene 2001;20:1860–72.
264. Daniel C, Schroder O, Zahn N, et al. The TGFbeta/Smad 3-signaling pathway is involved in butyrate-mediated vitamin D receptor (VDR)-expression. J Cell Biochem 2007;102:1420–31.
265. Gaschott T, Werz O, Steinmeyer A, et al. Butyrate-induced differentiation of Caco-2 cells is mediated by vitamin D receptor. Biochem Biophys Res Commun 2001;288:690–6.
266. Gaschott T, Wachtershauser A, Steinhilber D, et al. 1,25-Dihydroxycholecalciferol enhances butyrate-induced p21(Waf1/Cip1) expression. Biochem Biophys Res Commun 2001;283:80–5.
267. Malinen M, Saramaki A, Ropponen A, et al. Distinct HDACs regulate the transcriptional response of human cyclin-dependent kinase inhibitor genes to Trichostatin A and 1alpha,25-dihydroxyvitamin D3. Nucleic Acids Res 2008;36:121–32.
268. Roberts L, Davenport RJ, Pennisi E, et al. A history of the human genome project. Science 2001;291:1195.
269. Birney E. The making of ENCODE: lessons for big-data projects. Nature 2012;489:49–51.
270. ENCODE Project Consortium, Birney E, Stamatoyannopoulos JA, Dutta A, et al. Identification and analysis of functional elements in 1% of the human genome by the ENCODE pilot project. Nature 2007;447:799–816.
271. Roadmap Epigenomics Consortium, Kundaje A, Meuleman W, Ernst J, et al. Integrative analysis of 111 reference human epigenomes. Nature 2015;518:317–30.

272. Sanli K, Karlsson FH, Nookaew I, et al. FANTOM: functional and taxonomic analysis of metagenomes. BMC Bioinformatics 2013;14:38.

273. Bujold D, Morais DA, Gauthier C, et al. The International human epigenome consortium data portal. Cell Syst 2016;3:496–9.e2.

274. Chen L, Ge B, Casale FP, et al. Genetic drivers of epigenetic and transcriptional variation in human immune cells. Cell 2016;167:1398–414.e24.

275. Cancer Genome Atlas Research Network, Weinstein JN, Collisson EA, et al. The Cancer Genome Atlas Pan-Cancer analysis project. Nat Genet 2013;45:1113–20.

276. Mele M, Ferreira PG, Reverter F, et al. Human genomics. The human transcriptome across tissues and individuals. Science 2015;348:660–5.

277. GTEx Consortium. The Genotype-Tissue Expression (GTEx) project. Nat Genet 2013;45:580–5.

278. Martelotto LG, De Filippo MR, Ng CK, et al. Genomic landscape of adenoid cystic carcinoma of the breast. J Pathol 2015;237:179–89.

279. Ho AS, Kannan K, Roy DM, et al. The mutational landscape of adenoid cystic carcinoma. Nat Genet 2013;45:791–8.

280. Cerami E, Gao J, Dogrusoz U, et al. The cBio cancer genomics portal: an open platform for exploring multidimensional cancer genomics data. Cancer Discov 2012;2:401–4.

281. Gao J, Aksoy BA, Dogrusoz U, et al. Integrative analysis of complex cancer genomics and clinical profiles using the cBioPortal. Sci Signal 2013;6:pl1.

282. Novershtern N, Subramanian A, Lawton LN, et al. Densely interconnected transcriptional circuits control cell states in human hematopoiesis. Cell 2011;144:296–309.

283. Fuhrken PG, Chen C, Apostolidis PA, et al. Gene Ontology-driven transcriptional analysis of CD34+ cell-initiated megakaryocytic cultures identifies new transcriptional regulators of megakaryopoiesis. Physiol Genomics 2008;33:159–69.

284. Yetgin S, Ozsoylu S. Myeloid metaplasia in vitamin D deficiency rickets. Scand J Haematol 1982;28:180–5.

285. Koeffler HP. Induction of differentiation of human acute myelogenous leukemia cells: therapeutic implications. Blood 1983;62:709–21.

286. Mvubu NE, Pillay B, Gamieldien J, et al. Canonical pathways, networks and transcriptional factor regulation by clinical strains of Mycobacterium tuberculosis in pulmonary alveolar epithelial cells. Tuberculosis (Edinb) 2016;97:73–85.

287. Sims AC, Tilton SC, Menachery VD, et al. Release of severe acute respiratory syndrome coronavirus nuclear import block enhances host transcription in human lung cells. J Virol 2013;87:3885–902.

288. Zhou Y, Gong W, Xiao J, et al. Transcriptomic analysis reveals key regulators of mammogenesis and the pregnancy-lactation cycle. Sci China Life Sci 2014;57:340–55.

289. Zinser GM, Welsh J. Accelerated mammary gland development during pregnancy and delayed postlactational involution in vitamin D3 receptor null mice. Mol Endocrinol 2004;18:2208–23.

290. Zinser G, Packman K, Welsh J. Vitamin D(3) receptor ablation alters mammary gland morphogenesis. Development 2002;129:3067–76.

291. Pellacani D, Bilenky M, Kannan N, et al. Analysis of normal human mammary epigenomes reveals cell-specific active enhancer states and associated transcription factor networks. Cell Rep 2016;17:2060–74.

292. Suo C, Hrydziuszko O, Lee D, et al. Integration of somatic mutation, expression and functional data reveals potential driver genes predictive of breast cancer survival. Bioinformatics 2015;31:2607–13.

293. Ciriello G, Gatza ML, Beck AH, et al. Comprehensive molecular portraits of invasive lobular breast cancer. Cell 2015;163:506–19.

294. Keenan T, Moy B, Mroz EA, et al. Comparison of the genomic landscape between primary breast cancer in African American versus white women and the association of racial differences with tumor recurrence. J Clin Oncol 2015; 33:3621–7.

295. Robinson DR, Wu YM, Vats P, et al. Activating ESR1 mutations in hormone-resistant metastatic breast cancer. Nat Genet 2013;45:1446–51.

296. Cancer Genome Atlas Research Network. Comprehensive molecular characterization of urothelial bladder carcinoma. Nature 2014;507:315–22.

297. Cancer Genome Atlas Network. Comprehensive molecular portraits of human breast tumours. Nature 2012;490:61–70.

298. Cancer Genome Atlas Network. Comprehensive molecular characterization of human colon and rectal cancer. Nature 2012;487:330–7.

299. Cancer Genome Atlas Network. Comprehensive genomic characterization of head and neck squamous cell carcinomas. Nature 2015;517:576–82.

300. Ahn SM, Jang SJ, Shim JH, et al. Genomic portrait of resectable hepatocellular carcinomas: implications of RB1 and FGF19 aberrations for patient stratification. Hepatology 2014;60:1972–82.

301. Long MD, Thorne JL, Russell J, et al. Cooperative behavior of the nuclear receptor superfamily and its deregulation in prostate cancer. Carcinogenesis 2014;35: 262–71.

302. Long MD, Campbell MJ. Pan-cancer analyses of the nuclear receptor superfamily. Nucl Receptor Res 2015;2 [pii:101182].

303. Satelli A, Rao PS, Thirumala S, et al. Galectin-4 functions as a tumor suppressor of human colorectal cancer. Int J Cancer 2011;129:799–809.

304. Belo AI, van der Sar AM, Tefsen B, et al. Galectin-4 reduces migration and metastasis formation of pancreatic cancer cells. PLoS One 2013;8:e65957.

305. Kim SW, Park KC, Jeon SM, et al. Abrogation of galectin-4 expression promotes tumorigenesis in colorectal cancer. Cell Oncol (Dordr) 2013;36:169–78.

306. Tsai CH, Tzeng SF, Chao TK, et al. Metastatic progression of prostate cancer is mediated by autonomous binding of galectin-4-O-glycan to cancer cells. Cancer Res 2016;76(19):5756–67.

307. Pena C, Garcia JM, Silva J, et al. E-cadherin and vitamin D receptor regulation by SNAIL and ZEB1 in colon cancer: clinicopathological correlations. Hum Mol Genet 2005;14:3361–70.

308. Pereira F, Barbachano A, Silva J, et al. KDM6B/JMJD3 histone demethylase is induced by vitamin D and modulates its effects in colon cancer cells. Hum Mol Genet 2011;20:4655–65.

309. Boyle AP, Hong EL, Hariharan M, et al. Annotation of functional variation in personal genomes using RegulomeDB. Genome Res 2012;22:1790–7.

310. Singh P, van den Berg PR, Long MD, et al. Integration of VDR genome wide binding and GWAS genetic variation data reveals co-occurrence of VDR and NF-κB binding that is linked to immune phenotypes. BMC Genomics 2017; 18(1):132.

311. Peterlik M, Cross HS. Vitamin D and calcium deficits predispose for multiple chronic diseases. Eur J Clin Invest 2005;35:290–304.

312. Dougherty U, Mustafi R, Sadiq F, et al. The renin-angiotensin system mediates EGF receptor-vitamin d receptor cross-talk in colitis-associated colon cancer. Clin Cancer Res 2014;20:5848–59.

313. Giardina C, Madigan JP, Tierney CA, et al. Vitamin D resistance and colon cancer prevention. Carcinogenesis 2012;33:475–82.

314. Kaler P, Augenlicht L, Klampfer L. Macrophage-derived IL-1beta stimulates Wnt signaling and growth of colon cancer cells: a crosstalk interrupted by vitamin D3. Oncogene 2009;28:3892–902.

315. Liu W, Chen Y, Golan MA, et al. Intestinal epithelial vitamin D receptor signaling inhibits experimental colitis. J Clin Invest 2013;123:3983–96.

316. Long MD, Campbell MJ. Integrative genomic approaches to dissect clinically-significant relationships between the VDR cistrome and gene expression in primary colon cancer. J Steroid Biochem Mol Biol 2016. [Epub ahead of print].

317. Michalak M, Warnken U, Andre S, et al. Detection of proteome changes in human colon cancer induced by cell surface binding of growth-inhibitory human galectin-4 using quantitative SILAC-based proteomics. J Proteome Res 2016; 15(12):4412–22.

318. Solmi R, De Sanctis P, Zucchini C, et al. Search for epithelial-specific mRNAs in peripheral blood of patients with colon cancer by RT-PCR. Int J Oncol 2004;25: 1049–56.

319. Long MD, van den Berg PR, Russell JL, et al. Integrative genomic analysis in K562 chronic myelogenous leukemia cells reveals that proximal NCOR1 binding positively regulates genes that govern erythroid differentiation and Imatinib sensitivity. Nucleic Acids Res 2015;43:7330–48.

Role of Vitamin D in Cardiovascular Diseases

Vikrant Rai, MBBS, MS,
Devendra K. Agrawal, PhD (Biochem), PhD (Med Sciences), MBA, MS (ITM), FIACS*

KEYWORDS

- Vitamin D deficiency • Cardiovascular disease • Myocardial infarction
- Left ventricular hypertrophy • Cardiomyopathy • Cardiac failure and fibrosis
- Atherosclerosis • Peripheral vascular disease

KEY POINTS

- Vitamin D deficiency is associated with cardiovascular diseases, including coronary artery disease, myocardial infarction, cardiac failure and fibrosis, cardiomyopathy, atherosclerosis, hypertension, and peripheral arterial disease.
- Increased inflammation in diabetes and/or obesity lowers circulating vitamin D levels, thereby increasing the prevalence for cardiovascular diseases.
- Vitamin D supplementation attenuates inflammation and proinflammatory cytokines and, thus, may play a therapeutic role in the treatment of cardiovascular diseases.
- Cardiomyopathy in hypocalcemic patients is reversible with vitamin D supplementation.
- Vitamin D supplementation attenuates atherosclerosis and plaque formation.

INTRODUCTION

Vitamin D is a fat-soluble vitamin that also functions as a steroid hormone. Other than the dietary sources, vitamin D is produced nonenzymatically under the skin on exposure to ultraviolet sunlight and metabolized in liver and kidney involving cytochrome P450 enzymes (CYP2R1, CYP27B1, CYP24A1, CYP27B1)[1] (**Fig. 1**). Vitamin D plays a crucial role in mineral homeostasis and skeletal health. As a steroid hormone and immunomodulator, vitamin D regulates the immune response of the body. Deficiency of vitamin D has been associated with diseases, such as rickets, osteomalacia,

Disclosure: The authors have nothing to disclose.
This work was supported by research grants R01 HL112597, R01 HL116042 and R01 HL120659 to D.K. Agrawal from the National Heart, Lung, and Blood Institute, National Institutes of Health, USA. The content of this review article is solely the responsibility of the authors and does not necessarily represent the official views of the National Institutes of Health.
Department of Clinical and Translational Science, Creighton University School of Medicine, CRISS II Room 510, 2500 California Plaza, Omaha, NE 68178, USA
* Corresponding author.
E-mail address: dkagr@creighton.edu

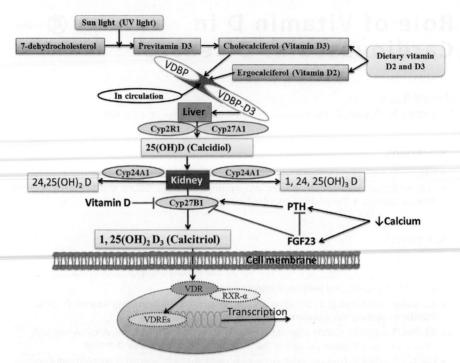

Fig. 1. Synthesis and regulation of vitamin D. Dietary vitamin D (vitamin D) and provitamin D synthesized in skin under UV light reaches the liver via the blood stream after binding with vitamin D binding protein (VDBP). Hydroxylation of vitamin D mainly with Cyp2R1 (vitamin D 25 hydroxylase) results in the formation of calcidiol (25[OH]D), which is further hydroxylated with Cyp27B1 (1 α-hydroxylase) in the kidney to form calcitriol (1,25 [OH]$_2$D$_3$), the biologically active form of vitamin D. The activity of Cyp27B1 is regulated by the plasma levels of calcium, phosphate, parathyroid hormone (PTH), fibroblast growth factor-23 (FGF23), and 1,25(OH)$_2$D$_3$ itself. RXR-α, retinoid X receptor-α; VDR, vitamin D receptor; VDREs, vitamin D response elements.

osteoporosis, skin diseases, and cardiovascular diseases (CVDs).[1–3] Currently, vitamin D deficiency exceeding 50% worldwide[4] warrants further investigations to explore the role of vitamin D in CVD and other diseases.

Vitamin D deficiency is associated with inflammation in the metabolic syndrome, a risk factor for CVD. Low levels of vitamin D have been associated with increased risk of CVD, such as coronary artery disease (CAD),[5] myocardial infarction (MI),[6,7] hypertrophy,[8] cardiomyopathy,[9,10] fibrosis,[11,12] and heart failure (HF).[13,14] In addition, deficiency of vitamin D has been found in arterial diseases, including aneurysm,[15,16] peripheral arterial disease (PAD),[17–19] arterial calcification,[20] hypertension (HTN),[21,22] and atherosclerosis[23] (**Figs. 2** and **3**). The low levels of vitamin D in these studies may be due to different confounding factors, such as environment, age, sex, socioeconomic status, and nutritional status. Daraghmeh and colleagues[24] conducted a National Health and Nutrition Examination Survey III follow-up study on extended mortality and found that low vitamin D levels are inversely associated with CAD and all-cause mortality adjusting for multiple confounders. In animals, Assalin and colleagues[25] studied the effect of vitamin D deficiency on cardiac metabolism, morphology, and function using male weanling Wistar rats. These investigators found a significant association

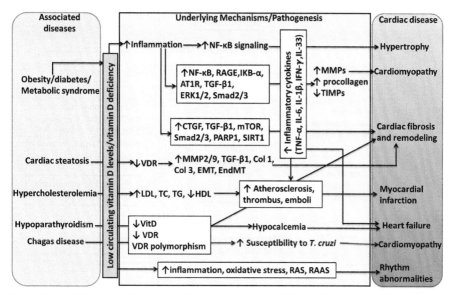

Fig. 2. Role of vitamin D deficiency in the pathogenesis of CVDs. Vitamin D deficiency is associated with many diseases, such as diabetes, obesity, metabolic syndrome, hypercholesterole-
mia, hypoparathyroidism, and CVDs. Vitamin D deficiency results in increased inflammation,
increased expression of inflammatory cytokines, and decreased expression and activity of
vitamin D receptor (VDR). These events result in enhanced signaling of downstream inflammatory signaling cascades leading to collagen loss, fibrosis, increased oxidative stress,
increased inflammation, increased sensitivity to infections, and decreased protective mechanisms. The cumulative effect of this results in various CVDs, such as cardiomyopathy, hypertrophy, MI, HF, cardiac fibrosis, and rhythm abnormalities. Hence, vitamin D supplementation
might decrease these mediators and attenuate the progression and development of CVD.
AT1R, angiotensin II type 1 receptor; col 1, collagen 1; col 3, collagen 3; CTGF, connective tissue
growth factor; EMT, epithelial-myofibroblast transformation; EndMT, endothelial myofibroblast transformation; ERK1/2, protein-serine/threonine kinases; HDL, high-density lipoprotein; IFN-γ, interferon-gamma; IKB-α, α subunit of inhibitor of κB; IL-1β, interleukin-1 beta;
IL-33, interleukin-33; IL-6, interleukin-6; LDL, low-density lipoprotein; MMPs, matrix metalloproteinases; mTOR, mechanistic target of rapamycin; NF-κB, nuclear-factor kappa
beta; PARP1, poly (ADP-ribose) polymerase 1; RAAS, renin-angiotensin-aldosterone system;
RAGE, receptor for advanced glycation end products; RAS, renin-angiotensin system; SIRT1,
sirtuin1; SMAD2/3, Sma- and mad-related protein 2/3; TC, total cholesterol; TG, triglycerides;
TGF-β1, transforming growth factor-beta 1; TIMPs, tissue inhibitors of metalloproteinases;
TNF-α, tumor necrosis factor-alpha; VDR, vitamin D receptor.

between vitamin D deficiency and cardiac inflammation, oxidative stress, energetic
metabolic changes, cardiac hypertrophy, alterations in the left auricle and left ventricle
(LV) of the heart with fibrosis and apoptosis, and systolic dysfunction.[25] These findings
were associated with increased secretion of cytokines, including tumor necrosis factor-
alpha (TNF-α) and interferon-gamma (IFN-γ). These reports suggest an important role
of vitamin D deficiency in the pathogenesis of CVD; hence, vitamin D supplementation
might be beneficial.

The association between vitamin D deficiency and CVD, the mechanistic basis of
low vitamin D and CVD, autocrine and paracrine effects of vitamin D, and the effect
of the renin-angiotensin-aldosterone system have been discussed previously.[3,26]

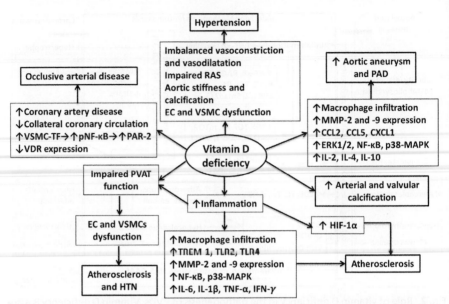

Fig. 3. Vitamin D deficiency and development of vascular diseases. Vitamin D deficiency is associated with increased inflammation, increased expression of inflammatory cytokines, endothelial cell and vascular smooth muscle cells dysfunction, and decreased expression and activity of VDR. These events enhance and aid in the development of vascular diseases, such as atherosclerosis, aneurysms, calcification, stiffness, and HTN. Because vitamin D deficiency is associated with the pathogenesis of development and progression of vascular diseases, vitamin D supplementation might help in attenuating the development and progression of these vascular diseases. CCL2, chemokine (C-C motif) ligand 2; CCL5, chemokine (C-C motif) ligand 5; CXCL1, chemokine (C-X-C motif) ligand 1; EC, endothelial cells; ERK1/2, protein-serine/threonine kinases; HIF-1α, hypoxia-induced factor-1 alpha; IFN-γ, interferon-gamma; IL-1β, interleukin-1 beta; IL-2, IL-4, IL-6, IL-10, interleukin-2, interleukin-4, interluekin-6, interleukin-10; MMP2 and MMP9, matrix metalloproteinases 2 and 9; p38-MAPK, p38 mitogen-activated protein kinases; PAR-2, protease-activated protein 2; pNF-κB, phosphorylated nuclear-factor kappa beta; PVAT, perivascular adipose tissue; RAS, renin-angiotensin system; TLR2, toll-like receptor 2; TLR4, toll-like receptor 4; TNF-α, tumor necrosis factor-alpha; TREM-1, triggering receptor expressed on myeloid cells 1; VDR, vitamin D receptor; VSMC-TF, vascular smooth muscle cells-tissue factor.

However, because of various confounding factors, there are discrepancies in studies on the low vitamin D and CVD association. Further, Aleksova and colleagues[27] found a U-shaped curve between levels of vitamin D and MI, suggesting the association of both low and high levels of vitamin D and CVD. Therefore, further understanding and research studies are needed. In this article, the authors critically review the recent literature on the association of vitamin D levels with cardiac and vascular diseases and the potential therapeutic role of vitamin D.

CARDIAC DISEASES
Cardiac Hypertrophy

LV hypertrophy (LVH) and myocardial performance have an association with low levels of vitamin D.[8] Ameri and colleagues,[28] in a vitamin D–deficient population-based study, found a significant association between HTN, vitamin D levels, and LVH, with the most favorable LV geometry at intermediate vitamin D levels. Further, LVH and car-diomyopathy in Fabry disease have been attributed to vitamin D deficiency because of less exposure to sunlight.[29] Diabetes, a chronic inflammatory disease, is a risk factor for LVH.[30] Reversal of LVH in diabetic rats[31] and attenuation of TNF-α expression by inhibition of nuclear factor-kappa beta (NF-κB/p65) signaling in hypertrophied rat hearts with vitamin D[32] suggest the role of vitamin D in reversal of LVH. These studies suggest a pathogenic role of vitamin D deficiency in LVH and vitamin D supplementa-tion is cardioprotective. However, Pandit and colleagues[33] found no association of vitamin D deficiency with LVH and LV dysfunction (see **Fig. 2**). Such discrepancy could be due to the comorbidities and other confounding factors and warrants further investigation.

Cardiomyopathy

The pathogenesis of dilated cardiomyopathy (DCM) is usually idiopathic; however, it may arise secondary to infections or metabolic or genetic causes. Various studies have reported vitamin D deficiency–induced hypocalcemia in infants and hypoparathyroidism-induced hypocalcemia in adults as a cause for DCM and HF. Low maternal vitamin D levels were suggested as a cause for infant hypocalcemia. These studies suggest severe hypocalcemia associated with rickets in infants and hy-poparathyroidism as causes of DCM, cardiac remodeling, HF, and impaired cardiac function. Improvement in clinical symptoms after vitamin D and calcium supplemen-tation for the treatment of hypovitaminosis and hypocalcemia signifies the importance and protective role of vitamin D in cardiomyopathy[9,10,34–39] (**Table 1**). Gruson and col-leagues[40] suggested that serum $1,25(OH)_2D_3$ and its ratio to parathyroid hormone (PTH) (1–84) strongly and independently predict cardiovascular mortality in chronic HF. Additionally, Leon Rodriguez and colleagues[41] suggested that vitamin D receptor (VDR) polymorphisms may also be a risk factor for increased susceptibility for cardio-myopathy and reported the increased probability of cardiac complications, such as chronic Chagas cardiomyopathy with rs2228570*A VDR allele due to impaired im-mune response against *Trypanosoma cruzi*. These studies suggest that low vitamin D levels and reduced VDR expression may be a potential risk factor for cardiomyop-athy and HF (see **Fig. 2**).

Low circulating levels of vitamin D have been correlated with cardiac steatosis. Further, the whole animal VDR gene knockout (VDR$^{-/-}$) as well as the myocyte-specific VDR gene deletion are associated with impairment in cardiac structure and function. Glenn and colleagues[42] performed a study of VDR deficiency (VDR$^{-/-}$ mouse) in a murine model of cardiac steatosis expressing terminal enzyme diacylglycerol acyltransferase 1 selectively in the cardiac myocyte. In this study, the mice display cardiac dysfunction, late cardiomyopathy, and HF with an increase in interstitial fibrosis and increased expression of collagen $1\alpha1$, collagen $3\alpha1$, matrix metalloproteinase (MMP)-2, and osteopontin. Further, increased expression of MMPs, activated transforming growth factor-beta (TGF-β), epithelial-mesenchymal transition, and endothelial-mesenchymal transition mediate cardiac fibrosis[43]; and vitamin D attenuates expression of endothelial cell transition.[44] These results suggest an association of deficient vitamin D signaling with enhanced cardiomyopathy and an important role for vitamin D in modulating disease severity (see **Fig. 2**).

Obesity is a chronic inflammatory disease associated with low vitamin D levels. Low vitamin D levels associated with obesity could be due to an increase in total body clearance of vitamin D and increased consumption of vitamin D in fighting against obesity-associated inflammation.[45] Chronic inflammation in obesity is a risk factor for diabetes and together is a risk factor for cardiac diseases, such as

Table 1
Cardioprotective role of vitamin D supplementation in clinical studies

	Disease	Intervention	Mechanism	Beneficial Effect
Human	DCM with HF[34]	Vitamin D + calcium supplementation × 1 wk	NA	Rapid improvement in cardiac morphology and function
	DCM[35]	Vitamin D + calcium supplementation × few days	NA	Rapid improvement in clinical symptoms and cardiac function
	DCM with HF[37]	Oral calcium and calcitriol in dosages of 3 g/d and 1.5 μg/d × 2 mo, 47-y-old pt	Treated secondary hyperparathyroidism	Improvement in clinical symptoms and cardiac function
	DCM with HF[37]	10% calcium gluconate (IV 2 mL/kg × 30 min + 80 mg/kg/d × 48 h) Oral calcium carbonate 100 mg/kg/d + calcitriol 0.125 μg/d × 3 mo, 2-m-old pt	Treatment of vitamin D deficiency and hypocalcemia	Improvement in clinical symptoms and cardiac function
	Chronic HF[90]	100 μg daily vitamin D₃ supplementation × 1 y, 229 pts	NA	Significant improvement in cardiac function with reversal of LV remodeling
	Chronic HF[91]	2000 IU oral vitamin D₃ daily × 6 wk, 101 pts	NA	Larger decrease in plasma renin concentration
	Anginal episodes[113]	Vitamin D supplementation (60,000 IU/wk × 8 wk) to 20 pts	NA	Significant 20% reduction in anginal episodes and 17.24% reduction in use of sublingual nitrates
	AAA[116]	Paricalcitol 1 μg daily × 2–4 wk	VDR activation	Decreased calcineurin-mediated inflammation in the arterial wall
In vitro	Arterial thrombosis[112]	Calcitriol (10⁻⁸M) and paricalcitol (3 × 10⁻⁸M) to HAVSMCs	Reduce expression of TF induced by TNF-α in HAVSMCs	Reduced prothrombotic state
	Cardiac fibrosis[64]	Calcitriol-1 μM to HCF-av 24–48 h	Inhibition of TGFβ1-mediated cell contraction	Prevention of biochemical and functional profibrotic changes in human primary cardiac fibroblasts

Vitamin D supplementation with or without calcium with improvement in clinical symptoms and cardiac morphology and function in these clinical studies suggest cardioprotective role of vitamin D.

Abbreviations: AAA, abdominal aortic aneurysm; HAVSMCs, human aortic smooth muscle cells; HCF-av, primary human adult ventricular cardiac fibroblasts; IV, intravenous; NA, not available/not mentioned; pts, patient(s); TGF-β1, transforming growth factor-beta 1; VDR, vitamin D receptor; VSMCs-TF, vascular smooth muscle cells-tissue factor.

cardiomyopathies, CAD, MI, fibrosis, arrhythmias, and HF.[46,47] Increased expression of the myocardial receptor for advanced glycation end products (RAGE), TNF-α, p65 subunit of NF-κB, α subunit of inhibitor of κB, subunits of nicotinamide adenine dinucleotide phosphate oxidase (NOX4 and p22^{phox}), angiotensin II type 1 receptor (AT1R), TGF-β1, TGF-β receptor I, total and phosphorylated Sma- and mad-related protein 2/3 (SMAD2/3) and protein serine/threonine kinase ERK, MMP2, and procollagen I and decreased expression of tissue inhibitors of metalloproteinases 2 were observed in diabetic mice. Treatment of the diabetic mice with calcitriol resulted in decreased expression of myocardial RAGE, TNF-α, p22^{phox}, AT1R, TGF-β1, p-SMAD2/3 and p-ERK signaling, and procollagen I. These results suggest the beneficial role of vitamin D in decreasing the effect of diabetes on myocardial RAGE and fibrosis by modulating the AT1R and further signify the antiinflammatory, antioxidative, and cardioprotective effects of vitamin D[48] (see **Fig. 2**).

Myocardial Infarction

Low levels of vitamin D are associated with the status and incident events of CVDs.[7] Analysis of 478 subjects diagnosed with acute MI showed a high prevalence of vitamin D deficiency in all seasons, though lower in summer than winter.[6] Low plasma vitamin D levels are independently associated with poor outcomes in the hospital and 1-year follow-up in acute coronary syndrome (ACS)[49] and patients with acute MI.[50] Further, hyperlipidemia is a risk factor for CVD; serum vitamin D has an inverse association with the levels of total cholesterol, low-density lipoprotein (LDL), homocysteine, and triglycerides and a positive association with high-density lipoprotein. Because hyperlipidemia is a risk factor for CVD and vitamin D has an inverse relationship with these lipid levels, vitamin D supplementation might be protective against CVD.[51]

Atherosclerosis and the formation of thrombus and embolus are major risk factors for MI. Inflammation plays a major role in the pathogenesis of these risk factors as well as in postmyocardial remodeling. Further, vitamin D deficiency is associated with increased inflammation, proinflammatory cytokines, and atherosclerosis; vitamin D supplementation may reduce these factors.[52,53] Thus, vitamin D deficiency may play a role in MI. It is further supported by a high prevalence of vitamin D deficiency in patients with acute MI.[54,55] However, studies have reported no association between vitamin D levels, inflammatory markers, and patients with ACS.[56,57] These results suggest the need of further research to elucidate the role of vitamin D in the pathogenesis of atherosclerosis and MI (see **Fig. 2**).

Polymorphisms or genetic variations of the VDR gene (eg, rs7968585) could be a positive predictor for MI.[58] Further, the upregulation of endogenous VDR expression in the mouse heart after the myocardial ischemia/reperfusion by natural and synthetic agonists and reduction in the myocardial infarct size with improved cardiac function suggest the protective role of upregulated VDR. The cardioprotective effect of VDR activation is attributed to inhibited endoplasmic reticulum stress, attenuated mitochondrial impairment, decreased autophagy dysfunction, and reduced cardiomyocyte apoptosis.[59] Further, reduced expression of myocardial vitamin D receptors in obstructive nephropathy rats is related to the myocardial remodeling with fibrosis with an increase in arrhythmogenesis. Protection against these changes by restoring myocardial VDR levels with paricalcitol suggests the protective role of vitamin D.[60]

Cardiac Fibrosis and Remodeling

Diabetes is a risk factor for cardiac diseases, including cardiac fibrosis. Increased expression of connective TGF (CTGF), TGF-β1, SMAD3, poly (ADP-ribose) polymerase 1 (PARP1), sirtuin 1 (SIRT1), and mechanistic target of rapamycin (mTOR) in diabetes mediates cardiac fibrosis.[61–63] The negative regulation of the activity of TGF-β1, SMAD3, CTGF, and PARP1/SIRT1/mTOR pathway with vitamin D suggests the protective role of vitamin D on fibrosis[63–66] (see **Table 1**). Wang and colleagues,[67] using the rat model, reported that diabetes induces the cardiac weight index, plasma glucose, lactic dehydrogenase, and creatine kinase with the reduced body and cardiac weights and pathologic changes of fibrosis. Further, reduction of these parameters and minimal pathologic changes with supplementation with vitamin D suggest the beneficial role of vitamin D in cardiac fibrosis. Furthermore, inflammation plays a major role in postinfarction remodeling[68]; vitamin D being an antiinflammatory agent may play a crucial role[69] (see **Fig. 2**).

Because vitamin D deficiency is associated with the development of cardiac hypertrophy and fibrosis, genomics of VDR may also play a role in the development of cardiac fibrosis. Dorsch and colleagues[12] suggested that the biomarker for collagen type III synthesis, PIIINP, is associated with the CGA haplotype of *Bsml*, *Apal,* and *Taql* single nucleotide polymorphisms in the VDR. Further, decreased cardiac fibrosis[11] and attenuated cardiac remodeling and dysfunction in polycystic ovarian syndrome[70] with vitamin D supplementation and/or VDR activation suggest the role of vitamin D in treating cardiac fibrosis.[71] Furthermore, the cardioprotective effects of VDR activators and modulators suggest the potential therapeutic role of vitamin D.[72,73]

Heart Failure

Vitamin D deficiency is associated with MI, post-MI HF, as well as new-onset HF.[74] Bae and colleagues[13] suggested that vitamin D deficiency after MI in VDR knockout mice leads to a decreased survival rate and cardiac function and vitamin D signaling promotes cardioprotection through antiinflammatory, antiapoptotic, and antifibrotic mechanisms. Further, vitamin D deficiency is associated with increased inflammation and inflammatory cytokines, such as TNF-α, interleukin (IL)-6, and IL-1beta (IL-1β), involved in mediating the cardiac diseases and HF.[14] Vitamin D supplementation reduces these cytokines in chronic HF.[75] IL-33 is a member of the IL-1 family of cytokines. IL-33, through its receptor ST2, prevents cardiomyocyte apoptosis and improves cardiac function and survival after MI[76] (see **Fig. 2**). An increase in the circulating levels of the soluble decoy receptor of ST2 (sST2) is associated with cardiac remodeling, fibrosis, and HF.[77] Further, low levels of vitamin D and hypoparathyroidism are associated with cardiomyopathy remodeling and worsening of HF.[78] Furthermore, calcitriol, the biologically active form of vitamin D, regulates cardiac function and might modulate ST2.[79] Thus, interrelations of the vitamin D/PTH axis and sST2 regulating inflammation and fibrosis in the heart may also regulate HF. Studies have suggested the strong relationship between low vitamin D levels, sST2, and the vitamin D/PTH (1–84) axis and HF. It was proposed that sST2 levels and a low plasma $1,25(OH)_2D_3$/PTH (1–84) ratio are strong predictors of worsening HF, hospitalization, reduced survival, and mortality due to cardiac disease.[80–83] However, there was no association between plasma levels of calcidiol, calcitriol, or PTH and risk of developing HF.[74]

Further, as discussed earlier, vitamin D deficiency associates with HF; vitamin D supplementation may be beneficial.[84] However, there are reports of no improvement or beneficial effect of vitamin D in HF with vitamin D supplementation; the discrepancies between the studies may be due to the genetic variations in the VDR (eg, Fok1) gene.[85–89] Improvement and beneficial effects of vitamin D on LV structure and function in the VitamIN D treatIng patients with Chronic heArT failure (VINDICATE) study in HF[90] and decreased renin activity with short-term vitamin D supplementation in patients with chronic HF[91] suggest the therapeutic role of vitamin D (see **Table 1**).

Rhythm Abnormalities

Vitamin D deficiency is associated with CVDs, including cardiac fibrosis, which is a hallmark for the arrhythmias. Low vitamin D levels are associated with HF and atrial fibrillations (AFs) in patients with HF.[92] Low levels of vitamin D are significantly associated with more extensive left atrial fibrosis in patients with lone paroxysmal AF as well as with recurrence of AF after cryoablation[93] and after coronary artery bypass graft surgery.[94] These results suggest that low vitamin D levels are associated with an increased incidence of AF. Increased inflammation, oxidative stress, and activation of the renin-angiotensin system (RAS) may cause increased arrhythmic events in HF. Furthermore, antiinflammatory and antioxidative properties of vitamin D, its binding to VDR on myocyte, along with negative regulation of RAS mediate the amelioration of inflammation and proarrhythmic substrate formation leading to decreased chances of fibrillation. These findings suggest the protective role of vitamin D[95] (see **Fig. 2**). However, no independent association was found between low vitamin D levels and AF after coronary artery bypass surgery.[96] Similarly, the Atherosclerosis Risk in Communities (ARIC) study did not find any significant association between low levels of vitamin D and incident AF in a community-based cohort and in a meta-analysis of prospective studies comprising 12,303 subjects. However, the investigators recommended further studies for an association in younger patients.[97]

VASCULAR DISEASE
Atherosclerosis

Obesity is a major risk factor for CVD. In human patients, there is a known association between vitamin D deficiency and HTN, metabolic syndrome, and related risk factors of CVD. Perivascular adipose tissue (PVAT) in obesity produces factors that affect atherogenesis and smooth muscle cell proliferation, thereby affecting the contractile function. Pelham and colleagues[98] demonstrated an association between vitamin D deficiency, impaired normal ability of PVAT to suppress contractile responses of the underlying mesenteric resistance artery to angiotensin II and serotonin, and enhanced angiotensin II–induced vasoconstriction. Vitamin D deficiency was also associated with the increased expression of TNF-α and heat-induced factor-1 alpha. These results suggest a protective role of vitamin D through regulating the mediators of inflammation and hypoxia signaling against vascular dysfunction, hypertension, and CVD. Lin and colleagues[99] reported similar effects of VDR agonists and retinoid X receptor agonists in alleviating atherosclerosis through inhibition of oxidative stress in a diabetic mice model (see **Fig. 3**). An inverse correlation between the vitamin D level and the stage of coronary atherosclerosis along with the levels of total cholesterol, LDL, and triglycerides in women and men older than 70 years has been reported.[100] Similarly, low levels of vitamin D have been associated with subclinical atherosclerosis and increased expression of high-sensitivity cardiac troponin T and N-terminal pro–brain natriuretic peptide (markers of subclinical myocardial damage and wall stress).[101] In addition, the role of vitamin D binding protein (VDBP) and its polymorphism in relation to atherosclerosis and the role of VDBP in resistance to atherosclerosis leading to the longevity of patients has also been examined.[102] However, no significant association between the serum vitamin D level and carotid atherosclerosis in patients with chronic kidney disease found by Ng and colleagues[103] indicates the need for further research.

Inflammation plays a crucial role in the pathogenesis of plaque development and progression involving mediators, such as triggering receptor expressed on myeloid cells 1, toll-like receptor 4 (TLR4), and cytokines (such as IL-6, TNF-α, IL-1β, and IFN-γ) and macrophages[104,105] (see **Fig. 3**). Low intraplaque VDR expression, the prevalence of VDR expression in M1 compared with M2 macrophages, and increased VDR expression in M1 macrophages incubated with 1,25(OH)$_2$D$_3$ with suppression of TLR4 expression suggest that low intraplaque VDR expression predicts an adverse cardiovascular event in patients with carotid stenosis. These findings signify the possible important therapeutic role for vitamin D and VDR in the treatment of arterial plaque.[106] Further, the protective role of vitamin D in atherosclerosis via regulation of macrophage polarization and cholesterol efflux and reducing intimal hyperplasia and restenosis has been documented in a swine model.[52,107] Vitamin D has a protective effect on the endothelial cells by reducing endoplasmic reticulum stress and oxidative stress thereby reducing the risk of atherosclerosis.[108] Furthermore, significant inhibition of atherosclerosis in ApoE-deficient mice with intravenous transfusion of endothelial progenitor cells with overexpressed VDR suggests the role of vitamin D and VDR in this disorder and a potential method for angiogenic therapy.[109]

Arterial Calcification

Subclinical atherosclerosis is precipitated by calcification of the arteries. A significant positive association between the low levels of vitamin D and coronary artery calcification has been reported by a population-based cross-sectional study.[110] Increased calcification and higher expression of osteogenic key factors, such as Msx2, Bmp2, and Runx2, in VDR knockout (VDR$^{-/-}$) mice as well as in LDL receptor knockout mice fed on a Western diet with low vitamin D (50 IU/kg) suggest the role of VDR and vitamin D deficiency as risk factors for aortic valve and aortic vessel calcification.[20]

Occlusive Arterial Disease

Arterial thrombosis is a major cause of anginal episodes, and rupture of the thrombus results in embolus formation leading to MI. Coronary occlusion precipitates MI, and coronary collaterals circulation (CCC) protects the myocardium from acute events in cases of the total coronary occlusive disease. Dogan and colleagues[111] found low vitamin D levels as the strong predictor of and associated with poor CCC. Further, increased expression of the vascular smooth muscle cell (VSMC)–derived tissue factor (TF) plays an important role in thrombus formation involving TNF-α and NF-κB. Phosphorylation of NF-κB is accompanied by upregulation of TF signaling because of increased expression of protease-activated receptor-2 (PAR-2) and downregulation of VDR (see **Fig. 3**). This results in increased inflammation and progression of thrombus formation. Attenuation in the expression of PAR-2, TNF-α, and NF-κB with vitamin D suggests the beneficial role of vitamin D in thrombosis.[112] Further, the significant reduction in the anginal episodes and reduction in the use of sublingual nitrates with vitamin D supplementation suggest the beneficial role of vitamin D in CVD[113] (see **Table 1**).

Aneurysm and Peripheral Arterial Disease

Vitamin D deficiency plays a role in the pathogenesis of vascular disease atherosclerosis. However, the presence of VDR in the vascular endothelium and VSMCs[1] suggests that vitamin D may play a role in other vascular diseases, such as aneurysm, PAD, and calcification. A study on 490 patients by van de Luijtgaarden and colleagues[16] suggests that vitamin D deficiency is associated with the severity of arterial diseases, such as abdominal and/or thoracic aneurysm and PAD, and the underlying mechanism for these occlusive and aneurysmal diseases is different from atherosclerosis. Vitamin D deficiency is a risk factor for severity of arterial disease irrespective of the type of arterial disease and independent of traditional cardiovascular risk factors.[15,16] Similarly, the study by Wong and colleagues[114] with 311 patients also found the association of low vitamin D with the severity of the abdominal aortic aneurysm (AAA) and suggested a graded inverse relationship between vitamin D concentrations and AAA diameter.

Further, inflammation plays a key role in the pathogenesis of aneurysm development; being an antiinflammatory agent, vitamin D may reduce the inflammation and progression. Reduction in AAA dissection, induced by angiotensin-II in ApoE$^{-/-}$ mice, by VDR activation with oral vitamin D suggests the potential therapeutic role of vitamin D to decrease the AAA progression.[115] The reduction in the progression of AAA was attributed to a decrease in many parameters, including macrophage infiltration, neo-vessel formation, MMP-2 and MMP-9 activation, chemokines (CCL2, CCL5, CXCL1) expression, and extracellular signal–regulated kinases 1/2, p38 mitogen-activated protein kinase, and NF-κB activity (see **Fig. 3**). Furthermore, the antiinflammatory effect of vitamin D by reducing the expression of inflammatory mediators, CD4+ T-helper cells, and cytokines IL-2, IL-4, and IL-10 with paricalcitol and reduction in the local inflammation in patients with AAA suggest the therapeutic role of vitamin D in arterial aneurysms. The antiinflammatory action of vitamin D was suggested to be mediated by an effect on calcineurin-mediated responses[116] (see **Table 1**). Further, a meta-analysis comprising 6 case-control studies assessing 6418 patients with PAD suggests the association of low levels of circulating vitamin D with PAD and with chronic limb ischemia.[17] Li and colleagues[18] and Oh and colleagues[19] also reported similar association in their studies with 1028 diabetic patients and 8960 subjects, respectively. The association of low levels of vitamin D with the prevalence of PAD supports the role of vitamin D deficiency as an independent risk factor for CVD.

Hypertension

The imbalance between the vasoconstriction and vasodilatation due to various genetic and epigenetic factors (vitamin D deficiency) results in vasoconstriction leading to essential HTN. Chen and colleagues[117] reported a clinically significant antihypertensive effect of vitamin D in vitamin D-deficient essential hypertensive patients. Similarly, significantly low vitamin D levels are associated with nondipper HTN as compared with dipper HTN.[118] Hypertensive patients with a nocturnal reduction in average daytime systolic and diastolic blood pressure of less than 10% are classed as nondippers and of 10% to 20% as dippers. In addition, impaired RAS is a risk factor for HTN, and low vitamin D levels are associated with impaired RAS. Negative regulation of RAS with vitamin D supplementation suggests the beneficial role of vitamin D in the treatment of HTN.[95] Aortic stiffness, decreased vessel compliance, and atherosclerosis are associated with HTN. The association between the low circulating vitamin D levels and aortic stiffness independent of classic risk factors and inflammatory markers in prediabetic patients suggests vitamin D deficiency as a risk factor for CVD and HTN.[119] However, Kang and colleagues[120] reported that the association between levels of vitamin D and blood pressure, lipid profiles, glycemic index, brachial-ankle pulse wave velocity, and carotid artery intima-media wall thickness are sex dependent and serum vitamin D level may not be a risk factor related to subclinical atherosclerosis and arterial stiffness.

Vitamin D regulates the proliferation of endothelial cells (ECs) and VSMCs,[121] and VDR is present in these cells.[1] Endothelial dysfunction plays a key role in vascular diseases, such as HTN. Vitamin D deficiency affecting the ECs may precipitate HTN[22] (see **Fig. 3**). Significant impairment in the acetylcholine-induced aortic relaxation, increased sensitivity to the hypertensive effects of angiotensin II, and increased expression of angiotensin II infusion–induced hypertrophy-sensitive myocardial genes in endothelial-specific VDR knockout mice compared with control mice suggest the potential role of endothelial VDR in EC function and blood pressure control and the therapeutic role of VDR agonists in the management of EC dysfunction-related CVD.[21]

FUTURE DIRECTIONS

Studying the microbiota for disease pathogenesis is an emerging field of research. Studies have hypothesized that a change in the microbiota results in an immune response and may result in a proinflammatory environment.[122,123] Altered intestinal microbiome due to vitamin D deficiency also impairs the B vitamins because of altered intestinal bacteria. This impairment may result in an increased risk of atherosclerosis, HTN, tachycardia, atrial arrhythmias, and a hyperadrenergic state predisposing to heart disease and stroke mediated by a proinflammatory state and lack of pantothenic acid. Improvement of the intestinal microbiota with the vitamin D supplementation along with B vitamins support the therapeutic benefit of vitamin D.[124] Thus, studying the intestinal and plaque microbiome might elucidate the novel therapeutic options for CVD.

The $1,25(OH)_2D_3$/PTH ratio plays an important role in CVD. Further, PTH, fibroblast growth factor 23 (FGF23), and 25(OH)D itself regulate the enzymes involved in the calcitriol synthesis. FGF23 negatively regulates the PTH. PTH has a positive and FGF23 has a negative effect on CYP27B1. The $1,25(OH)_2D_3$ has a feedback inhibitory effect on CYP27B1[125] (see **Fig. 1**). FGF23 also regulates vitamin D metabolism by regulating the urinary secretion of phosphate in the presence of FGF receptor 1 and its coreceptor Klotho.[126] Increased FGF23 along with increased PTH in kidney disease increase the cardiovascular events and mortality; calcium supplementation reduces FGF23, CVD events, and mortality.[127] Increased levels of FGF23 decrease serum $1,25(OH)_2D_3$ without any change in PTH and antiaging protein Klotho after MI in a mouse model.[128] Increased FGF23 is also associated with incident AF, LVH, and systolic and diastolic dysfunction.[129] Furthermore, inactive Klotho is associated with increased atherosclerosis, vascular calcification, and CVD events, whereas the activation of Klotho is associated with decreased atherosclerosis and vascular calcification.[126] Furthermore, soluble α-Klotho has a cardioprotective effect via inhibition of TRPC6 channel-mediated abnormal Ca^{2+} signaling in the heart[130]; higher PTH levels are associated with LVH and increased risk of incident HF.[131] These results suggest that interactions between PTH, FGF23, Klotho, calcium, and vitamin D levels play a crucial role in the pathogenesis of CVD. Thus, supplementation of vitamin D and calcium might be cardioprotective. However, Kopecky and colleagues[132] suggested a lack of evidence between calcium with or without vitamin D intake from food or supplements and the risk for CVD mortality or all-cause mortality in generally healthy adults. Thus, interactions between PTH, FGF23, Klotho, calcium levels, vitamin D levels, and the underlying signaling mechanism need further research.

Further, RAS and AT1R play important roles in the pathogenesis of CVD. Angiotensin-converting enzyme (ACE) inhibitors and angiotensin II receptor blockers (ARBs) are used to treat HTN, and they act differently on RAS.[133] ACE inhibitors block both AT1R and angiotensin II type 2 receptors (AT2R), whereas ARB blocks only

AT1R. Thus, ARB therapy results in a decrease in blood pressure as well as an over-expressed AT2R.[133] Although the beneficial effect of AT1R is well established in treating HTN, HF, atherosclerosis, and aortic aneurysms, the beneficial effect of AT2R is under investigation.[133,134] The beneficial role of the AT2R agonist, Compound 21, in diabetes-associated atherosclerosis[135] and increased AT2R expression by targeting intron 2 enhancer element to increase satellite cell proliferation and potentiating skeletal muscle regenerative capacity in patients with congestive heart failure has been discussed.[136] However, the protective role of AT2R and the underlying mechanism and interaction with vitamin D levels in CVD warrant further investigation.

SUMMARY

CAD, stroke, and sudden cardiac death remain the leading causes of morbidity and mortality worldwide. For screening, the assessment of at-risk individuals is based on the Framingham Risk Score or the American Heart Association/American College of Cardiology's pooled cohort equations/guidelines. However, scoring the risk with traditional risk factors using these methods may underestimate or overestimate the risk. Thus, the need to consider the inclusion of additional factors associated with the CVDs to decrease the morbidity and mortality and improve the outcome has been warranted.[137,138] Further, reduced C-reactive protein levels in 2 clinical trials,[139,140] relaxation of VSMCs, decreased renin production by kidney, and reduced mortality in patients with renal failure with $1,25(OH)_2D_3$[141] suggest the protective role of vitamin D. Because the studies discussed earlier suggest strong evidence for the role of vitamin D deficiency in the pathogenesis of CVD, inclusion of low levels of vitamin D in the risk stratification may be beneficial in identifying high-risk individuals and can help in guiding personalized risk assessment. Although, as discussed, the interaction between PTH, FGF23, Klotho, calcium, and serum 25(OH)D levels is associated with CVD. Vitamin D deficiency may serve as a novel marker and predictor of the severity of CVD. However, the beneficial role of vitamin D supplementation in CVD remains inconclusive and needs further research.

REFERENCES

1. Holick MF. Vitamin D deficiency. N Engl J Med 2007;357(3):266–81.
2. Wadhwa B, Relhan V, Goel K, et al. Vitamin D and skin diseases: a review. Indian J Dermatol Venereol Leprol 2015;81(4):344–55.
3. Norman PE, Powell JT. Vitamin D and cardiovascular disease. Circ Res 2014; 114(2):379–93.
4. Durup D, Jorgensen HL, Christensen J, et al. A reverse J-shaped association of all-cause mortality with serum 25-hydroxyvitamin D in general practice: the CopD study. J Clin Endocrinol Metab 2012;97(8):2644–52.
5. Chen S, Swier VJ, Boosani CS, et al. Vitamin D deficiency accelerates coronary artery disease progression in swine. Arterioscler Thromb Vasc Biol 2016;36(8): 1651–9.
6. Aleksova A, Belfiore R, Carriere C, et al. Vitamin D deficiency in patients with acute myocardial infarction: an Italian single-center study. Int J Vitam Nutr Res 2015;85(1–2):23–30.
7. Anderson JL, May HT, Horne BD, et al. Relation of vitamin D deficiency to cardiovascular risk factors, disease status, and incident events in a general health-care population. Am J Cardiol 2010;106(7):963–8.

8. Seker T, Gur M, Ucar H, et al. Lower serum 25-hydroxyvitamin D level is associated with impaired myocardial performance and left ventricle hypertrophy in newly diagnosed hypertensive patients. Anatol J Cardiol 2015;15(9):744–50.

9. Yilmaz O, Olgun H, Ciftel M, et al. Dilated cardiomyopathy secondary to rickets-related hypocalcaemia: eight case reports and a review of the literature. Cardiol Young 2015;25(2):261–6.

10. Polat V, Bozcali E, Uygun T, et al. Low vitamin D status associated with dilated cardiomyopathy. Int J Clin Exp Med 2015;8(1):1356–62.

11. Charytan DM, Padera RF, Helfand AM, et al. Association of activated vitamin D use with myocardial fibrosis and capillary supply: results of an autopsy study. Ren Fail 2015;37(6):1067–9.

12. Dorsch MP, Nemerovski CW, Ellingrod VL, et al. Vitamin D receptor genetics on extracellular matrix biomarkers and hemodynamics in systolic heart failure. J Cardiovasc Pharmacol Ther 2014;19(5):439–45.

13. Bae S, Singh SS, Yu H, et al. Vitamin D signaling pathway plays an important role in the development of heart failure after myocardial infarction. J Appl Physiol (1985) 2013;114(8):1070–07.

14. Gullestad L, Ueland T, Vinge LE, et al. Inflammatory cytokines in heart failure: mediators and markers. Cardiology 2012;122(1):23–35.

15. Demir M, Uyan U, Melek M. The relationship between vitamin D deficiency and thoracic aortic dilatation. Vasa 2012;41(6):419–24.

16. van de Luijtgaarden KM, Voute MT, Hoeks SE, et al. Vitamin D deficiency may be an independent risk factor for arterial disease. Eur J Vasc Endovasc Surg 2012; 44(3):301–6.

17. Nsengiyumva V, Fernando ME, Moxon JV, et al. The association of circulating 25-hydroxyvitamin D concentration with peripheral arterial disease: a meta-analysis of observational studies. Atherosclerosis 2015;243(2):645–51.

18. Li DM, Zhang Y, Li Q, et al. Low 25-hydroxyvitamin D level is associated with peripheral arterial disease in type 2 diabetes patients. Arch Med Res 2016;47(1): 49–54.

19. Oh SH, Kweon SS, Choi JS, et al. Association between vitamin D status and risk of peripheral arterial disease: the Dong-gu study. Chonnam Med J 2016;52(3): 212–6.

20. Schmidt N, Brandsch C, Kuhne H, et al. Vitamin D receptor deficiency and low vitamin D diet stimulate aortic calcification and osteogenic key factor expression in mice. PLoS One 2012;7(4):e35316.

21. Ni W, Watts SW, Ng M, et al. Elimination of vitamin D receptor in vascular endothelial cells alters vascular function. Hypertension 2014;64(6):1290–8.

22. Oruc CU, Akpinar YE, Amikishiyev S, et al. Hypovitaminosis D is associated with endothelial dysfunction in patients with metabolic syndrome. Curr Vasc Pharmacol 2016;15(2):152–7.

23. Lupton JR, Faridi KF, Martin SS, et al. Deficient serum 25-hydroxyvitamin D is associated with an atherogenic lipid profile: the very large database of lipids (VLDL-3) study. J Clin Lipidol 2016;10(1):72–81.e1.

24. Daraghmeh AH, Bertoia ML, Al-Qadi MO, et al. Evidence for the vitamin D hypothesis: the NHANES III extended mortality follow-up. Atherosclerosis 2016; 255:96–101.

25. Assalin HB, Rafacho BP, dos Santos PP, et al. Impact of the length of vitamin D deficiency on cardiac remodeling. Circ Heart Fail 2013;6(4):809–16.

26. Wang TJ. Vitamin D and cardiovascular disease. Annu Rev Med 2016;67: 261–72.

27. Aleksova A, Beltrami AP, Belfiore R, et al. U-shaped relationship between vitamin D levels and long-term outcome in large cohort of survivors of acute myocardial infarction. Int J Cardiol 2016;223:962–6.
28. Ameri P, Canepa M, Milaneschi Y, et al. Relationship between vitamin D status and left ventricular geometry in a healthy population: results from the Baltimore longitudinal study of aging. J Intern Med 2013;273(3):253–62.
29. Drechsler C, Schmiedeke B, Niemann M, et al. Potential role of vitamin D deficiency on Fabry cardiomyopathy. J Inherit Metab Dis 2014;37(2):289–95.
30. Somaratne JB, Whalley GA, Poppe KK, et al. Screening for left ventricular hypertrophy in patients with type 2 diabetes mellitus in the community. Cardiovasc Diabetol 2011;10:29.
31. Fan Y, Zhang SX, Ren M, et al. Impact of 1, 25-(OH)2D3 on left ventricular hypertrophy in type 2 diabetic rats. Chin Med Sci J 2015;30(2):114–20.
32. Al-Rasheed NM, Bassiouni YA, Hasan IH, et al. Vitamin D attenuates proinflammatory TNF-alpha cytokine expression by inhibiting NF-small ka, Cyrillic B/p65 signaling in hypertrophied rat hearts. J Physiol Biochem 2015;71(2):289–99.
33. Pandit A, Mookadam F, Boddu S, et al. Vitamin D levels and left ventricular diastolic function. Open Heart 2014;1(1):e000011.
34. Yilmaz O, Kilic O, Ciftel M, et al. Rapid response to treatment of heart failure resulting from hypocalcemic cardiomyopathy. Pediatr Emerg Care 2014;30(11):822–3.
35. Batra CM, Agarwal R. Hypocalcemic cardiomyopathy and pseudohypoparathyroidism due to severe vitamin D deficiency. J Assoc Physicians India 2016;64(6):74–6.
36. Laranjo S, Trigo C, Pinto FF. Dual etiology of dilated cardiomyopathy: the synergistic role of vitamin D deficiency. Rev Port Cardiol 2014;33(3):179.e1-4.
37. Bansal B, Bansal M, Bajpai P, et al. Hypocalcemic cardiomyopathy-different mechanisms in adult and pediatric cases. J Clin Endocrinol Metab 2014;99(8):2627–32.
38. Venugopalan G, Navinath M, Pradeep B, et al. Hypocalcemic cardiomyopathy due to vitamin D deficiency in a very old man. J Am Geriatr Soc 2015;63(8):1708–9.
39. Loncar G, Bozic B, Cvetinovic N, et al. Secondary hyperparathyroidism prevalence and prognostic role in elderly males with heart failure. J Endocrinol Invest 2017;40(3):297–304.
40. Gruson D, Ferracin B, Ahn SA, et al. 1,25-dihydroxyvitamin D to PTH(1-84) ratios strongly predict cardiovascular death in heart failure. PLoS One 2015;10(8):e0135427.
41. Leon Rodriguez DA, Carmona FD, Gonzalez CI, et al. Evaluation of VDR gene polymorphisms in Trypanosoma cruzi infection and chronic chagasic cardiomyopathy. Sci Rep 2016;6:31263.
42. Glenn DJ, Cardema MC, Gardner DG. Amplification of lipotoxic cardiomyopathy in the VDR gene knockout mouse. J Steroid Biochem Mol Biol 2016;164:292–8.
43. Rai V, Sharma P, Agrawal S, et al. Relevance of mouse models of cardiac fibrosis and hypertrophy in cardiac research. Mol Cell Biochem 2017;424(1–2):123–45.
44. Lai CC, Liu CP, Cheng PW, et al. Paricalcitol attenuates cardiac fibrosis and expression of endothelial cell transition markers in isoproterenol-induced cardiomyopathic rats. Crit Care Med 2016;44(9):e866–74.
45. Cartier JL, Kukreja SC, Barengolts E. Lower serum 25-hydroxyvitamin D is associated with obesity but not common chronic conditions: an observational study

of African American and Caucasian male veterans. Endocr Pract 2017;23(3): 271–8.

46. Seferovic PM, Paulus WJ. Clinical diabetic cardiomyopathy: a two-faced disease with restrictive and dilated phenotypes. Eur Heart J 2015;36(27): 1718–27, 1727a–c.

47. Luft VC, Schmidt MI, Pankow JS, et al. Chronic inflammation role in the obesity-diabetes association: a case-cohort study. Diabetol Metab Syndr 2013;5(1):31.

48. Lee TW, Kao YH, Lee TI, et al. Calcitriol modulates receptor for advanced glycation end products (RAGE) in diabetic hearts. Int J Cardiol 2014;173(2): 236–41.

49. De Metrio M, Milazzo V, Rubino M, et al. Vitamin D plasma levels and in-hospital and 1-year outcomes in acute coronary syndromes: a prospective study. Medicine (Baltimore) 2015;94(19):e857.

50. Roy A, Lakshmy R, Tarik M, et al. Independent association of severe vitamin D deficiency as a risk of acute myocardial infarction in Indians. Indian Heart J 2015;67(1):27–32.

51. Glueck CJ, Jetty V, Rothschild M, et al. Associations between serum 25-hydroxyvitamin D and lipids, lipoprotein cholesterols, and homocysteine. N Am J Med Sci 2016;8(7):284–90.

52. Gupta GK, Agrawal T, Rai V, et al. Vitamin D supplementation reduces intimal hyperplasia and restenosis following coronary intervention in atherosclerotic swine. PLoS One 2016;11(6):e0156857.

53. Satilmis S, Celik O, Biyik I, et al. Association between serum vitamin D levels and subclinical coronary atherosclerosis and plaque burden/composition in young adult population. Bosn J Basic Med Sci 2015;15(1):67–72.

54. Tokarz A, Kusnierz-Cabala B, Kuzniewski M, et al. Seasonal effect of vitamin D deficiency in patients with acute myocardial infarction. Kardiol Pol 2016;74(8): 786–92.

55. Gondim F, Caribe A, Vasconcelos KF, et al. Vitamin D deficiency is associated with severity of acute coronary syndrome in patients with type 2 diabetes and high rates of sun exposure. Clin Med Insights Endocrinol Diabetes 2016;9: 37–41.

56. Eren E, Ellidag HY, Yilmaz A, et al. No association between vitamin D levels and inflammation markers in patients with acute coronary syndrome. Adv Med Sci 2015;60(1):89–93.

57. Brondum-Jacobsen P, Benn M, Afzal S, et al. No evidence that genetically reduced 25-hydroxyvitamin D is associated with increased risk of ischaemic heart disease or myocardial infarction: a Mendelian randomization study. Int J Epidemiol 2015;44(2):651–61.

58. Zostautiene I, Jorde R, Schirmer H, et al. Genetic variations in the vitamin D receptor predict type 2 diabetes and myocardial infarction in a community-based population: the TROMSO study. PLoS One 2015;10(12):e0145359.

59. Yao T, Ying X, Zhao Y, et al. Vitamin D receptor activation protects against myocardial reperfusion injury through inhibition of apoptosis and modulation of autophagy. Antioxid Redox Signal 2015;22(8):633–50.

60. Diez ER, Altamirano LB, Garcia IM, et al. Heart remodeling and ischemia-reperfusion arrhythmias linked to myocardial vitamin d receptors deficiency in obstructive nephropathy are reversed by paricalcitol. J Cardiovasc Pharmacol Ther 2015;20(2):211–20.

61. Lipson KE, Wong C, Teng Y, et al. CTGF is a central mediator of tissue remodeling and fibrosis and its inhibition can reverse the process of fibrosis. Fibrogenesis Tissue Repair 2012;5(Suppl 1):S24.

62. Biernacka A, Cavalera M, Wang J, et al. Smad3 signaling promotes fibrosis while preserving cardiac and aortic geometry in obese diabetic mice. Circ Heart Fail 2015;8(4):788–98.

63. Qu H, Lin K, Wang H, et al. 1,25(OH)2 D3 improves cardiac dysfunction, hypertrophy, and fibrosis through PARP1/SIRT1/mTOR-related mechanisms in type 1 diabetes. Mol Nutr Food Res 2017;61(5).

64. Meredith A, Boroomand S, Carthy J, et al. 1,25 dihydroxyvitamin D3 Inhibits TGFbeta1-mediated primary human cardiac myofibroblast activation. PLoS One 2015;10(6):e0128655.

65. Tian Y, Lv G, Yang Y, et al. Effects of vitamin D on renal fibrosis in diabetic nephropathy model rats. Int J Clin Exp Pathol 2014;7(6):3028–37.

66. Ito I, Waku T, Aoki M, et al. A nonclassical vitamin D receptor pathway suppresses renal fibrosis. J Clin Invest 2013;123(11):4579–94.

67. Wang L, Yuan T, Du G, et al. The impact of 1,25-dihydroxyvitamin D3 on the expression of connective tissue growth factor and transforming growth factor-beta1 in the myocardium of rats with diabetes. Diabetes Res Clin Pract 2014;104(2):226–33.

68. Saxena A, Chen W, Su Y, et al. IL-1 induces proinflammatory leukocyte infiltration and regulates fibroblast phenotype in the infarcted myocardium. J Immunol 2013;191(9):4838–48.

69. Hlaing SM, Garcia LA, Contreras JR, et al. 1,25-vitamin D3 promotes cardiac differentiation through modulation of the WNT signaling pathway. J Mol Endocrinol 2014;53(3):303–17.

70. Gao L, Cao JT, Liang Y, et al. Calcitriol attenuates cardiac remodeling and dysfunction in a murine model of polycystic ovary syndrome. Endocrine 2016;52(2):363–73.

71. Panizo S, Barrio-Vazquez S, Naves-Diaz M, et al. Vitamin D receptor activation, left ventricular hypertrophy and myocardial fibrosis. Nephrol Dial Transplant 2013;28(11):2735–44.

72. Fujii H, Nakai K, Yonekura Y, et al. The vitamin D receptor activator maxacalcitol provides cardioprotective effects in diabetes mellitus. Cardiovasc Drugs Ther 2015;29(6):499–507.

73. Mizobuchi M, Ogata H, Yamazaki-Nakazawa A, et al. Cardiac effect of vitamin D receptor modulators in uremic rats. J Steroid Biochem Mol Biol 2016;163:20–7.

74. Meems LM, Brouwers FP, Joosten MM, et al. Plasma calcidiol, calcitriol, and parathyroid hormone and risk of new onset heart failure in a population-based cohort study. ESC Heart Fail 2016;3(3):189–97.

75. Schleithoff SS, Zittermann A, Tenderich G, et al. Vitamin D supplementation improves cytokine profiles in patients with congestive heart failure: a double-blind, randomized, placebo-controlled trial. Am J Clin Nutr 2006;83(4):754–9.

76. Seki K, Sanada S, Kudinova AY, et al. Interleukin-33 prevents apoptosis and improves survival after experimental myocardial infarction through ST2 signaling. Circ Heart Fail 2009;2(6):684–91.

77. Yao HC, Li XY, Han QF, et al. Elevated serum soluble ST2 levels may predict the fatal outcomes in patients with chronic heart failure. Int J Cardiol 2015;186:303–4.

78. Schierbeck LL, Jensen TS, Bang U, et al. Parathyroid hormone and vitamin D–markers for cardiovascular and all cause mortality in heart failure. Eur J Heart Fail 2011;13(6):626–32.

79. Pfeffer PE, Chen YH, Woszczek G, et al. Vitamin D enhances production of soluble ST2, inhibiting the action of IL-33. J Allergy Clin Immunol 2015;135(3): 824–7.e3.

80. Gruson D, Ferracin B, Ahn SA, et al. Soluble ST2, the vitamin D/PTH axis and the heart: new interactions in the air? Int J Cardiol 2016;212:292–4.

81. Masson S, Barlera S, Colotta F, et al. A low plasma 1,25(OH)2 vitamin D/PTH (1-84) ratio predicts worsening of renal function in patients with chronic heart failure. Int J Cardiol 2016;224:220–5.

82. Belen E, Sungur A, Sungur MA. Vitamin D levels predict hospitalization and mortality in patients with heart failure. Scand Cardiovasc J 2016;50(1):17–22.

83. Gotsman I, Shauer A, Zwas DR, et al. Vitamin D deficiency is a predictor of reduced survival in patients with heart failure; vitamin D supplementation improves outcome. Eur J Heart Fail 2012;14(4):357–66.

84. Jiang WL, Gu HB, Zhang YF, et al. Vitamin D supplementation in the treatment of chronic heart failure: a meta-analysis of randomized controlled trials. Clin Cardiol 2016;39(1):56–61.

85. Robbins J, Petrone AB, Gaziano JM, et al. Dietary vitamin D and risk of heart failure in the physicians' health study. Clin Nutr 2016;35(3):650–3.

86. Hsia J, Heiss G, Ren H, et al. Calcium/vitamin D supplementation and cardiovascular events. Circulation 2007;115(7):846–54.

87. Abu El Maaty MA, Hassanein SI, Gad MZ. Genetic variation in vitamin D receptor gene (Fok1:rs2228570) is associated with risk of coronary artery disease. Biomarkers 2016;21(1):68–72.

88. Donneyong MM, Hornung CA, Taylor KC, et al. Risk of heart failure among postmenopausal women: a secondary analysis of the randomized trial of vitamin D plus calcium of the women's health initiative. Circ Heart Fail 2015;8(1):49–56.

89. Vaidya A, Sun B, Forman JP, et al. The Fok1 vitamin D receptor gene polymorphism is associated with plasma renin activity in Caucasians. Clin Endocrinol (Oxf) 2011;74(6):783–90.

90. Witte KK, Byrom R, Gierula J, et al. Effects of vitamin D on cardiac function in patients with chronic HF: the VINDICATE study. J Am Coll Cardiol 2016; 67(22):2593–603.

91. Schroten NF, Ruifrok WP, Kleijn L, et al. Short-term vitamin D3 supplementation lowers plasma renin activity in patients with stable chronic heart failure: an open-label, blinded end point, randomized prospective trial (VitD-CHF trial). Am Heart J 2013;166(2):357–64.e2.

92. Belen E, Aykan AC, Kalaycioglu E, et al. Low-level vitamin D is associated with atrial fibrillation in patients with chronic heart failure. Adv Clin Exp Med 2016; 25(1):51–7.

93. Canpolat U, Aytemir K, Hazirolan T, et al. Relationship between vitamin D level and left atrial fibrosis in patients with lone paroxysmal atrial fibrillation undergoing cryoballoon-based catheter ablation. J Cardiol 2017;69(1):16–23.

94. Emren SV, Aldemir M, Ada F. Does deficiency of vitamin d increase new onset atrial fibrillation after coronary artery bypass grafting surgery? Heart Surg Forum 2016;19(4):E180–4.

95. Li YC, Qiao G, Uskokovic M, et al. Vitamin D: a negative endocrine regulator of the renin-angiotensin system and blood pressure. J Steroid Biochem Mol Biol 2004;89-90(1–5):387–92.

96. Cerit L, Kemal H, Gulsen K, et al. Relationship between vitamin D and the development of atrial fibrillation after on-pump coronary artery bypass graft surgery. Cardiovasc J Afr 2016;27:1–4.

97. Alonso A, Misialek JR, Michos ED, et al. Serum 25-hydroxyvitamin D and the incidence of atrial fibrillation: the atherosclerosis risk in communities (ARIC) study. Europace 2016;18(8):1143–9.

98. Pelham CJ, Drews EM, Agrawal DK. Vitamin D controls resistance artery function through regulation of perivascular adipose tissue hypoxia and inflammation. J Mol Cell Cardiol 2016;98:1–10.

99. Lin LM, Peng F, Liu YP, et al. Coadministration of VDR and RXR agonists synergistically alleviates atherosclerosis through inhibition of oxidative stress: an in vivo and in vitro study. Atherosclerosis 2016;251:273–81.

100. Dziedzic EA, Przychodzen S, Dabrowski M. The effects of vitamin D on severity of coronary artery atherosclerosis and lipid profile of cardiac patients. Arch Med Sci 2016;12(6):1199–206.

101. Michos ED, Selvin E, Misialek JR, et al. 25-hydroxyvitamin D levels and markers of subclinical myocardial damage and wall stress: the atherosclerosis risk in communities study. J Am Heart Assoc 2016;5(11) [pii:e003575].

102. Stakisaitis D, Lesauskaite V, Girdauskaite M, et al. Investigation of vitamin D-binding protein polymorphism impact on coronary artery disease and relationship with longevity: own data and a review. Int J Endocrinol 2016;2016: 8347379.

103. Ng YM, Lim SK, Kang PS, et al. Association between serum 25-hydroxyvitamin D levels and carotid atherosclerosis in chronic kidney disease patients. BMC Nephrol 2016;17(1):151.

104. Rai V, Rao VH, Shao Z, et al. Dendritic cells expressing triggering receptor expressed on myeloid cells-1 correlate with plaque stability in symptomatic and asymptomatic patients with carotid stenosis. PLoS One 2016;11(5):e0154802.

105. Rao VH, Rai V, Stoupa S, et al. Tumor necrosis factor-alpha regulates triggering receptor expressed on myeloid cells-1-dependent matrix metalloproteinases in the carotid plaques of symptomatic patients with carotid stenosis. Atherosclerosis 2016;248:160–9.

106. Carbone F, Satta N, Burger F, et al. Vitamin D receptor is expressed within human carotid plaques and correlates with pro-inflammatory M1 macrophages. Vascul Pharmacol 2016;85:57–65.

107. Yin K, You Y, Swier V, et al. Vitamin D protects against atherosclerosis via regulation of cholesterol efflux and macrophage polarization in hypercholesterolemic swine. Arterioscler Thromb Vasc Biol 2015;35(11):2432–42.

108. Haas MJ, Jafri M, Wehmeier KR, et al. Inhibition of endoplasmic reticulum stress and oxidative stress by vitamin D in endothelial cells. Free Radic Biol Med 2016; 99:1–10.

109. Xiang W, Hu ZL, He XJ, et al. Intravenous transfusion of endothelial progenitor cells that overexpress vitamin D receptor inhibits atherosclerosis in ApoE-deficient mice. Biomed Pharmacother 2016;84:1233–42.

110. Lee S, Ahuja V, Masaki K, et al. A significant positive association of vitamin D deficiency with coronary artery calcification among middle-aged men: for the ERA JUMP study. J Am Coll Nutr 2016;35(7):614–20.

111. Dogan Y, Sarli B, Baktir AO, et al. 25-Hydroxy-vitamin D level may predict presence of coronary collaterals in patients with chronic coronary total occlusion. Postepy Kardiol Interwencyjnej 2015;11(3):191–6.

112. Martinez-Moreno JM, Herencia C, Montes de Oca A, et al. Vitamin D modulates tissue factor and protease-activated receptor 2 expression in vascular smooth muscle cells. FASEB J 2016;30(3):1367–76.
113. Sagarad SV, Sukhani N, Machanur B, et al. Effect of vitamin D on anginal episodes in vitamin D deficient patients with chronic stable angina on medical management. J Clin Diagn Res 2016;10(8):OC24–6.
114. Wong YY, Flicker L, Yeap BB, et al. Is hypovitaminosis D associated with abdominal aortic aneurysm, and is there a dose-response relationship? Eur J Vasc Endovasc Surg 2013;45(6):657–64.
115. Martorell S, Hueso L, Gonzalez-Navarro H, et al. Vitamin D receptor activation reduces angiotensin-II-induced dissecting abdominal aortic aneurysm in apolipoprotein E-knockout mice. Arterioscler Thromb Vasc Biol 2016;36(8):1587–97.
116. Nieuwland AJ, Kokje VB, Koning OH, et al. Activation of the vitamin D receptor selectively interferes with calcineurin-mediated inflammation: a clinical evaluation in the abdominal aortic aneurysm. Lab Invest 2016;96(7):784–90.
117. Chen S, Sun Y, Agrawal DK. Vitamin D deficiency and essential hypertension. J Am Soc Hypertens 2015;9(11):885–901.
118. Yilmaz S, Sen F, Ozeke O, et al. The relationship between vitamin D levels and nondipper hypertension. Blood Press Monit 2015;20(6):330–4.
119. Zagami RM, Di Pino A, Urbano F, et al. Low circulating vitamin D levels are associated with increased arterial stiffness in prediabetic subjects identified according to HbA1c. Atherosclerosis 2015;243(2):395–401.
120. Kang JY, Kim MK, Jung S, et al. The cross-sectional relationships of dietary and serum vitamin D with cardiometabolic risk factors: metabolic components, subclinical atherosclerosis, and arterial stiffness. Nutrition 2016;32(10):1048–56.e1.
121. Kassi E, Adamopoulos C, Basdra EK, et al. Role of vitamin D in atherosclerosis. Circulation 2013;128(23):2517–31.
122. Belkaid Y, Hand TW. Role of the microbiota in immunity and inflammation. Cell 2014;157(1):121–41.
123. Wu HJ, Wu E. The role of gut microbiota in immune homeostasis and autoimmunity. Gut Microbes 2012;3(1):4–14.
124. Gominak SC. Vitamin D deficiency changes the intestinal microbiome reducing B vitamin production in the gut. The resulting lack of pantothenic acid adversely affects the immune system, producing a "pro-inflammatory" state associated with atherosclerosis and autoimmunity. Med Hypotheses 2016;94:103–7.
125. Henry HL. Regulation of vitamin D metabolism. Best Pract Res Clin Endocrinol Metab 2011;25(4):531–41.
126. Ding HY, Ma HX. Significant roles of anti-aging protein Klotho and fibroblast growth factor23 in cardiovascular disease. J Geriatr Cardiol 2015;12(4):439–47.
127. Moe SM, Chertow GM, Parfrey PS, et al. Cinacalcet, fibroblast growth factor-23, and cardiovascular disease in hemodialysis: the evaluation of cinacalcet HCl therapy to lower cardiovascular events (EVOLVE) trial. Circulation 2015;132(1):27–39.
128. Andrukhova O, Slavic S, Odörfer KI, et al. Experimental myocardial infarction upregulates circulating fibroblast growth factor-23. J Bone Miner Res 2015;30(10):1831–9.
129. Mathew JS, Sachs MC, Katz R, et al. Fibroblast growth factor-23 and incident atrial fibrillation: the multi-ethnic study of atherosclerosis (MESA) and the cardiovascular health study (CHS). Circulation 2014;130(4):298–307.
130. Xie J, Wu YL, Huang CL. Deficiency of soluble alpha-Klotho as an independent cause of uremic cardiomyopathy. Vitam Horm 2016;101:311–30.

131. Bansal N, Zelnick L, Robinson-Cohen C, et al. Serum parathyroid hormone and 25-hydroxyvitamin D concentrations and risk of incident heart failure: the multiethnic study of atherosclerosis. J Am Heart Assoc 2014;3(6):e001278.
132. Kopecky SL, Bauer DC, Gulati M, et al. Lack of evidence linking calcium with or without vitamin D supplementation to cardiovascular disease in generally healthy adults: a clinical guideline from the national osteoporosis foundation and the American Society for Preventive Cardiology. Ann Intern Med 2016; 165(12):867–8.
133. Levy BI. Can angiotensin II type 2 receptors have deleterious effects in cardiovascular disease? Implications for therapeutic blockade of the renin-angiotensin system. Circulation 2004;109(1):8–13.
134. Singh KD, Karnik SS. Angiotensin receptors: structure, function, signaling and clinical applications. J Cell Signal 2016;1(2) [pii:111].
135. Chow BS, Koulis C, Krishnaswamy P, et al. The angiotensin II type 2 receptor agonist Compound 21 is protective in experimental diabetes-associated atherosclerosis. Diabetologia 2016;59(8):1778–90.
136. Yoshida T, Delafontaine P. An intronic enhancer element regulates angiotensin II type 2 receptor expression during satellite cell differentiation, and its activity is suppressed in congestive heart failure. J Biol Chem 2016;291(49):25578–90.
137. Michos ED, Lutsey PL. 25-hydroxyvitamin D levels and coronary heart disease risk reclassification in hypertension–is it worth the "hype"? Atherosclerosis 2016; 245:237–9.
138. Rai V, Agrawal DK. Role of risk stratification and genetics in sudden cardiac death. Can J Physiol Pharmacol 2017;95(3):225–38.
139. Timms PM, Mannan N, Hitman GA, et al. Circulating MMP9, vitamin D and variation in the TIMP-1 response with VDR genotype: mechanisms for inflammatory damage in chronic disorders? QJM 2002;95(12):787–96.
140. Van den Berghe G, Van Roosbroeck D, Vanhove P, et al. Bone turnover in prolonged critical illness: effect of vitamin D. J Clin Endocrinol Metab 2003;88(10): 4623–32.
141. Teng M, Wolf M, Ofsthun MN, et al. Activated injectable vitamin D and hemodialysis survival: a historical cohort study. J Am Soc Nephrol 2005;16(4):1115–25.

Regulation of Immune Function by Vitamin D and Its Use in Diseases of Immunity

An-Sofie Vanherwegen, MSc, Conny Gysemans, PhD*,
Chantal Mathieu, MD, PhD

KEYWORDS

- Vitamin D_3 • Macrophage • Dendritic cells • Neutrophils • B cell T cells
- Autoimmunity • Infections

KEY POINTS

- Vitamin D deficiency, owing to low dietary intake or low sunlight exposure, is an environmental risk factor for autoimmune and infectious diseases.
- The bioactive form of vitamin D has a wide variety of immunomodulatory effects in innate and adaptive immune cells.
- Vitamin D enhances the antimicrobial activity in macrophages relevant for defense against infectious diseases.
- The role of vitamin D supplementation in a situation of vitamin D sufficiency remains unclear.
- Beneficial effects on disease risk and severity in animal studies and some human trials has been shown.

INTRODUCTION

The immune system, innate and adaptive, is a highly evolved and complex network, essential for promoting survival in an environment full of potential pathogens, while maintaining self-tolerance. It is now well-established that vitamin D_3 plays a prominent role in immune health on top of its classical effects on calcium and bone homeostasis. The VDR is expressed in all immune cells, and several of these cells are also capable of synthesizing and/or responding to the bioactive metabolite, allowing for autocrine and paracrine actions of vitamin D.[1] It is not surprising that vitamin D insufficiency and deficiency seem to increase susceptibility to bacterial and viral infections and, in genetically susceptible individuals, to autoimmunity. Vitamin D insufficiency and deficiency

Disclosure Statement: The authors have nothing to disclose.
Laboratory of Clinical and Experimental Endocrinology (CEE), KU Leuven, O&N1 Herestraat 49 - bus 902, Leuven 3000, Belgium
* Corresponding author.
E-mail address: conny.gysemans@kuleuven.be

are increasing globally and can be attributed to changes in diet and behavior.[2] Despite improved sanitation and lifestyle, epidemiologic studies also point to a strong increase in the prevalence of autoimmune diseases like type 1 diabetes (T1D), multiple sclerosis (MS), rheumatoid arthritis (RA), systemic lupus erythematosus (SLE), and inflammatory bowel disease (IBD) worldwide over the past decades.[3] Each of these conditions has a strong genetic predisposition, and environmental factors like diet and viruses are proposed triggers. Current treatments are insufficient and mainly comprise general immunosuppression. This review summarizes and critically evaluates genetic, epidemiologic, preclinical, and interventional studies to unravel the role and mode of action of vitamin D and the bioactive metabolite $1,25(OH)_2D$ in disorders of the immune system, such as infections, inflammation, and autoimmune diseases.

METABOLISM AND MODE OF ACTION OF $1,25(OH)_2D_3$ IN A NUTSHELL

Vitamin D, or cholecalciferol, is a secosteroidal prohormone that can be obtained from diet (eg, fatty fish, cod liver oil, egg yolk, and fortified dairy products); however, its main source is endogenous production in the skin through ultraviolet B (UV-B)–mediated photosynthesis. The form produced in animals and humans is vitamin D_3, whereas fungi and some plants produce vitamin D_2. In the present work, the focus is on vitamin D_3.

Vitamin D requires 2 sequential hydroxylation steps to become the bioactive metabolite 1,25-dihydroxyvitamin D_3 ($1,25(OH)_2D_3$, also called calcitriol). In the liver, vitamin D is hydroxylated by 25-hydroxylases (eg, CYP2R1, CYP2D11, CYP2D25, and CYP3A4) resulting in the formation of 25-hydroxyvitamin D_3 ($25(OH)D_3$). $25(OH)D_3$ is the major circulating form of vitamin D and is therefore used to determine the vitamin D status. Interestingly, whereas serum concentrations of vitamin D required to achieve calcium homeostasis and bone health are around 20 ng/mL (50 nmol/L),[4] serum concentrations of vitamin D to reach most of the immunomodulatory benefits will probably be much higher (40–80 ng/mL or 100–200 nmol/L). Data in diabetes-prone nonobese diabetic mice even suggest that $25(OH)D$ concentrations of more than 90 ng/mL (225 nmol/L) would be required to modulate immune dysregulation, but these doses will most likely induce calcemic side effects when administered long-term. Vitamin D deficiency (<20 ng/mL or 50 nmol/L) can lead to clinical diseases, the most prominent being the typical bow-legged musculoskeletal condition known as rickets.[5] More recent publications also describe associations with other disorders like cardiovascular disease, cancer, autoimmune manifestations, and impaired antimicrobial protection.[6]

The vitamin D binding protein transports $25(OH)D_3$ to the kidneys, where it undergoes a second hydroxylation step mediated by the 1α-hydroxylase enzyme CYP27B1 to form the bioactive form $1,25(OH)_2D_3$, a crucial step for bone health.[7] Interestingly, these vitamin D metabolizing enzymes are also found in other tissues including placenta, skin, and immune cells.[8] Importantly, the control enzyme for the breakdown of vitamin D, 24-hydroxylase (CYP24A1), is also expressed by different immune cells, allowing these cells to balance the concentration of $1,25(OH)_2D_3$ in the direct microenvironment (autocrine effects) as well as to influence $1,25(OH)_2D_3$ actions on adjacent cells (paracrine effects). Systemic levels of $1,25(OH)_2D_3$ are mainly determined by renal CYP27B1 activity. Parathyroid hormone and the phosphaturic hormone fibroblast growth factor 23 regulate the delicate balance between CYP27B1 and CYP24A1 and thereby control systemic levels of $1,25(OH)_2D_3$.

Through binding to the VDR, $1,25(OH)_2D_3$ exerts its genomic actions. The VDR is a ligand-regulated transcription factor and member of the nuclear receptor superfamily, which is widely expressed in almost all body tissues and cell types, including immune cells.[1,9] Upon ligand binding, the VDR will form a heterodimer with the retinoid X receptor. This VDR–retinoid X receptor complex can bind specific DNA sequences, also referred to as vitamin D responsive elements (VDREs), in the promotor region of vitamin D–regulated genes to recruit coregulatory proteins to activate or repress gene transcription.[10,11] Currently, more than 250 coregulatory proteins (ie, coactivators [gene activation] or corepressors [gene repression]) have been identified, but their precise functions and interactions with DNA-bound VDR are only partially understood.[12] In addition, $1,25(OH)_2D_3$ can exert rapid, nongenomic actions that occur within seconds to minutes after addition of the hormone mediated by a membrane-bound form of the VDR.[13,14]

VITAMIN D AS A MODULATOR OF THE IMMUNE SYSTEM

The widespread expression of the nuclear receptor VDR and vitamin D–metabolizing enzymes in practically all cells of the innate and adaptive immune system, such as macrophages, dendritic cells (DCs) and activated B and T cells, indicate an important immunomodulatory role for $1,25(OH)_2D_3$.[9,15,16] Through local production of $1,25(OH)_2D_3$, these cells are able to obtain supraphysiologic doses of the bioactive metabolite, which are necessary for subsequent immune modulation. Herein, we discuss the modulating effects of $1,25(OH)_2D_3$ on different cellular subsets of the innate and adaptive immune systems.

Neutrophils

Neutrophils are the most abundant white blood cell in humans and contribute to the first line of defense against microbial pathogens. Neutrophils can clear microbes through phagocytosis, generation of reactive oxygen species, and the production of biologically active antimicrobial molecules from granules. In addition, they release structures called neutrophil extracellular traps (NETs) through a process called NETosis, and these can capture and kill microbes. Although the original observation of NET formation placed this process within the setting of innate immune responses to infectious agents, current evidence suggests that this phenomenon is also implicated in autoantigen modification and triggering of the autoimmune system, with induction of tissue destruction.[17] The effects of vitamin D and its bioactive metabolite on neutrophils are poorly understood. Neutrophils express functional VDRs,[18] but unlike monocytes/macrophages they do not seem to express CYP27B1 and are consequently not subject to autocrine activation of innate immune responses by $1,25(OH)_2D_3$. Nevertheless, exogenously administered $1,25(OH)_2D_3$ has been shown to reduce the production of inflammatory mediators and formation of reactive oxygen species in neutrophils through the induction of the 5-lipoxygenase gene and suppression of the cyclooxygenase-2 gene. This study also demonstrated that $1,25(OH)_2D_3$ can downregulate neutrophil function and decrease neutrophil activity, but data are scarce on the particular role of $1,25(OH)_2D_3$ in NETosis.[19] Some investigators have shown that $1,25(OH)_2D_3$ can inhibit NETosis activity, which could have implications on the battle against infections but also in the development of autoimmune diseases and tissue damage.[20] Another study reported that $1,25(OH)_2D_3$ can affect the activation of the mitogen-activated protein kinase phospho-p38 and lead to decreased neutrophil apoptosis.[21]

Macrophages

Macrophages are highly phagocytic antigen-presenting cells (APCs), which add to the first line of innate defense against pathogens.[22] During microbial infections, macrophages will be activated by pathogen-associated molecular patterns such as lipopolysaccharide to become inflammatory M1 macrophages, which are characterized by the secretion of proinflammatory cytokines and induction of antimicrobial activities. M2 macrophages are activated by the cytokines interleukin (IL)-4 and IL-13 to promote wound repair, tissue homeostasis, and immunomodulatory activities. Interestingly, 1,25(OH)$_2$D$_3$ has different roles in macrophage differentiation and activation. Exposure to 1,25(OH)$_2$D$_3$ can enhance the differentiation of macrophages from monocytes.[23] Inflammatory immune signals (eg, T-cell–derived interferon [IFN]-γ or Toll-like receptor [TLR; eg, TLR1/2, TLR4, and TLR coreceptor CD14) triggering can stimulate the expression of CYP27B1, allowing the macrophage to locally produce the bioactive metabolite 1,25(OH)$_2$D$_3$.[24–27] Interestingly, CYP27B1 activity is not regulated by parathyroid hormone or fibroblast growth factor 23 in macrophages, unlike in renal tubules, and these cells synthesize an alternative splice variant of CYP24A1, leading to the generation of a dominant negative-acting protein that is catalytically dysfunctional.[28] This lack of feedback machinery may allow for the local production of high concentrations of 1,25(OH)$_2$D$_3$ necessary for immune modulation. Then again, IL-15, which is produced after TLR activation of human monocytes, upregulates CYP27B1 and the VDR, allowing for the bioconversion of 25(OH)D$_3$ to 1,25(OH)$_2$D$_3$.[29] Obtained via this pathway, 1,25(OH)$_2$D$_3$ can induce autophagy, phagosomal maturation, and the production of antimicrobial peptides such as cathelicidins (eg, hCAP18/LL-37/FALL39 in humans and CRAMP/CNLP/MCLP in mice)[30] and defensins (eg, DEFB-4 and -7).[31] The hCAP18 is the sole cathelicidin in humans and encodes the cathelicidin antimicrobial peptide cyclic AMP (CAMP) necessary for the intracellular killing of bacteria like *Mycobacterium tuberculosis*. Whereas in activated macrophages cathelicidin gene transcription is directly regulated by 1,25(OH)$_2$D$_3$, DEFB4 gene transcription also requires the convergence of the 1,25(OH)$_2$D$_3$ and IL-1β pathways.[32,33] In addition, 1,25(OH)$_2$D$_3$ can regulate TLR signaling by stimulating suppressor of cytokine signaling 1 through inhibition of miR-155 in macrophages, which provides a new negative feedback mode of action for vitamin D to control innate immunity.[34]

In addition, 1,25(OH)$_2$D$_3$ can reduce the surface expression of costimulatory molecules such as CD80 and CD86 as well as the production of the proinflammatory cytokine IL-12, hereby reducing the T-cell stimulatory capacity of the macrophage.[23] In addition, 1,25(OH)$_2$D$_3$ is acknowledged as a natural endoplasmic reticulum stress reliever[35] and can inhibit essential effector functions of IFN-γ–activated macrophages.[36] Furthermore, 1,25(OH)$_2$D$_3$ can reduce the production of proinflammatory mediators from M1 macrophages, including the proinflammatory cytokines (eg, IL-1β, IL-6, IL-12p40 and tumor necrosis factor [TNF]-α) and chemokines (eg, CXCL9, CXCL10, CXCL11, and CCL2) in an IL-10–dependent manner.[24,37,38] Also, 1,25(OH)$_2$D$_3$ can enhance phagocytosis and CCL22 production, a chemokine able to promote immune tolerance. However, neither 1,25(OH)$_2$D$_3$ administration nor VDR ablation can fully modulate macrophage polarization to the antiinflammatory M2 phenotype.[39]

Dendritic Cells

DCs are APCs that permanently survey the peripheral microenvironment and are specialized in antigen uptake and processing. Upon exposure to inflammatory signals, DCs mature, migrate to the lymph nodes, and present the captured antigens to T cells, thereby priming an antigen-specific adaptive immune response. Moreover, DCs are crucial regulators of the delicate balance between immunogenicity and immune tolerance.[40] In the DC, 1,25(OH)$_2$D$_3$ is able to interfere with the differentiation and maturation process,[41,42] resulting in an altered morphology, phenotype, and function corresponding with a semimature or tolerogenic state. Exposure to 1,25(OH)$_2$D$_3$

allows the DC to become adherent and form large spindle-shaped dendrites.[43] The tolerogenic phenotype is characterized by a reduced surface expression of antigen-presenting molecules (eg, MHC-II, CD1a) and costimulatory molecules (eg, CD40 CD80, CD86). In addition, the secretion of proinflammatory cytokines (eg, IL-12, IL-23) is strongly diminished, whereas IL-10 and TNF-α production are enhanced in the 1,25(OH)$_2$D$_3$–modulated tolerogenic DCs (tDCs).[41,43–46] Moreover, the surface expression of several T-cell inhibitory molecules, such as immunoglobin-like transcript and programmed death-1 ligand, are upregulated by 1,25(OH)$_2$D$_3$.[47,48] In this way, the tDC is able to influence T-cell behavior through induction of hyporesponsiveness and allows a shift in the T-cell polarization from T helper (Th)1- and Th17-mediated inflammatory responses (eg, IFN-γ and IL-17) toward more tolerogenic responses with Th2 (eg, IL-4) and regulatory T cells (Tregs; eg, IL-10 and tumor growth factor-β).[41,43,45,48,49]

The presence of programmed death-1 ligand on the tDC is crucial to establish the phenotype of Tregs as well as their IL-10 production.[47,48] Interestingly, the establishment of the tolerogenic profile induced by 1,25(OH)$_2$D$_3$ is accompanied by an early and transcriptionally mediated metabolic reprogramming. Treatment with the active metabolite strongly impacts the expression profile of genes implicated in several metabolic pathways like glycolysis, tricarboxylic acid cycle and oxidative phosphorylation.[50] These observations are in line with a proteomics study in which 1,25(OH)$_2$D$_3$ or its structural, but less calcemic analogue TX527, were found to induce major alterations in proteins involved in cytoskeletal organization, protein biosynthesis and proteolysis, and metabolic pathways.[45,51] Although both aerobic glycolysis and oxidative phosphorylation metabolism are enhanced simultaneously by 1,25(OH)$_2$D$_3$, only glucose availability and glycolysis seem to be essential to establish and maintain the tolerogenic phenotype and function of the 1,25(OH)$_2$D$_3$–modulated tDC.[50] Importantly, these phenotypic and functional changes of the tDC induced by 1,25(OH)$_2$D$_3$ treatment are stable after removal of the compound.[48,52]

B Cells

B cells express clonally different plasma membrane immunoglobulin (Ig) receptors recognizing specific antigenic epitopes. They are particularly known for their production of autoantibodies, the formation of B-cell follicles with germinal center activity, antigen presentation, and production of proinflammatory cytokines, but also for their immunomodulatory activities (Bregs). B cells can upregulate the expression of the VDR and vitamin D–metabolizing enzyme CYP27B1 upon activation, indicating a direct effect of 1,25(OH)$_2$D$_3$ on the B cell. Interestingly, VDR expression increases further in the presence of 1,25(OH)$_2$D$_3$.[53] In contrast with the kidney, where 1,25(OH)$_2$D$_3$ itself provides negative feedback regulation of CYP27B1,[1] 1,25(OH)$_2$D$_3$ does not directly inhibit CYP27B1 gene expression levels in the B cell.[53] In contrast, CYP24A1 is only expressed in the presence of 1,25(OH)$_2$D$_3$, implying that B cells can perfectly adapt their local concentrations of 1,25(OH)$_2$D$_3$.[54] In addition, 1,25(OH)$_2$D$_3$ is able to induce apoptosis, inhibits memory B-cell formation, and prevents the differentiation of B cells into Ig-producing plasma cells.[55,56] This is reflected in a decreased production of IgG and IgM after 1,25(OH)$_2$D$_3$ exposure in vitro. Although these inhibitory effects of 1,25(OH)$_2$D$_3$ on Ig production have not been confirmed in vivo, 1,25(OH)2D3 has been shown to influence antigen-specific antibody production.[57]

Literature on the effect of 1,25(OH)$_2$D$_3$ on APC capacity of B cells is limited. Upon CD40 activation, B cells express costimulatory molecules like CD80 and CD86 and consequently provide naive T-cell activation. The $1,25(OH)_2D_3$-primed B cells display a diminished costimulatory activation (CD40 L) profile, which results in reduced expansion and proinflammatory cytokine production of autologous T cells.[58]

Interestingly, $1,25(OH)_2D_3$ can also induce the production of IL-10 by naïve B cells and increase the expression of CCR10 on terminally differentiated human B cells.[53,54,59] Although IL-10 is primarily produced by naive B cells, it may be that $1,25(OH)_2D_3$ also dictates the formation of Bregs that are known to help in the tolerization of autoreactive T cells.

T Cells

As described, $1,25(OH)_2D_3$ is able to modulate T-cell behavior in an indirect manner through effects on APC phenotype and function. However, the presence of the VDR in activated T cells also indicates that the T cell is a direct target of $1,25(OH)_2D_3$.

CD4+ T cells

During T-cell receptor (TCR) activation in a distinct cytokine milieu, naive CD4+ T cells differentiate into one of several lineages of Th cells, including Th1, Th2, Th9, Th17, and inducible Tregs, and will acquire particular functions to combat specific pathogens, and can also adapt their functions in response to changing milieu.

Upon exposure to several activation stimuli, gene expression of both the VDR and vitamin D–metabolizing enzymes is upregulated in human CD4+ T cells.[9,60] Initial TCR signaling via mitogen-activated protein kinase p38 leads to successive induction of the VDR and phospholipase C-γ1, which are required for subsequent classical TCR signaling and T-cell activation.[61] Phospholipase C-γ1 induction seemed to be VDR dependent. Thus, $1,25(OH)_2D_3$ is able to decrease the production of multiple inflammatory cytokines IFN-γ, IL-9, and IL-17 by CD4+ Th1, Th9, and Th17 cells, respectively, thereby modifying the T-cell phenotype and function.[62–67] In Th1 cells, $1,25(OH)_2D_3$ suppresses the gene transcription of IFN-γ through VDR–retinoid X receptor binding to a silencer sequence in its promoter region.[63,68] Ultimately, $1,25(OH)_2D_3$ prevents Th17 differentiation through inhibition of the transcription factor retinoic acid–related orphan receptor C as well as IL-17 cytokine production by blocking nuclear factor of activated T cells, a transcription factor that binds to the IL-17 promoter.[62,69] The direct effects of $1,25(OH)_2D_3$ on Th2 cytokines are contradictory. Some report an induction of GATA-binding protein 3 (GATA3) and c-maf, Th2-specific transcription factors, and production of the Th2 cytokines IL-4 and IL-5. Other investigators did not observe effects on cytokine production.[63,67,70,71] By reversing the inhibitory effects of the Th17 polarizing cytokines on T lymphocyte-associated protein (CTLA)-4, $1,25(OH)_2D_3$ may induce CTLA-4 upregulation.[72] In Th9 polarized memory T cells, $1,25(OH)_2D_3$ is able to inhibit the production of the IL-8 and IL-9 cytokines, whereas IL-5 production was unaffected. In addition, $1,25(OH)_2D_3$ slightly downregulated the Th9-associated transcription factors PU.1 and IRF-4.[73]

To date, the antiproliferative effects of $1,25(OH)_2D_3$ on T cells are still under debate.[63,66,74] Yet, $1,25(OH)_2D_3$ can stimulate the formation of IL-10–producing Tregs in the absence of an APC.[66,74,75] Moreover, $1,25(OH)_2D_3$ and its structural analogue TX527 are able to induce a stable CD4+CD25^highCD127^low Treg phenotype with IL-10 production and functional suppressive capacity.[74,76] Moreover, $1,25(OH)_2D_3$ (and TX527) can upregulate the T-cell expression of the skin-homing receptor CCR10 as well as the inflammation-associated homing receptors CCR5, CXCR3, and CXCR6. In contrast, it downregulates the expression of the lymph node-homing molecules (CD62 L, CCR7, and CXCR4) on T cells. In this way $1,25(OH)_2D_3$ can modulate cellular tropism for specific tissues.[74] Also, other incestigators found that $1,25(OH)_2D_3$ can upregulate the gut-homing receptor CCR9 and inhibit CXCR3 on T cells, potentially changing the homing properties of the Th cells.[77]

The $1,25(OH)_2D_3$-modulated Tregs also express higher levels of CTLA-4, programmed cell-death protein-1, and CD25, and display enhanced suppressive capacity.[78] Because there are several VDREs in the conserved noncoding sequence of the Foxp3 promoter, $1,25(OH)_2D_3$ may directly control Foxp3 gene transcription.[79] Interestingly, Foxp3 seems to be increased at high concentrations of $1,25(OH)_2D_3$, whereas IL-10 is induced at more moderate levels, with little coexpression of these molecules.[78]

CD8+ T cells

Upon activation, CD8+ T cells will rapidly proliferate and kill infected cells through induction of apoptosis. In addition, these cytotoxic T cells will secrete cytokines such as perforin, granzyme B, IFN-γ, and TNF-α.[80] The highest expression levels of the VDR were found in CD8+ cytotoxic T cells, suggesting that $1,25(OH)_2D_3$ is able to exert direct actions in these cells.[15] Transfer of VDR knockout CD8+ T cells into RAG knockout recipients induced colitis, indicating that inability to signal through the VDR results in the generation of pathogenic CD8+ T cells. In addition, VDR-mediated signaling is required to sustain CD8+ T-cell quiescence, because increased proliferation was observed in VDR knockout cells.[81] In addition, $1,25(OH)_2D_3$ exposure significantly alters the cytokine profile of Epstein-Barr virus–specific CD8+ T cells with a decreased secretion of IFN-γ and TNF-α, although IL-5 and tumor growth factor-β production was increased.[82]

Moreover, one of the $1,25(OH)_2D_3$ analogues, calcipotriol, reduces the frequency of CD8+ IL-17+ T cells in psoriatic skin lesions.[83] The intraepithelial intestinal lymphocyte population contains large numbers of CD8αα+ T cells, which are shown to maintain tolerance in the gut. VDR knockout mice present lower numbers of CD8αα+ T cells. A reduction in maturation and proliferation of these cells results in a reduced fraction of functional cells, which might contribute to the excessive gastrointestinal inflammation in VDR knockout mice.[84]

VITAMIN D AND DISEASES OF IMMUNITY

Inflammation is a common factor in many chronic disorders, and concern has been raised about the impact of vitamin D deficiency on several inflammatory immune processes. There is a clear link between infections, inflammation, and autoimmunity. In addition to genetic factors, environmental triggers (more specifically viruses, bacteria, and other infectious pathogens) are thought to play a key role in the development and progression of autoimmune diseases. Genetic studies show an association between polymorphisms in vitamin D–related genes such as the VDR and vitamin D metabolism genes and certain diseases (**Fig. 1**). In addition, epidemiologic studies indicate a strong correlation between vitamin D deficiency and the increased incidence of autoimmune and chronic inflammatory diseases. These findings, together with the in vitro and in vivo immunomodulatory effects of $1,25(OH)_2D_3$, form the basis to suggest that using vitamin D supplementation might provide protection against these immune diseases.

So far, there is limited evidence for this proposal. A 2010 Institute of Medicine report clearly supports a key role for calcium and vitamin D in bone health, but outcomes related to cancer, cardiovascular disease, diabetes, and autoimmune disorders could not be linked reliably with calcium and vitamin D intake, and the evidence was inconsistent, inconclusive as to causality, and insufficient to inform on dietary

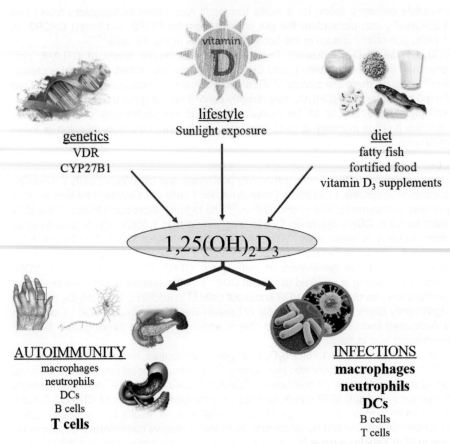

Fig. 1. Genetic polymorphisms in vitamin D-related genes, such as the vitamin D receptor (VDR) or 25-hydroxylase CYP27B1, lifestyle differences (eg, sunlight exposure, outdoor activities, sunscreen use) and diet can influence vitamin D levels and subsequent vitamin D actions. Bioactive vitamin D, 1,25(OH)$_2$D$_3$, exerts immunomodulatory effects on various, almost all, cells of the innate (macrophages, neutrophils, dendritic cells [DCs]) and adaptive (T and B cells) immune systems, hereby playing an important role in autoimmune and infectious diseases.

recommendations.[85] Moreover, higher vitamin D intake in large populations may also carry the possible risk of overdosing in specific patient groups. Because supraphysiologic doses are required to modulate the dysregulated immune responses, clinical application of vitamin D and its bioactive form 1,25(OH)$_2$D$_3$ is impeded by their hypercalcemic toxicity. Still, no toxic effects have been found in humans with doses of up to 50,000 IU vitamin D weekly for 12 weeks, or 100,000 IU weekly for 1 month followed by 100,000 IU monthly for 5 months.[57,86] Presently, there is no international consensus on the optimal level for vitamin D supplementation, especially on a safe upper level. Alternatively, structural analogues of 1,25(OH)$_2$D$_3$ with immunomodulatory properties and reduced calcemic effects or combination immunotherapies that also aim at restoring the dysregulated vitamin D metabolism may form a suitable alternative for clinical application. In this review, we mainly focused on the effects of vitamin D or its active metabolite on Th1-driven autoimmune diseases and chronic infections, but there are also associations between vitamin D levels and Th2-mediated disorders like asthma, allergic disorders, and atopic dermatitis (reviewed in[87]).

Vitamin D and Autoimmune Diseases

There are more than 100 different autoimmune syndromes, including T1D, MS, RA, and IBD. In these chronic immune disorders, the immune system reacts against harmless self-antigens. Strikingly, there has been a steep increase in the incidence of especially T1D and MS but also of other autoimmune diseases in the last half century.

Vitamin D and type 1 diabetes

T1D is a chronic autoimmune disease characterized by the selective destruction of the insulin-producing beta cells in the pancreatic islets, resulting in absolute insulin deficiency and subsequent hyperglycemia.[88] The exact pathogenic mechanisms underlying T1D are not fully understood, but it is thought to be a complex interplay between genetic susceptibility (eg, HLA-DR4 and DQ8 alleles) and environmental triggers like viral infections (eg, enteroviruses) and diet (eg, cow's milk). There is some evidence that Coxsackie virus B4 may cause T1D via molecular mimicry, although bystander activation may be a more likely explanation. Several genetic studies investigating the correlation between polymorphisms in the VDR gene (ie, *ApaI*, *BsmI*, *TaqI*, and *FokI*) and T1D incidence provide conflicting results. A metaanalysis performed by Zhang and colleagues[89] found an association between VDR polymorphisms and an increased risk for T1D in the Asian population, whereas 2 other, independent studies could not find any association between VDR and T1D risk in general or in any subpopulation.[90,91] Interestingly, the *FokI* restriction site is a functional polymorphism of the VDR gene, resulting in VDR proteins with different structures, a long f-VDR or a shorter F-VDR.[92] The *FokI* polymorphisms can also alter the amount of VDR produced, and the presence of the shorter F-VDR results in higher nuclear factor-κB– and nuclear factor of activated T cell–driven transcription in addition to higher IL-12p40 promoter-driven transcription, which could have implications on the immune system.[93] A study described that nonstimulated and 25(OH)D$_3$-stimulated Th cells isolated from T1D patients had lower VDR expression. Moreover, a significantly lower percentage of CD4$^+$ cells were observed in T1D patients carrying the "FF" genotype compared with those with the genotypes "Ff/ff."[94] Then again, genetic association with T1D has been found for the vitamin D-metabolizing genes CYP2R1, CYP27B1, and DHCR7.[95–97] These polymorphisms are thought to reduce the (local) bioconversion of 25(OH)D$_3$ into 1,25(OH)$_2$D$_3$. Intriguing observations allude to an epistatic interaction between VDR and HLA-DR alleles in T1D. This interaction is mediated by a VDRE present in the promoter region of HLA-DRB1*0301 allele, which may be unfavorable for the manifestation of T1D in the absence of 1,25(OH)$_2$D$_3$ in early childhood owing to poor expression of DRB1*0301 in the thymus, ensuing in autoimmunity.[98] Alleles without the putative VDRE were linked with disease resistance.

Epidemiologic studies show an inverse correlation between T1D prevalence and sunlight exposure, and more specifically UV-B radiation, with an evident north–south gradient and seasonal onset of disease.[98–101] Also, a higher prevalence of vitamin D deficiency can be found in patients with T1D.[102,103] Moreover, low serum 25(OH)D$_3$ levels were associated with an increased risk to develop T1D in some studies,[104,105] suggesting that in the case of prediabetic children with multiple autoantibodies, it may be sensible avoid vitamin D deficiency and consider recommending vitamin D supplementation at an early stage of T1D. To support this proposal, animal studies indicate that vitamin D deficiency in utero and during early life is a strong risk factor for T1D development in the offspring.[106] Still, these observations could only be partially confirmed in human studies.[107,108] In diabetes-prone nonobese diabetic mice, treatment with high doses of vitamin D, $1,25(OH)_2D_3$ or with less calcemic analogues could prevent insulitis and diabetes or delay disease onset.[109–112] In some clinical studies, vitamin D supplementation in pregnant women and young children significantly reduces the risk to develop T1D in the later life of the offspring.[113–116] However, clinical intervention trials in which $1,25(OH)_2D_3$ was administered in newly diagnosed patients with T1D were to date rather disappointing, because vitamin D (2,000 IU/d) or calcitriol (0.25 μg/2 days) supplementation was not able to preserve or improve beta cell function.[117,118]

T1D is a Th1-mediated autoimmune disease involving cytotoxic $CD8^+$ T cells and innate immune cells.[119] Either $1,25(OH)_2D_3$ or one of its analogues inhibits full differentiation and maturation of DCs, thereby impairing their proper T-cell stimulatory capacity.[45,46,49,51,120] In addition, DC modulation with the active form of vitamin D allows the DC to redirect and block the proliferation of a committed T cell clone from a T1D patient.[121] Further, $1,25(OH)_2D_3$ can also affect the T cell in a direct manner. Administration of $1,25(OH)_2D_3$, increases the number of $CD4^+$ $CD25^+$ $Foxp3^+$ Treg cells with functional suppressive function in both the nonobese diabetic mouse model as in human subjects supplemented with vitamin D.[112,122–125] This restoration of Tregs will likely suppress the autoreactive effector T cells, thereby arresting the beta cell destruction.[112] Moreover, bioactive vitamin D decreased Th1 infiltration into the pancreas and mediated a shift from Th1 toward Th2 phenotype in pancreas and pancreas-draining lymph nodes.[123,125] Interestingly, the VDR is also expressed in the beta cell itself, allowing $1,25(OH)_2D_3$ to exert direct effects in these cells as well. Here, $1,25(OH)_2D_3$ inhibits the expression of several proinflammatory cytokines and chemokines (eg, IL-1β, IL-15 and CXCL10), thereby reducing infiltration of monocytes, macrophages, and T cells into the islets. This results in a preserved beta cell function and enhanced insulin synthesis and secretion.[111,126]

Vitamin D and multiple sclerosis

MS is an autoimmune-mediated neurodegenerative disease of the central nervous system characterized by demyelination and axon injury in the spinal cord and the brain. Clinical symptoms are determined by the site of lesions and can include numbness, pain, muscle weakness, and cognitive problems. Although disease etiology is not well-known, a combination of individual genetic and environmental factors are believed to contribute to disease susceptibility.[127,128] Although the exact triggers for the development of MS are unknown, it is well-established that relapses or disease flares in patients diagnosed with relapsing–remitting MS are often associated with exogenous infections, particularly upper respiratory infections. In addition, there is a clear link that can be found between inflammation, infections, and autoimmune responses.

Genetic studies have reported conflicting results on the association of polymorphisms in vitamin D–associated genes with an increased risk for MS.[129–136] Interestingly, $1,25(OH)_2D_3$ was found to interact with gene transcription of the principal MS susceptibility gene HLA-DRB1*1501 through a functional VDRE in its promoter region.[137] Moreover, an important MS-associated genetic polymorphism is able to influence the gene expression of CYP27B1 and the VDR.[138] This strongly points toward vitamin D as an important environmental factor in MS etiology. Moreover, the geographic distribution of the prevalence of MS, with a low prevalence near the equator and increasing rates with higher altitudes,[139] together with the month of birth effect,[140] supports the importance of sunlight exposure as a source of vitamin D. Indeed, poor vitamin D status has been associated with increased risk for the development of MS and MS relapses, as well as an elevated rate of disability progression.[141–144] Similar to T1D, lower levels of vitamin D during the neonatal period (from birth to 1 month of age) are associated with an increased risk of MS later in life. The risk was greatest for people with the lowest vitamin D levels during that period.[145] In line with this, high childhood sunlight exposure is correlated with decreased risk of MS.[146] Supplementation with $1,25(OH)_2D_3$ in experimental autoimmune encephalitis (EAE), an animal model of MS, can prevent disease development[147–149] or ameliorate disease progression when administered at clinical onset.[150] In contrast, the beneficial effects of vitamin D supplementation on clinical disease in MS are not as clear. Administration of vitamin D or its analogues could induce several beneficial effects, including a reduction in lesions, reduced rate of relapses, a decreased disability progression, and an improved quality of life.[151–154] High-dose vitamin D supplementation with 10,400 IU/d exhibited pleiotropic immunomodulatory effects in MS, which included reduction of IL-17 production by CD4$^+$ T cells and decreased proportion of effector memory CD4$^+$ T cells with a concomitant increase in central memory CD4$^+$ T cells and naive CD4$^+$ T cells,[155] and this without inducing toxicity. However, other trials reported no differences in any of these parameters.[156,157]

The immunologic distortion underlying autoimmunity in MS and murine EAE comprises abnormalities in immune cell subsets of both innate and adaptive immunity. T-cell activation during relapses is mediated by accumulated APCs such as macrophages, CD11c$^+$ myeloid DCs, CD8$^+$ DCs, and plasmacytoid DCs in the central nervous system.[158] The CD4$^+$ T cell subsets Th1 and Th17 are the main drivers of the pathologies in EAE and MS. The number of Th17 cells increases strongly in patients with MS during relapse.[159] Moreover, the production of IL-17 damages the blood–brain barrier, reinforcing the entry of immune cells into the central nervous system.[160] Myelin-targeted CD8$^+$ cytotoxic T cells can directly injure neural cells via the production of cytotoxic mediators such as perforin and granzyme B. In addition, through the production of cytokines, these CD8$^+$ T cells enhance the ongoing inflammation.[161,162] Owing to its broad immunomodulatory capacity, $1,25(OH)_2D_3$ can intervene at several of these immune processes implicated in the pathology of MS and EAE. Through inhibition of chemokine production (eg, CCL2, CCL3, CXCL10), $1,25(OH)_2D_3$ is able to modulate leukocyte migration into the central nervous system, thereby decreasing the accumulation of monocytes and macrophages.[163,164] Studies in knockout mice showed that suppression of EAE by $1,25(OH)_2D_3$ requires the presence of the VDR in T cells[165] and depends on the IL-10 signaling pathway.[166] These observations indicate that $1,25(OH)_2D_3$ is able to suppress EAE through direct effects on T cells and more specifically through the induction of Treg cells and the suppression of Th1 and Th17 cell differentiation and function.[167] Indeed, higher serum levels of $25(OH)D_3$ are correlated with improved Treg function in patients with MS.[168] Moreover, $1,25(OH)_2D_3$ prevents the migration of CD4$^+$ Th cells into the central nervous system.[169] CD8$^+$ cytotoxic T cells were dispensable for EAE prevention by $1,25(OH)_2D_3$.[170]

A significant role for B cells in the pathology of MS became evident because B-cell–depleting therapies reduce the number of relapses.[171] In the B cell, $1,25(OH)_2D_3$ is able to induce the expression of IL-10 through direct binding of the VDR to the IL-10 promoter region.[54] However, no correlation between vitamin D_3 status and IL-10–producing B cells was found in patients with MS and healthy controls.[172] Interestingly, the VDR is highly expressed in MS plaques with not only expression in microglia and macrophages, but also in neurons, astrocytes, and oligodendrocyte progenitor cells.[173] As such, vitamin D deficiency in patients with MS may be a contributor to remyelination failure. Previous studies have already indicated a role for vitamin D in myelination and remyelination.[174,175]

Vitamin D and rheumatoid arthritis

RA is a chronic immune-mediated disease characterized by inflammation of the synovial joints and destruction of bone and cartilage, leading to disability and increased mortality.[176] Genetic studies involving patients with RA indicate an association between VDR polymorphisms and the susceptibility to develop RA. The "F" allele of the VDR *FokI* polymorphism is associated with RA in the European population.[177] In addition, VDR polymorphism *BsmI* seems to correlate with disease severity.[178] Moreover, VDREs were identified in multiple RA susceptibility gene loci.[179] Although not as pronounced as the geographic distribution in T1D or MS, a lower vitamin D status as well as an increased risk for RA is observed at higher lattitudes.[180,181] In line with this, higher doses of UV-B radiation can reduce the risk to develop RA.[182] In general, patients with RA have lower serum $25(OH)D_3$ levels compared with healthy controls.[183] A metaanalysis performed by Lin and colleagues[184] confirmed the previous observation that low serum $25(OH)D_3$ levels are inversely correlated with RA susceptibility and RA disease activity as determined by Disease Activity Score in 28 Joints.[183] Oral supplementation with $1,25(OH)_2D_3$ prevents the initiation and progression of arthritis in the collagen-induced arthritis mouse model as well as in the Lyme arthritis model, where mice are infected with *Borrelia burgdorferi*.[185] In humans, a prospective cohort study of 29,368 women showed that additional vitamin D intake through diet over an 11-year follow-up period is inversely related to the risk of developing RA.[186] In addition, the beneficial effect of vitamin D supplementation (50,000 IU vitamin D or $25(OH)D_3$ per week) as an add-on to the standard therapy on disease activity, including tender and swollen joints, and relapse rate were shown.[187,188] Supplementation with an oral high dose of 2 μg/d alphacalcidiol provides a positive effect on disease activity in 89% of the patients with 45% of the patients in complete remission.[189] Although significance is often not reached owing to the relative low sample sizes, these changes might be clinically relevant.

The pathogenesis of RA is associated with the production of the proinflammatory cytokines IL-1β, IL-6, and TNF-α by activated macrophages present in the synovial fluid. These cytokines are able to induce synovitis together with the production of matrix metalloproteinases, resulting in articular damage.[190] In addition, both Th1 and Th17 responses play an important role in the acute phase of RA, and IFN-γ and IL-17 also contribute to the synovial inflammation.[191] In patients with RA, the number of Th17 cells are increased and correlate with disease severity. These Th17 cells are able to induce osteoclastogenesis while activating synovial fibroblasts thereby enhancing the local inflammation and joint destruction.[191,192] Treatment with $1,25(OH)_2D_3$ has been shown to inhibit IFN-γ and IL-17 cytokine production form Th1 and Th17 cells, respectively, and is able to induce a shift toward Th2 phenotype, with increased IL-4 levels in peripheral blood mononuclear cells from patients with RA.[193] Here, Th2 cells act as regulators, and IL-4 is able to prevent bone erosion through inhibition of IL-17 production.[194] Several groups reported that the peripheral Treg function is impaired in patients with RA owing to inhibition by TNF-α, because TNF-α blockade improves Treg function.[195–197] Either $1,25(OH)_2D_3$ or its analogue TX527 can promote the establishment of a stable $CD4^+CD25^{high}CD127^{low}$ Treg phenotype and functional suppressive capacity.[74,76] As a result of VDR expression in the synovial fibroblast, $1,25(OH)_2D_3$ is also able to directly modulate these cells and inhibits the IL-1β–induced production of MMP1 while reducing the invasion of RA fibroblasts.[198] Moreover, treatment with $1,25(OH)_2D_3$ or one of its analogues, calcipotriol, causes a long-lasting inhibition of proliferation and secretion of inflammatory factors, such as IL-6 and IFN-γ, in vitro.[199]

Vitamin D and systemic lupus erythematosus

SLE is a systemic autoimmune disease characterized by the production of autoantibodies against chromatin. SLE occurs predominantly in women and is accompanied by multiorgan inflammatory manifestations, including lupus nephritis, arthritis, fatigue, and skin lesions.[200] Although its etiology in not yet clear, disease onset has been linked to a combination of genetic, environmental, and hormonal factors. Genetic association studies on VDR polymorphisms and the risk to develop SLE reported conflicting results. A metaanalysis performed by Mao and Huang[201] shows an association between the *BsmI* "B" allele and the onset of SLE in the overall population. In addition, the *FokI* "FF" genotype correlated with SLE susceptibility in Asians only. Epidemiologic data show significantly lower serum $25(OH)D_3$ levels in recently diagnosed patients with SLE as well as in patients with a longer disease course.[202–204] A higher prevalence of vitamin D deficiency among patients was observed.[203] This is consistent with the fact that 70% of patients with SLE are photosensitive and therefore avoid sunlight exposure.[205] Moreover, an increased prevalence of SLE was observed among non-white compared with white individuals, which can be explained by the reduced penetration of UV light through the pigmented skin.[206] Autoantibodies against vitamin D were only found in 4% of patients with SLE and do not substantially contribute to the general vitamin D deficiency observed.[207] In addition, several studies reported an inverse correlation between serum $25(OH)D_3$ levels and disease activity.[208–210] Treatment with $1,25(OH)_2D_3$ or one of its synthetic analogues, 22-oxa-$1,25(OH)_2D_3$, could exert beneficial effects in the MRL/l mouse model, which spontaneously develops an SLE-like syndrome, sharing many immunologic features with human disease. The effects mediated by $1,25(OH)_2D_3$ include a prolonged lifespan of the mice, and a reduction in proteinuria, renal arteritis, and knee joint arthritis.[211,212] Several human trials have also investigated the therapeutic potential of vitamin D supplementation in patients with SLE. A clinical trial with oral vitamin D supplementation (2,000 IU/d for 12 months) showed an improvement in inflammatory markers as well as in disease activity, assessed by a reduction in autoantibody levels and SLE disease activity scores.[213] This beneficial effect on disease activity and fatigue was confirmed by another trial supplementing patients with SLE with 50,000 IU/wk oral vitamin D for 24 weeks.[214] In contrast, Aranow and colleagues[215] did not observe any effects when patients with SLE with inactive disease were treated with either a low (2,000 IU/d) or a high (4,000 IU/d) dose of vitamin D for 12 weeks. SLE is a T- and B-cell–mediated autoimmune disease. Antinuclear autoantibodies are found in almost all of patients with SLE. In addition, $1,25(OH)_2D_3$ has direct inhibiting effects on B-cell proliferation and memory B-cell formation, and induces apoptosis of the activated B cells from patients with SLE. Moreover, active vitamin D reduces the polyclonal and anti–double-stranded DNA Ig production by the B cells, resulting in reduced autoantibody titers.[57,216] During active disease, an increase in Th17 cells is observed in patients with SLE.[217] Also, $1,25(OH)_2D_3$ is able to inhibit the differentiation of Th17 cells and IL-17 cytokine production, thereby inducing a shift from Th17 cells toward Th2 and Tregs in patients with SLE.[57,218,219] Although Treg numbers are increased in the peripheral blood of patients with SLE, they have a deficient suppressive function caused by the high IFN-α production by APCs.[220] In addition, $1,25(OH)_2D_3$ is able to exert regulatory effects on DCs from both healthy individuals and patients with SLE.[43,208] In these cells, $1,25(OH)_2D_3$ interferes with the expression of IFN-α–regulated genes.[208] In addition, $1,25(OH)_2D_3$ treatment increases Foxp3 expression and tumor growth factor-β production in the Treg population.[221,222]

Vitamin D and inflammatory bowel disease

IBD is a group of idiopathic autoimmune diseases characterized by inflammation of the gastrointestinal tract and includes Crohn's disease (CD) and ulcerative colitis (UC). Both diseases are very distinct in clinical and pathologic features. Although disease etiology is not clear, it is believed that excessive inflammation is triggered by intestinal bacteria and that genetic predisposition and environmental factors play an important role.[223] Several genetic studies have investigated the association of VDR polymorphisms with the susceptibility of CD or UC. A metaanalysis showed that a higher risk for CD correlates with the *TaqI* "tt" genotype in Europeans, whereas the *ApaI* "a" allele seems to have a protective role in CD.[224] However, another metaanalysis observed an association between *ApaI* and increased CD risk and *TaqI* and higher UC risk.[225] The *FokI* "ff" genotype was associated with an increased risk for UC in Asians.[224] A relationship between geographic latitude, sunlight exposure, and disease prevalence has also been described for IBD. A higher latitude, corresponding with lower sunshine exposure, is associated with a higher prevalence of IBD in general[226] as well as an enhanced risk for CD[227–229] or UC[229] separately. In line with this, the majority of patients with IBD are vitamin D deficient.[230–232] Here, malabsorption of nutrients owing to the intestinal inflammation as well as a poor dietary intake might be additional risk factors contributing to the observed vitamin D deficiency. Moreover, vitamin D deficiency is associated with an enhanced disease activity[233–235] with lower serum $25(OH)D_3$ levels in active patients compared with patients in clinical remission.[236] In addition, $25(OH)D_3$ levels are inversely correlated with intestinal inflammation.[237]

In an IL-10 knockout mouse model, which spontaneously develops an IBD-like syndrome, oral $1,25(OH)_2D_3$ treatment (0.2 µg/d) significantly blocked the progression of disease and ameliorated IBD symptoms.[238] These beneficial effects of $1,25(OH)_2D_3$ were also observed in a dextran sodium sulfate–induced colitis mouse model, where oral administration of $1,25(OH)_2D_3$ (0.2 µg/25 g/d) or intrarectal administration of the $1,25(OH)_2D_3$ analogue BXL-60 (1 µg/kg) improved inflammation in the colon.[239,240] In humans, a supplementation trial giving 1200 IU of cholecalciferol per day for 1 year to CD patients in remission showed a trend toward a lower relapse rate among patients treated with vitamin D.[241] In another clinical study, 2,000 IU vitamin D per day for 3 months could stabilize the intestinal permeability. Here, additional beneficial effects were observed when serum $25(OH)D_3$ concentrations reached more than 30 ng/mL or 75 nmol/L, including a reduction in disease activity, lower serum levels of C-reactive protein (which is a marker of inflammation), and a better quality of life.[242] In contrast, supplementation with a low (400 IU/d) or a high (2,000 IU/d) dose of cholecalciferol in children with CD did not affect disease activity.[243] Interestingly, normalization of vitamin D status also reduced the probability of IBD-related surgery.[244] In IBD, abnormalities of innate immunity lead to an adaptive immune disorder with dysregulated responses toward gut microbiota. Immune cells in the intestinal mucosa produce inflammatory cytokines like TNF-α and IFN-γ, which induce epithelial cell apoptosis, thereby increasing the permeability of the intestinal barrier. This allows for the translocation of bacteria and immune cell activation of DCs, macrophages, T cells, and B cells.[245] In addition, $1,25(OH)_2D_3$ increases the expression of the pathogen recognition receptor NOD2, which is a known susceptibility gene in IBD, in human monocytes,[246] resulting in the production of antimicrobial peptides such as cathelicidin, which are important in the mucosal barrier. Indeed, an increase in the concentration of CAMP was observed in CD patients after vitamin D treatment.[242] In DCs originating from CD patients, both $25(OH)D_3$ and $1,25(OH)_2D_3$ reduce maturation markers CD80 and HLA-DR while decreasing their TNF-α production. This indicates that $1,25(OH)_2D_3$ modulates DC function in CD, thereby contributing to the suppression of the ongoing immune response.[247] Moreover, oral vitamin D supplementation decreased serum TNF-α levels.[248] In IBD, Th1 and Th17 cells accumulate in the gut, secreting IFN-γ and IL-17, respectively. Ex vivo treatment of peripheral blood mononuclear cells from UC patients with $1,25(OH)_2D_3$ reduced IFN-γ, while increasing IL-10 production.[249] In addition, the percentage of $CD4^+CD25^{high}$ Tregs increased 3-fold in the presence of vitamin D, and their suppressive function was confirmed.[250] In the intestine, other regulatory cell populations are present, including $CD8\alpha\alpha^+$ $TCR\alpha\beta^+$ cells to limit inflammation in the gastrointestinal tract.[251] Vitamin D deficiency was shown to decrease the maturation and proliferation of $CD8\alpha\alpha^+$ $TCR\alpha\beta^+$ cells, resulting in a lower number of functional cells.[84]

Presently, it is clear that vitamin D is an important environmental factor that seems to play an important role in autoimmune disease onset in genetically susceptible individuals. Although larger intervention trials are required to determine the therapeutic potential of vitamin D supplementation or $1,25(OH)_2D_3$ therapy in autoimmunity, we advocate that vitamin D deficiency should be avoided.

Vitamin D and Infectious Diseases

Since the early 1990s, researchers proposed a link between vitamin D deficiency and susceptibility to infections, with the initial observation that rachitic children experienced more infections of the upper respiratory system.[252] Moreover, cod liver oil (a rich source of vitamin D) or UV-B light were systematically used for the treatment of pulmonary tuberculosis (TB). It is also well-known that $1,25(OH)_2D_3$ can inhibit the growth of *M tuberculosis* in human macrophages in vitro.[253] Also epidemiologic studies demonstrated associations between seasonal variations in vitamin D concentrations and the incidence of various infectious disorders.[254–256] The World Health Organization global burden of disease estimated that infectious diseases caused by either bacteria or viruses are yearly responsible for around 3 million deaths of children under the age of 5 years. Especially in low-income countries, in particular in the regions of South-East Asia and sub-Saharan Africa exposure to these pathogens is very high and leads to long-lasting activation of inflammatory processes. Neutrophils and macrophages play an active role in the control of infections. Although these cells are necessary for the containment and clearance of infectious pathogens, they are also recognized as tissue-destructive cells responsible for inflammatory tissue damage when their activity is prolonged. To serve as potent innate immune cells against invading microbes, these cells harbor numerous granules enriched with different antimicrobial molecules (eg, CAMP and some β-defensins). Several of these antimicrobial peptides are directly regulated by $1,25(OH)_2D_3$.[31] Moreover, the ability to mount a suitable immune reaction to intracellular pathogens is highly dependent on a competent VDR. Moreover, as discussed in previous paragraphs, infectious pathogens are also linked to the development of autoimmune disorders. Either through molecular mimicry; expression of modified, cryptic, or new antigenic determinants; or bystander activation autoimmune cells may eventually become activated. Vitamin D may combat infections via different mechanisms. On the one hand, it impacts directly on the production of antimicrobial peptides, but it can also influence cytokine profiles during infection via the innate and adaptive immune system.

Vitamin D and bacterial infections
Mycobacterium tuberculosis Pulmonary TB is a global epidemic. More than 2 billion people (about one-third of the world population) are estimated to be infected with *M tuberculosis*. Before appropriate antibiotics were available, clinicians motivated

people with TB to get sufficient sunlight exposure or consume sufficient amounts of vitamin D. Niels Ryberg Finsen received in 1903 the Nobel Prize for Medicine for demonstrating that UV-B radiation could alleviate the epidermal form of TB, also known as *Lupus vulgaris*. Genetic studies of various populations have demonstrated that the *FokI* "ff" genotype is more commonly observed in patients with TB,[257,258] but other studies could not confirm these observations.[259,260] Potential selection bias exists in most analyses using human immunodeficiency virus-positive patients with TB. A more recent metaanalysis study demonstrated that the VDR *FokI* polymorphism can contribute to TB risk, especially in human immunodeficiency virus-negative patients with TB and in Asians,[261] whereas no evidence of difference in distribution and association between human immunodeficiency virus infection and the genotypes of the *BsmI*, *FokI*, and *TaqI* VDR polymorphisms were found.[262] Still, large and well-designed studies are needed to strengthen these conclusions. Additionally, analysis of a large cohort of white Caucasians identified an association between polymorphisms in the vitamin D binding protein gene and the risk of serum vitamin D insufficiency.[16,263] Thus, in the setting of TB, genetic differences in the vitamin D binding protein and epigenetic rather than genetic variations in the VDR gene may be linked with disease susceptibility. Epidemiologic studies have shown that circulating levels of vitamin D of less than 30 ng/mL or 75 nmol/L are a risk factor for active TB and impaired antimycobacterial activity.[264–266] Vitamin D supplementation during TB therapy is controversial; a few studies reported clinical benefit in pulmonary TB[267]; however, 1 study reported no effect.[268]

The current interest in the benefits of vitamin D for TB comes from studies describing the cellular and molecular mode of actions of vitamin D on *M tuberculosis*. Although macrophages play an imperative role in controlling and eradicating the intracellular mycobacteria, large amounts of neutrophils are recruited to the lungs in the early stages of the *M tuberculosis* infection. Neutrophils activated by *M tuberculosis* form NETs, containing chromatin and several cytosolic and granular proteins. Apoptotic neutrophils prevent the growth of extracellular mycobacteria. Elimination of apoptotic neutrophils by macrophages results in decreased viability of intracellular mycobacteria through the antimicrobial peptides from the ingested neutrophils.[269] Little information is available on the effect of vitamin D on these processes, but $1,25(OH)_2D_3$ has been shown to decrease NETosis activity in patients with SLE.[20] Whether this is also the case during a *M tuberculosis* infection needs to be explored. Moreover, $1,25(OH)_2D_3$ can inhibit neutrophil migration, but its consequence in infectious diseases remains to be determined. As described, the activation of the vitamin D pathway via immune or TLR signals clearly provides a means for macrophages to prevent the suppression of the antimicrobial CAMP gene and to contribute in the killing of intracellular *M tuberculosis*.[30] Thus, $1,25(OH)_2D_3$–mediated CAMP induction offers a potential mechanism to neutralize pathogen-mediated suppression and modulate innate immunity. The contribution of additional signaling pathways like IL-1β in the induction of antimicrobial peptide gene expression is especially imperative for DEFB4 gene transcription. In the condition of vitamin D deficiency, infected macrophages will not be able to generate sufficient amounts of $1,25(OH)_2D_3$ to upregulate the production of cathelicidin or β-defensins.[270] Interestingly, lung airway cells also can produce high levels of CYP27B1 leading to the local bioconversion of $25(OH)D_3$ into $1,25(OH)_2D_3$. Locally produced $1,25(OH)_2D_3$ was able to induce expression of CAMP and CD14. This finding suggests that these cells may use vitamin D as part of their defense system against infections.

The link between vitamin D deficiency and lung disease does not seem to be limited to pulmonary TB, and the vitamin D–induced antimicrobial activity is probably a characteristic of cells at multiple so-called barrier sites. Indeed, $1,25(OH)_2D_3$ was able to enhance DC maturation and expression of the migration marker CCR7 in *Streptococcus pneumoniae*-stimulated cells. It also enhanced expression of key pattern recognition receptors (eg, TLR2, NOD2) and induced a synergistic upregulation of IL-1β and the β-defensin hBD3. Furthermore, $1,25(OH)_2D_3$ skewed the DC-mediated Th response to *S pneumoniae* from an proinflammatory Th1/Th17 phenotype toward a Treg phenotype.[271] In another setting, in the placenta, $1,25(OH)_2D_3$ may boost the relatively high basal expression of antimicrobial peptides to combat infection by pathogens such as *Listeria monocytogenes* and *Streptococcus* species, which are known to have a role in adverse events associated with pregnancy.[272]

Also at the skin barrier, $1,25(OH)_2D_3$ plays an important role, where it synergizes with parathyroid hormone to induce the expression of cathelicidin peptides thereby playing a protective role against group A *Streptococcus* skin infections in vivo. Interestingly, vitamin D deficiency increased the susceptibility of skin infection with group A *Streptococcus* in CYP27B1 knockout mice.[273] Interestingly, upon a skin injury, the expression of CYP27B1 is induced in keratinocytes around the wound, enhancing the production of $1,25(OH)_2D_3$. This results in the induced gene transcription of microbial pathogen recognition receptors CD14 and TLR2 as well as the cathelicidin antimicrobial peptide through vitamin D–mediated epigenetic regulation.[274,275] Ablation of the VDR or CYP27B1 or limited $25(OH)D_3$ availability prevented the production of CD14, TLR2, and cathelicidin in human keratinocytes.[274]

Clinically, vitamin D deficiency has been associated with an increased risk for various infectious diseases. Moreover, vitamin D supplementation might be advantageous to the attenuation of bacterial infections, but robust clinical data are still missing.

Vitamin D and viral infections

Colds and influenza viruses Common colds or upper respiratory tract infections are the most widespread of infectious diseases, with more than 200 viruses contributing to the clinical symptoms. Influenza is a viral respiratory infection causing fever, cough, headache, and malaise. Indirect evidence initially pointed at the observation that wintertime low levels of vitamin D were related to the seasonal escalations in viral respiratory tract infections, such as those caused by influenza virus ("the flu") and rhinovirus ("the common cold"). Some small studies also found a link between vitamin D deficiency and a higher risk of respiratory infections. The Third National Health and Nutrition Examination Survey from October 1988 to October 1994 analyzed information on circulating vitamin D levels and upper respiratory infections in a population of nearly 19,000 adults and adolescents. Participants with the lowest $25(OH)D_3$ levels (<10 ng/mL or 25 nmol/L) were 36% more likely to report having a recent upper respiratory tract infection than those with higher levels ($\geq$30 ng/mL or 75 nmol/L). This correlation persevered during all seasons and was even clearer among those with a history of asthma or chronic obstructive pulmonary disease.[255] A metaanalysis and systemic review of prior studies demonstrated that vitamin D (D_2 or D_3) supplementation can prevent acute respiratory tract infections. In a subgroup analysis, beneficial effects were observed in those receiving daily or weekly vitamin D without additional bolus doses but not in those receiving one or more bolus doses of at least 30,000 IU of vitamin D. Among those receiving daily or weekly vitamin D, protective effects were stronger in those with baseline $25(OH)D_3$ <10 ng/mL or 25 nmol/L than in those with baseline $25(OH)D_3$ levels of 10 ng/mL or greater or 25 nmol/L or greater.[276] Patients who were very vitamin D deficient and those not receiving bolus doses experienced the most benefit. Randomized, controlled trials will be needed to examine the direct effect of vitamin D supplements and to determine the optimal serum concentrations of $25(OH)D_3$ needed to prevent upper respiratory tract infections.

Because these colds involve mostly innate immune responses, vitamin D can on one hand inhibit inflammatory cytokine production, but in contrast also stimulate production of antimicrobial peptides from innate immune cells. Although $1,25(OH)_2D_3$ does not consistently influence replication or clearance of rhinovirus or influenza A virus in human lung epithelial cells,[277] it can modulate the expression and secretion of proinflammatory cytokines like IL-6 and TNF-α but also of chemokines including CXCL8 and CXCL10.[277] Similar observations were found in experiments with primary human bronchial epithelial cells treated with $25(OH)D_3$ or $1,25(OH)_2D_3$ and subsequently infected with rhinovirus-16.[278] The antimicrobial peptides LL-37 and defensin $\beta2$ have antiviral properties against influenza virus, reducing disease severity and viral replication, inhibiting infectivity, and demonstrating counteracting activity.[279]

SUMMARY

In general, vitamin D deficiency is associated with an increased risk for various autoimmune and infectious diseases. However, whether this is a cause or a consequence, or just an association, is not yet clear. Although in vitro studies show that vitamin D and its metabolites play a crucial role in the modulation of phenotype and function of immune cells and animal studies provide substantial evidence for a therapeutic effect in autoimmunity and infection, human data for the potential clinical use of vitamin D supplementation in autoimmune diseases and infectious disorders is rather limited and sometimes conflicting. This might be attributed to the small sample size of some trials or the dose of vitamin D used in these studies, which might be adequate for bone health, but may not be insufficient for immune modulation. In contrast, vitamin D toxicity should be avoided. The use of safe, noncalcemic analogues are very promising tools to further investigate and exploit the therapeutic potential of vitamin D.

REFERENCES

1. Baeke F, Takiishi T, Korf H, et al. Modulator of the immune system. Curr Opin Pharmacol 2010;10(4):482–96.

2. Cantorna MT, Mahon BD. Mounting evidence for vitamin D as an environmental factor affecting autoimmune disease prevalence. Exp Biol Med (Maywood) 2004;229(11):1136–42.

3. Lerner A, Jeremias P, Matthias T. The world incidence and prevalence of autoimmune diseases is increasing. Int J Celiac Dis 2015;3(4):151–5.

4. Bouillon R, Van Schoor NM, Gielen E, et al. Optimal vitamin D status: a critical analysis on the basis of evidence-based medicine. J Clin Endocrinol Metab 2013;98(8):E1283–304.

5. Bouillon R, Carmeliet G, Verlinden L, et al. Vitamin D and human health: lessons from vitamin D receptor null mice. Endocr Rev 2008;29(6):726–76.

6. Bouillon R, Eelen G, Verlinden L, et al. Vitamin D and cancer. J Steroid Biochem Mol Biol 2006;102(1–5):156–62.

7. Christakos S, Dhawan P, Verstuyf A, et al. Metabolism, molecular mechanism of action, and pleiotropic effects. Physiol Rev 2016;96(1):365–408.

8. Jones G. Expanding role for vitamin D in chronic kidney disease: importance of blood 25-OH-D levels and extra-renal 1alpha-hydroxylase in the classical and nonclassical actions of 1alpha,25-dihydroxyvitamin D(3). Semin Dial 2007; 20(4):316–24.

9. Booth D, Ding N, Parnell G, et al. Cistromic and genetic evidence that the vitamin D receptor mediates susceptibility to latitude-dependent autoimmune diseases. Genes Immun 2016;1712(10):213–9.

10. Pike JW, Meyer MB, Bishop KA. Regulation of target gene expression by the vitamin D receptor - an update on mechanisms. Rev Endocr Metab Disord 2012;13(1):45–55.

11. Carlberg C, Campbell MJ. Vitamin D receptor signaling mechanisms: integrated actions of a well-defined transcription factor. Steroids 2013;78(2):127–36.

12. Lonard DM, O'Malley BW. Nuclear receptor coregulators: modulators of pathology and therapeutic targets. Nat Rev Endocrinol 2012;8(10):598–604.

13. Haussler MR, Jurutka PW, Mizwicki M, et al. Vitamin D receptor (VDR)-mediated actions of 1a,25(OH)2-vitamin D3: genomic and non-genomic mechanisms. Best Pract Res Clin Endocrinol Metab 2011;25(4):543–59.

14. Norman AW. Minireview: Vitamin D receptor: new assignments for an already busy receptor. Endocrinology 2006;147(12):5542–8.

15. Veldman CM, Cantorna MT, DeLuca HF. Expression of 1,25-dihydroxyvitamin D(3) receptor in the immune system. Arch Biochem Biophys 2000;374(2):334–8.

16. Hewison M, Freeman L, Hughes SV, et al. Differential regulation of vitamin D receptor and its ligand in human monocyte-derived dendritic cells. J Immunol 2003;170(11):5382–90.

17. Kaplan MJ, Radic M. Neutrophil extracellular traps: double-edged swords of innate immunity. J Immunol 2012;189(6):2689–95.

18. Takahashi K, Nakayama Y, Horiuchi H, et al. Human neutrophils express messenger RNA of vitamin D receptor and respond to 1alpha,25-dihydroxyvitamin D3. Immunopharmacol Immunotoxicol 2002;24(3):335–47.

19. Hirsch D, Archer FE, Joshi-Kale M, et al. Decreased anti-inflammatory responses to vitamin D in neonatal neutrophils. Mediators Inflamm 2011;2011:598345.

20. Handono K, Sidarta YO, Pradana BA, et al. Vitamin D prevents endothelial damage induced by increased neutrophil extracellular traps formation in patients with systemic lupus erythematosus. Acta Med Indones 2014;46(3):189–98.

21. Yang H, Long F, Zhang Y, et al. 1a,25-dihydroxyvitamin D3 induces neutrophil apoptosis through the p38 MAPK signaling pathway in chronic obstructive pulmonary disease patients. PLoS One 2015;10(4):e0120515.

22. Murray PJ, Wynn TA. Protective and pathogenic functions of macrophage subsets. Nat Rev Immunol 2011;11(11):723–37.

23. Xu H, Soruri A, Gieseler RKH, et al. 1,25-Dihydroxyvitamin D3 exerts opposing effects to IL-4 on MHC class-II antigen expression, accessory activity, and phagocytosis of human monocytes. Scand J Immunol 1993;38(6):535–40.

24. Korf H, Wenes M, Stijlemans B, et al. 1,25-Dihydroxyvitamin D3 curtails the inflammatory and T cell stimulatory capacity of macrophages through an IL-10-dependent mechanism. Immunobiology 2012;217(12):1292–300.

25. Stoffels K, Overbergh L, Giulietti A, et al. Immune regulation of 25-hydroxyvitamin-D3-1alpha-hydroxylase in human monocytes. J Bone Miner Res 2006;21(1):37–47.

26. Stoffels K, Overbergh L, Bouillon R, et al. Immune regulation of 1alpha-hydroxylase in murine peritoneal macrophages: unravelling the IFNgamma pathway. J Steroid Biochem Mol Biol 2007;103(3–5):567–71.

27. Oberg F, Botling J, Nilsson K. Functional antagonism between vitamin D3 and retinoic acid in the regulation of CD14 and CD23 expression during monocytic differentiation of U-937 cells. J Immunol 1993;150(8 Pt 1):3487–95.

28. Ren S, Nguyen L, Wu S, et al. Alternative splicing of vitamin D-24-hydroxylase: a novel mechanism for the regulation of extrarenal 1,25-dihydroxyvitamin D synthesis. J Biol Chem 2005;280(21):20604–11.

29. Krutzik SR, Hewison M, Liu PT, et al. IL-15 Links TLR2/1-induced macrophage differentiation to the vitamin D-dependent antimicrobial pathway. J Immunol 2008;181(10):7115–20.

30. Liu PT, Stenger S, Li H, et al. Toll-like receptor triggering of a vitamin D-mediated human antimicrobial response. Science 2006;311(5768):1770–3.

31. Wang T-T, Nestel FP, Bourdeau V, et al. Cutting edge: 1,25-dihydroxyvitamin D3 is a direct inducer of antimicrobial peptide gene expression. J Immunol 2004; 173(5):2909–12.

32. Lee BNR, Kim TH, Jun JB, et al. Upregulation of interleukin-1β production by 1,25-dihydroxyvitamin D3 in activated human macrophages. Mol Biol Rep 2011;38(3):2193–201.

33. Verway M, Bouttier M, Wang TT, et al. Vitamin D induces interleukin-1beta expression: paracrine macrophage epithelial signaling controls M. tuberculosis infection. PLoS Pathog 2013;9(6):e1003407.

34. Chen Y, Liu W, Sun T, et al. 1,25-Dihydroxyvitamin D promotes negative feedback regulation of TLR signaling via targeting microRNA-155-SOCS1 in macrophages. J Immunol 2013;190(7):3687–95.

35. Riek AE, Oh J, Sprague JE, et al. Vitamin D suppression of endoplasmic reticulum stress promotes an antiatherogenic monocyte/macrophage phenotype in type 2 diabetic patients. J Biol Chem 2012;287(46):38482–94.

36. Helming L, Bose J, Ehrchen J, et al. 1alpha,25-Dihydroxyvitamin D3 is a potent suppressor of interferon gamma-mediated macrophage activation. Blood 2005; 106(13):4351–8.

37. Neve A, Corrado A, Cantatore FP. Immunomodulatory effects of vitamin D in peripheral blood monocyte-derived macrophages from patients with rheumatoid arthritis. Clin Exp Med 2014;14(3):275–83.

38. Heulens N, Korf H, Mathyssen C, et al. 1,25-dihydroxyvitamin D modulates antibacterial and inflammatory response in human cigarette smoke-exposed macrophages. PLoS One 2016;11(8):e0160482.

39. Song L, Papaioannou G, Zhao H, et al. The vitamin D receptor regulates tissue resident macrophage response to injury. Endocrinology 2016;157(10):4066–75.

40. Steinman RM. Some interfaces of dendritic cell biology. APMIS 2003;111(7–8): 675–97.

41. Penna G, Adorini L. 1 ,25-Dihydroxyvitamin D3 inhibits differentiation, maturation, activation, and survival of dendritic cells leading to impaired alloreactive T cell activation. J Immunol 2000;164(5):2405–11.

42. Adorini L, Penna G. Dendritic cell tolerogenicity: a key mechanism in immunomodulation by vitamin D receptor agonists. Hum Immunol 2009;70(5):345–52.

43. Ferreira GB, Kleijwegt FS, Waelkens E, et al. Differential protein pathways in 1,25-dihydroxyvitamin D 3 and dexamethasone modulated tolerogenic human dendritic cells. J Proteome Res 2012;11(2):941–71.

44. Kleijwegt FS, Laban S, Duinkerken G, et al. Critical role for TNF in the induction of human antigen-specific regulatory T cells by tolerogenic dendritic cells. J Immunol 2010;185(3):1412–8.

45. Ferreira GB, van Etten E, Verstuyf A, et al. 1,25-Dihydroxyvitamin D3 alters murine dendritic cell behaviour in vitro and in vivo. Diabetes Metab Res Rev 2011; 27(8):933–41.

46. Van Halteren AGS, Van Etten E, De Jong EC, et al. Redirection of human autoreactive T-cells upon interaction with dendritic cells modulated by TX527, an analog of 1,25 dihydroxyvitamin D3. Diabetes 2002;51(7):2119–25.

47. Penna G, Roncari A, Amuchastegui S, et al. Expression of the inhibitory receptor ILT3 on dendritic cells is dispensable for induction of CD4+Foxp3+ regulatory T cells by 1,25-dihydroxyvitamin D3. Blood 2005;106(10):3490–7.

48. Unger WWJ, Laban S, Kleijwegt FS, et al. Induction of Treg by monocyte-derived DC modulated by vitamin D3 or dexamethasone: differential role for PD-L1. Eur J Immunol 2009;39(11):3147–59.

49. van Etten E, Dardenne O, Gysemans C, et al. 1,25-Dihydroxyvitamin D3 alters the profile of bone marrow-derived dendritic cells of NOD mice. Ann N Y Acad Sci 2004;1037:186–92.

50. Ferreira GB, Vanherwegen A-S, Eelen G, et al. Vitamin D3 induces tolerance in human dendritic cells by activation of intracellular metabolic pathways. Cell Rep 2015;10(5):711–25.

51. Ferreira GB, Van Etten E, Lage K, et al. Proteome analysis demonstrates profound alterations in human dendritic cell nature by TX527, an analogue of vitamin D. Proteomics 2009;9(14):3752–64.

52. Naranjo-Gomez M, Raich-Regue D, Onate C, et al. Comparative study of clinical grade human tolerogenic dendritic cells. J Transl Med 2011;9:89.

53. Chen S, Sims GP, Chen XX, et al. Modulatory effects of 1,25-dihydroxyvitamin D3 on human B cell differentiation. J Immunol 2007;179(3):1634–47.

54. Heine G, Niesner U, Chang HD, et al. 1,25-dihydroxyvitamin D(3) promotes IL-10 production in human B cells. Eur J Immunol 2008;38:2210–8.

55. Lemire JM, Adams JS, Sakai R, et al. 1 alpha,25-dihydroxyvitamin D3 suppresses proliferation and immunoglobulin production by normal human peripheral blood mononuclear cells. J Clin Invest 1984;74(2):657–61.

56. Provvedini DM, Tsoukas CD, Deftos LJ, et al. 1 alpha,25-Dihydroxyvitamin D3-binding macromolecules in human B lymphocytes: effects on immunoglobulin production. J Immunol 1986;136(8):2734–40.

57. Terrier B, Derian N, Schoindre Y, et al. Restoration of regulatory and effector T cell balance and B cell homeostasis in systemic lupus erythematosus patients through vitamin D supplementation. Arthritis Res Ther 2012;14(5):R221.

58. Drozdenko G, Scheel T, Heine G, et al. Impaired T cell activation and cytokine production by calcitriol-primed human B cells. Clin Exp Immunol 2014;178(2):364–72.

59. Shirakawa A-K, Nagakubo D, Hieshima K, et al. 1,25-dihydroxyvitamin D3 induces CCR10 expression in terminally differentiating human B cells. J Immunol 2008;180(5):2786–95.

60. Baeke F, Korf H, Overbergh L, et al. Human T lymphocytes are direct targets of 1,25-dihydroxyvitamin D3 in the immune system. J Steroid Biochem Mol Biol 2010;121(1–2):221–7.

61. von Essen MR, Kongsbak M, Schjerling P, et al. Vitamin D controls T cell antigen receptor signaling and activation of human T cells. Nat Immunol 2010;11(4):344–9.

62. Palmer MT, Lee YK, Maynard CL, et al. Lineage-specific effects of 1,25-dihydroxyvitamin D3 on the development of effector CD4 T cells. J Biol Chem 2011;286(2):997–1004.

63. Staeva-Vieira TP, Freedman LP. 1,25-Dihydroxyvitamin D3 inhibits IFN-gamma and IL-4 levels during in vitro polarization of primary murine CD4+ T cells. J Immunol 2002;168(3):1181–9.

64. Lemire JM, Adams JS, Kermani-Arab V, et al. 1,25-Dihydroxyvitamin D3 suppresses human T helper/inducer lymphocyte activity in vitro. J Immunol 1985; 134(5):3032–5.

65. Tang J, Zhou R, Luger D, et al. Calcitriol suppresses antiretinal autoimmunity through inhibitory effects on the Th17 effector response. J Immunol 2009; 182(8):4624–32.

66. Jeffery LE, Burke F, Mura M, et al. 1,25-Dihydroxyvitamin D3 and IL-2 combine to inhibit T cell production of inflammatory cytokines and promote development of regulatory T cells expressing CTLA-4 and FoxP3. J Immunol 2009;183(9): 5458–67.

67. Borgogni E, Sarchielli E, Sottili M, et al. Elocalcitol inhibits inflammatory responses in human thyroid cells and T cells. Endocrinology 2008;149(7): 3626–34.

68. Cippitelli M, Santoni A. Vitamin D3: a transcriptional modulator of the interferon-gamma gene. Eur J Immunol 1998;28(10):3017–30.

69. Joshi S, Pantalena L-C, Liu XK, et al. 1,25-dihydroxyvitamin D(3) ameliorates Th17 autoimmunity via transcriptional modulation of interleukin-17A. Mol Cell Biol 2011;31(17):3653–69.

70. Boonstra A, Barrat FJ, Crain C, et al. 1alpha,25-Dihydroxyvitamin d3 has a direct effect on naive CD4(+) T cells to enhance the development of Th2 cells. J Immunol 2001;167(9):4974–80.

71. Mahon BD, Wittke A, Weaver V, et al. The targets of vitamin D depend on the differentiation and activation status of CD4 positive T cells. J Cell Biochem 2003;89(5):922–32.

72. Jeffery LE, Qureshi OS, Gardner D, et al. Vitamin D antagonises the suppressive effect of inflammatory cytokines on CTLA-4 expression and regulatory function. PLoS One 2015;10(7):e0131539.

73. Keating P, Munim A, Hartmann JX. Effect of vitamin D on T-helper type 9 polarized human memory cells in chronic persistent asthma. Ann Allergy Asthma Immunol 2014;112(2):154–62.

74. Baeke F, Korf H, Overbergh L, et al. The vitamin D analog, TX527, promotes a human CD4+CD25highCD127low regulatory T cell profile and induces a migratory signature specific for homing to sites of inflammation. J Immunol 2011; 186(1):132–42.

75. Barrat FJ, Cua DJ, Boonstra A, et al. In vitro generation of interleukin 10-producing regulatory CD4(+) T cells is induced by immunosuppressive drugs and inhibited by T helper type 1 (Th1)- and Th2-inducing cytokines. J Exp Med 2002; 195(5):603–16.

76. Van Belle TL, Vanherwegen A-S, Feyaerts D, et al. 1,25-Dihydroxyvitamin D3 and its analog TX527 promote a stable regulatory T cell phenotype in T cells from type 1 diabetes patients. PLoS One 2014;9(10):e109194.

77. Sigmundsdottir H, Pan J, Debes GF, et al. DCs metabolize sunlight-induced vitamin D3 to "program" T cell attraction to the epidermal chemokine CCL27. Nat Immunol 2007;8(3):285–93.

78. Urry Z, Chambers ES, Xystrakis E, et al. The role of 1alpha,25-dihydroxyvitamin D3 and cytokines in the promotion of distinct Foxp3+ and IL-10+ CD4+ T cells. Eur J Immunol 2012;42(10):2697–708.

79. Kang SW, Kim SH, Lee N, et al. 1,25-Dihyroxyvitamin D3 promotes FOXP3 expression via binding to vitamin D response elements in its conserved noncoding sequence region. J Immunol 2012;188(11):5276–82.
80. Zhang N, Bevan MJ. CD8+ T Cells: foot soldiers of the immune system. Immunity 2011;35(2):161–8.
81. Chen J, Bruce D, Cantorna MT. Vitamin D receptor expression controls proliferation of naive CD8+ T cells and development of CD8 mediated gastrointestinal inflammation. BMC Immunol 2014;15(1):6.
82. Lysandropoulos AP, Jaquiéry E, Jilek S, et al. Vitamin D has a direct immunomodulatory effect on CD8+ T cells of patients with early multiple sclerosis and healthy control subjects. J Neuroimmunol 2011;233(1–2):240–4.
83. Dyring-Andersen B, Bonefeld CM, Bzorek M, et al. The vitamin D analogue calcipotriol reduces the frequency of CD8+IL-17+ T cells in psoriasis lesions. Scand J Immunol 2015;82(1):84–91.
84. Bruce D, Cantorna MT. Intrinsic requirement for the vitamin D receptor in the development of CD8{alpha}{alpha}-expressing T cells. J Immunol 2011;186(5):2819–25.
85. Ross AC, Taylor CL, Yaktine AL, et al. Dietary reference intakes for calcium and vitamin D. Washington, DC: National Academies Press; 2011.
86. Smolders J, Peelen E, Thewissen M, et al. Safety and T cell modulating effects of high dose vitamin D3 supplementation in multiple sclerosis. PLoS One 2010;5(12):e15235.
87. Searing DA, Leung DYM. Vitamin D in atopic dermatitis, asthma and allergic diseases. Immunol Allergy Clin North Am 2010;30(3):397–409.
88. Herold KC, Vignali D, Cooke A, et al. Type 1 diabetes: translating mechanistic observations into effective clinical outcomes. Nat Rev Immunol 2013;13(4):243–56.
89. Zhang J, Li W, Liu J, et al. Polymorphisms in the vitamin D receptor gene and type 1 diabetes mellitus risk: an update by meta-analysis. Mol Cell Endocrinol 2012;355(1):135–42.
90. Kahles H, Morahan G, Todd JA, et al. Association analyses of the vitamin D receptor gene in 1654 families with type I diabetes. Genes Immun 2009;10(Suppl 1):S60–3.
91. Tizaoui K, Kaabachi W, Hamzaoui A, et al. Contribution of VDR polymorphisms to type 1 diabetes susceptibility: systematic review of case-control studies and meta-analysis. J Steroid Biochem Mol Biol 2014;143:240–9.
92. Arai H, Miyamoto K, Taketani Y, et al. A vitamin D receptor gene polymorphism in the translation initiation codon: effect on protein activity and relation to bone mineral density in Japanese women. J Bone Miner Res 1997;12(6):915–21.
93. van Etten E, Verlinden L, Giulietti A, et al. The vitamin D receptor gene FokI polymorphism: functional impact on the immune system. Eur J Immunol 2007;37(2):395–405.
94. Morán-Auth Y, Penna-Martinez M, Badenhoop K. VDR FokI polymorphism is associated with a reduced T-helper cell population under vitamin D stimulation in type 1 diabetes patients. J Steroid Biochem Mol Biol 2015;148:184–6.
95. Hussein AG, Mohamed RH, Alghobashy AA. Synergism of CYP2R1 and CYP27B1 polymorphisms and susceptibility to type 1 diabetes in Egyptian children. Cell Immunol 2012;279(1):42–5.
96. Frederiksen BN, Kroehl M, Fingerlin TE, et al. Association between vitamin D metabolism gene polymorphisms and risk of islet autoimmunity and progression

to type 1 diabetes: the diabetes autoimmunity study in the young (DAISY). J Clin Endocrinol Metab 2013;98(11):E1845–51.

97. Cooper JD, Smyth DJ, Walker NM, et al. Inherited variation in vitamin D genes is associated with predisposition to autoimmune disease type 1 diabetes. Diabetes 2011;60(5):1624–31.

98. Israni N, Goswami R, Kumar A, et al. Interaction of vitamin D receptor with HLA DRB1*0301 in type 1 diabetes patients from North India. PLoS One 2009;4(12): e8023.

99. Mohr SB, Garland CF, Gorham ED, et al. The association between ultraviolet B irradiance, vitamin D status and incidence rates of type 1 diabetes in 51 regions worldwide. Diabetologia 2008;51(8):1391–8.

100. Sloka S, Grant M, Newhook LA. The geospatial relation between UV solar radiation and type 1 diabetes in Newfoundland. Acta Diabetol 2010;47(1):73–8.

101. Karvonen M. Incidence and trends of childhood type 1 diabetes worldwide 1990-1999. Diabet Med 2006;23(8):857–66.

102. Feng R, Li Y, Li G, et al. Lower serum 25 (OH) D concentrations in type 1 diabetes: a meta-analysis. Diabetes Res Clin Pract 2015;108(3):e71–5.

103. Shen L, Zhuang Q-S, Ji H-F. Assessment of vitamin D levels in type 1 and type 2 diabetes patients: results from metaanalysis. Mol Nutr Food Res 2016;60(5): 1059–67.

104. Munger KL, Levin LI, Massa J, et al. Preclinical serum 25-hydroxyvitamin D levels and risk of type 1 diabetes in a cohort of US military personnel. Am J Epidemiol 2013;177(5):411–9.

105. Raab J, Giannopoulou EZ, Schneider S, et al. Prevalence of vitamin D deficiency in pre-type 1 diabetes and its association with disease progression. Diabetologia 2014;57(5):902–8.

106. Giulietti A, Gysemans C, Stoffels K, et al. Vitamin D deficiency in early life accelerates type 1 diabetes in non-obese diabetic mice. Diabetologia 2004;47(3): 451–62.

107. Miettinen ME, Reinert L, Kinnunen L, et al. Serum 25-hydroxyvitamin D level during early pregnancy and type 1 diabetes risk in the offspring. Diabetologia 2012; 55(5):1291–4.

108. Sørensen IM, Joner G, Jenum PA, et al. Maternal serum levels of 25-hydroxyvitamin D during pregnancy and risk of type 1 diabetes in the offspring. Diabetes 2012;61(1):175–8.

109. Mathieu C, Waer M, Laureys J, et al. Prevention of autoimmune diabetes in NOD mice by 1,25 dihydroxyvitamin D3. Diabetologia 1994;37(6):552–8.

110. Zella JB, McCary LC, DeLuca HF. Oral administration of 1,25-dihydroxyvitamin D3 completely protects NOD mice from insulin-dependent diabetes mellitus. Arch Biochem Biophys 2003;417(1):77–80.

111. Gysemans CA, Cardozo AK, Callewaert H, et al. 1,25-Dihydroxyvitamin D3 modulates expression of chemokines and cytokines in pancreatic islets: implications for prevention of diabetes in nonobese diabetic mice. Endocrinology 2005; 146(4):1956–64.

112. Takiishi T, Ding L, Baeke F, et al. Dietary supplementation with high doses of regular vitamin D3 safely reduces diabetes incidence in NOD mice when given early and long term. Diabetes 2014;63(6):2026–36.

113. Stene LC, Ulriksen J, Magnus P, et al. Use of cod liver oil during pregnancy associated with lower risk of type I diabetes in the offspring. Diabetologia 2000;43(9):1093–8.

114. Stene LC, Joner G. Use of cod liver oil during the first year of life is associated with lower risk of childhood-onset type 1 diabetes: a large, population-based, case-control study. Am J Clin Nutr 2003;78(6):1128–34.
115. Zipitis CS, Akobeng AK. Vitamin D supplementation in early childhood and risk of type 1 diabetes: a systematic review and meta-analysis. Arch Dis Child 2008; 93(6):512–7.
116. Hyppönen E, Läärä E, Reunanen A, et al. Intake of vitamin D and risk of type 1 diabetes: a birth-cohort study. Lancet 2001;358(9292):1500–3.
117. Gabbay MAL, Sato MN, Finazzo C, et al. Effect of cholecalciferol as adjunctive therapy with insulin on protective immunologic profile and decline of residual β-cell function in new-onset type 1 diabetes mellitus. Arch Pediatr Adolesc Med 2012;166(7):601–7.
118. Pitocco D, Crinò A, Di Stasio E, et al. The effects of calcitriol and nicotinamide on residual pancreatic beta-cell function in patients with recent-onset type 1 diabetes (IMDIAB XI). Diabet Med 2006;23(8):920–3.
119. Lehuen A, Diana J, Zaccone P, et al. Immune cell crosstalk in type 1 diabetes. Nat Rev Immunol 2010;10(7):501–13.
120. Ferreira GB, Gysemans CA, Demengeot J, et al. 1,25-Dihydroxyvitamin D3 promotes tolerogenic dendritic cells with functional migratory properties in NOD Mice. J Immunol 2014;192(9):4210–20.
121. Van Halteren AGS, Tysma OM, Van Etten E, et al. 1a,25-Dihydroxyvitamin D3 or analogue treated dendritic cells modulate human autoreactive T cells via the selective induction of apoptosis. J Autoimmun 2004;23(3):233–9.
122. Treiber G, Prietl B, Fröhlich-Reiterer E, et al. Cholecalciferol supplementation improves suppressive capacity of regulatory T-cells in young patients with new-onset type 1 diabetes mellitus - A randomized clinical trial. Clin Immunol 2015;161(2):217–24.
123. Overbergh L, Decallonne B, Waer M, et al. 1α,25-dihydroxyvitamin D3 induces an autoantigen-specific T-helper 1/T-helper 2 immune shift in NOD mice immunized with GAD65 (p524-543). Diabetes 2000;49(8):1301–7.
124. Bock G, Prietl B, Mader JK, et al. The effect of vitamin D supplementation on peripheral regulatory T cells and β cell function in healthy humans: a randomized controlled trial. Diabetes Metab Res Rev 2011;27(8):942–5.
125. Gregori S, Giarratana N, Smiroldo S, et al. 1a,25-dihydroxyvitamin D3 analog enhances regulatory T-cells and arrests autoimmune diabetes in NOD mice. Diabetes 2002;51(5):1367–74.
126. Wolden-Kirk H, Rondas D, Bugliani M, et al. Discovery of molecular pathways mediating 1,25-dihydroxyvitamin D3 protection against cytokine-induced inflammation and damage of human and male mouse islets of Langerhans. Endocrinology 2014;155(3):736–47.
127. Nylander A, Hafler DA. Multiple sclerosis. J Clin Invest 2012;122(4):1180–8.
128. Goverman J. Autoimmune T cell responses in the central nervous system. Nat Rev Immunol 2009;9(6):393–407.
129. Smolders J, Damoiseaux J, Menheere P, et al. Association study on two vitamin D receptor gene polymorphisms and vitamin D metabolites in multiple sclerosis. Ann N Y Acad Sci 2009;1173:515–20.
130. Ramagopalan SV, Dyment DA, Cader MZ, et al. Rare variants in the CYP27B1 gene are associated with multiple sclerosis. Ann Neurol 2011;70(6):881–6.
131. Jiang T, Li L, Wang Y, et al. The Association Between Genetic Polymorphism rs703842 in CYP27B1 and multiple sclerosis: a meta-analysis. Medicine (Baltimore) 2016;95(19):e3612.

132. Australia and New Zealand Multiple Sclerosis Genetics Consortium (ANZgene). Genome-wide association study identifies new multiple sclerosis susceptibility loci on chromosomes 12 and 20. Nat Genet 2009;41(7):824–8.

133. Agnello L, Scazzone C, Ragonese P, et al. Vitamin D receptor polymorphisms and 25-hydroxyvitamin D in a group of Sicilian multiple sclerosis patients. Neurol Sci 2016;37:261–7.

134. Barizzone N, Pauwels I, Luciano B, et al. No evidence for a role of rare CYP27B1 functional variations in multiple sclerosis. Ann Neurol 2013;73(3):433–7.

135. Ban M, Caillier S, Mero IL, et al. No evidence of association between mutant alleles of the CYP27B1 gene and multiple sclerosis. Ann Neurol 2013;73(3):430–2.

136. Reinthaler E, Machetanz G, Hotzy C, et al. No evidence for a role of rare CYP27B1 variants in Austrian multiple sclerosis patients. Mult Scler 2014; 20(3):391–2.

137. Ramagopalan SV, Maugeri NJ, Handunnetthi L, et al. Expression of the multiple sclerosis-associated MHC class II allele HLA-DRB1*1501 is regulated by vitamin D. PLoS Genet 2009;5(2):e1000369.

138. Karaky M, Alcina A, Fedetz M, et al. The multiple sclerosis-associated regulatory variant rs10877013 affects expression of CYP27B1 and VDR under inflammatory or vitamin D stimuli. Mult Scler 2015;22(8):999–1006.

139. Ascherio A, Munger KL. Environmental risk factors for multiple sclerosis. Part II: noninfectious factors. Ann Neurol 2007;61(6):504–13.

140. Dobson R, Giovannoni G, Ramagopalan S. The month of birth effect in multiple sclerosis: systematic review, meta-analysis and effect of latitude. J Neurol Neurosurg Psychiatr 2013;84:427–32.

141. Ascherio A, Munger KL, White R, et al. Vitamin D as an early predictor of multiple sclerosis activity and progression. JAMA Neurol 2014;71:306–14.

142. Mowry EM, Waubant E, McCulloch CE, et al. Vitamin D status predicts new brain magnetic resonance imaging activity in multiple sclerosis. Ann Neurol 2012; 72(2):234–40.

143. Simpson S, Taylor B, Blizzard L, et al. Higher 25-hydroxyvitamin D is associated with lower relapse risk in multiple sclerosis. Ann Neurol 2010;68(2):193–203.

144. Smolders J, Peelen E, Thewissen M, et al. Circulating vitamin D binding protein levels are not associated with relapses or with vitamin D status in multiple sclerosis. Mult Scler 2014;20(4):433–7.

145. Nielsen NM, Munger KL, Koch-Henriksen N, et al. Neonatal vitamin D status and risk of multiple sclerosis. Neurology 2016;88(1):44–51.

146. Islam T, Gauderman WJ, Cozen W, et al. Childhood sun exposure influences risk of multiple sclerosis in monozygotic twins. Neurology 2007;69(4):381–8.

147. Lemire JM, Archer DC. 1,25-dihydroxyvitamin D3 prevents the in vivo induction of murine experimental autoimmune encephalomyelitis. J Clin Invest 1991;87(3): 1103–7.

148. Sloka S, Silva C, Wang J, et al. Predominance of Th2 polarization by vitamin D through a STAT6-dependent mechanism. J Neuroinflammation 2011;8(1):56.

149. Van Etten E, Branisteanu DD, Overbergh L, et al. Combination of a 1,25-dihydroxyvitamin D3 analog and a bisphosphonate prevents experimental autoimmune encephalomyelitis and preserves bone. Bone 2003;32(4):397–404.

150. Cantorna MT, Hayes CE, Deluca HF. 1,25-Dihydroxyvitamin D3 reversibly blocks the progression of relapsing encephalomyelitis, a model of multiple sclerosis. Proc Natl Acad Sci U S A 1996;93(15):7861–4.

151. Achiron A, Givon U, Magalashvili D, et al. Effect of alfacalcidol on multiple sclerosis-related fatigue: a randomized, double-blind placebo-controlled study. Mult Scler 2015;21(6):767–75.

152. Burton JM, Kimball S, Vieth R, et al. A phase I/II dose-escalation trial of vitamin D3 and calcium in multiple sclerosis. Neurology 2010;74(23):1852–9.

153. Soilu-Hänninen M, Aivo J, Lindström B-M, et al. A randomised, double blind, placebo controlled trial with vitamin D3 as an add on treatment to interferon β-1b in patients with multiple sclerosis. J Neurol Neurosurg Psychiatr 2012; 83(5):565–71.

154. Naghavi Gargari B, Behmanesh M, Shirvani Farsani Z, et al. Vitamin D supplementation up-regulates IL-6 and IL-17A gene expression in multiple sclerosis patients. Int Immunopharmacol 2015;28(1):414–9.

155. Sotirchos ES, Bhargava P, Eckstein C, et al. Safety and immunologic effects of high-vs low-dose cholecalciferol in multiple sclerosis. Neurology 2016;86(4): 382–90.

156. Kampman MT, Steffensen LH, Mellgren SI, et al. Effect of vitamin D3 supplementation on relapses, disease progression, and measures of function in persons with multiple sclerosis: exploratory outcomes from a double-blind randomised controlled trial. Mult Scler 2012;18(8):1144–51.

157. Mosayebi G, Ghazavi A, Ghasami K, et al. Therapeutic effect of vitamin D3 in multiple sclerosis patients. Immunol Invest 2011;40(6):627–39.

158. Bailey SL, Schreiner B, McMahon EJ, et al. CNS myeloid DCs presenting endogenous myelin peptides "preferentially" polarize CD4+ T(H)-17 cells in relapsing EAE. Nat Immunol 2007;8(2):172–80.

159. Durelli L, Conti L, Clerico M, et al. T-helper 17 cells expand in multiple sclerosis and are inhibited by interferon-gamma. Ann Neurol 2009;65(5):499–509.

160. Waisman A, Hauptmann J, Regen T. The role of IL-17 in CNS diseases. Acta Neuropathol 2015;129(5):625–37.

161. Huseby ES, Huseby PG, Shah S, et al. Pathogenic CD8 T cells in multiple sclerosis and its experimental models. Front Immunol 2012;3:64.

162. Denic A, Wootla B, Rodriguez M. CD8(+) T cells in multiple sclerosis. Expert Opin Ther Targets 2013;17(9):1053–66.

163. Nashold FE, Miller DJ, Hayes CE. 1,25-Dihydroxyvitamin D3 treatment decreases macrophage accumulation in the CNS of mice with experimental autoimmune encephalomyelitis. J Neuroimmunol 2000;103(2):171–9.

164. Pedersen LB, Nashold FE, Spach KM, et al. 1,25-Dihydroxyvitamin D3 reverses experimental autoimmune encephalomyelitis by inhibiting chemokine synthesis and monocyte trafficking. J Neurosci Res 2007;85(11):2480–90.

165. Mayne CG, Spanier JA, Relland LM, et al. 1,25-Dihydroxyvitamin D3 acts directly on the T lymphocyte vitamin D receptor to inhibit experimental autoimmune encephalomyelitis. Eur J Immunol 2011;41(3):822–32.

166. Spach KM, Nashold FE, Dittel BN, et al. IL-10 signaling is essential for 1,25-dihydroxyvitamin D3-mediated inhibition of experimental autoimmune encephalomyelitis. J Immunol 2006;177(9):6030–7.

167. Cantorna MT, Waddell A. The vitamin D receptor turns off chronically activated T cells. Ann N Y Acad Sci 2014;1317(1):70–5.

168. Smolders J, Thewissen M, Peelen E, et al. Vitamin D status is positively correlated with regulatory T cell function in patients with multiple sclerosis. PLoS One 2009;4(8):e6635.

169. Grishkan IV, Fairchild AN, Calabresi PA, et al. 1,25-Dihydroxyvitamin D3 selectively and reversibly impairs T helper-cell CNS localization. Proc Natl Acad Sci U S A 2013;110(52):21101–6.

170. Meehan MA, Kerman RH, Lemire JM. 1,25-Dihydroxyvitamin D3 enhances the generation of nonspecific suppressor cells while inhibiting the induction of cytotoxic cells in a human MLR. Cell Immunol 1992;140(2):400–9.

171. Sorensen PS, Blinkenberg M. The potential role for ocrelizumab in the treatment of multiple sclerosis: current evidence and future prospects. Ther Adv Neurol Disord 2016;9(1):44–52.

172. Knippenberg S, Peelen E, Smolders J, et al. Reduction in IL-10 producing B cells (Breg) in multiple sclerosis is accompanied by a reduced naïve/memory Breg ratio during a relapse but not in remission. J Neuroimmunol 2011; 239(1–2):80–6.

173. de la Fuente AG, Errea O, van Wijngaarden P, et al. Vitamin D receptor-retinoid X receptor heterodimer signaling regulates oligodendrocyte progenitor cell differentiation. J Cell Biol 2015;211(5):975–85.

174. Goudarzvand M, Javan M, Mirnajafi-Zadeh J, et al. Vitamins e and D3 attenuate demyelination and potentiate remyelination processes of hippocampal formation of rats following local injection of ethidium bromide. Cell Mol Neurobiol 2010;30(2):289–99.

175. Montava M, Garcia S, Mancini J, et al. Vitamin D3 potentiates myelination and recovery after facial nerve injury. Eur Arch Otorhinolaryngol 2015;272(10): 2815–23.

176. Smolen JS, Aletaha D, McInnes IB. Rheumatoid arthritis. Lancet 2016;6736(16): 1–16.

177. Song GG, Bae S-C, Lee YH. Vitamin D receptor FokI, BsmI, and TaqI polymorphisms and susceptibility to rheumatoid arthritis. Z Rheumatol 2015;1–8.

178. Gomez-Vaquero C, Fiter J, Enjuanes A, et al. Influence of the BsmI polymorphism of the vitamin D receptor gene on rheumatoid arthritis clinical activity. J Rheumatol 2007;34(9):1823–6.

179. Yarwood A, Martin P, Bowes J, et al. Enrichment of vitamin D response elements in RA-associated loci supports a role for vitamin D in the pathogenesis of RA. Genes Immun 2013;14(5):325–9.

180. Cutolo M, Otsa K, Laas K, et al. Circannual vitamin d serum levels and disease activity in rheumatoid arthritis: Northern versus Southern Europe. Clin Exp Rheumatol 2006;24(6):702–4.

181. Vieira VM, Hart JE, Webster TF, et al. Association between residences in U.S. northern latitudes and rheumatoid arthritis: a spatial analysis of the nurses' health study. Environ Health Perspect 2010;118(7):957–61.

182. Arkema EV, Hart JE, Bertrand KA, et al. Exposure to ultraviolet-B and risk of developing rheumatoid arthritis among women in the Nurses' Health Study. Ann Rheum Dis 2013;72(4):506–11.

183. Lin J, Liu J, Davies ML, et al. Serum vitamin D level and rheumatoid arthritis disease activity: review and meta-analysis. PLoS One 2016;11(1):e0146351.

184. Song GG, Bae S-C, Lee YH. Association between vitamin D intake and the risk of rheumatoid arthritis: a meta-analysis. Clin Rheumatol 2012;31(12):1733–9.

185. Cantorna MT, Hayes CE, DeLuca HF. 1,25-Dihydroxycholecalciferol inhibits the progression of arthritis in murine models of human arthritis. J Nutr 1998;128(1): 68–72.

186. Merlino LA, Curtis J, Mikuls TR, et al. Vitamin D intake is inversely associated with rheumatoid arthritis: results from the Iowa Women's Health Study. Arthritis Rheum 2004;50(1):72–7.

187. Salesi M, Farajzadegan Z. Efficacy of Vitamin D in patients with active rheumatoid arthritis receiving methotrexate therapy. Rheumatol Int 2012;32(7):2129–33.

188. Dehghan A, Rahimpour S, Soleymani-Salehabadi H, et al. Role of vitamin D in flare ups of rheumatoid arthritis. Z Rheumatol 2014;73(5):461–4.

189. Andjelkovic Z, Vojinovic J, Pejnovic N, et al. Disease modifying and immunomodulatory effects of high dose 1 alpha (OH) D3 in rheumatoid arthritis patients. Clin Exp Rheumatol 1999;17(4):453–6.

190. Brzustewicz E, Bryl E. The role of cytokines in the pathogenesis of rheumatoid arthritis - practical and potential application of cytokines as biomarkers and targets of personalized therapy. Cytokine 2015;76(2):527–36.

191. Komatsu N, Takayanagi H. Arthritogenic T cells in autoimmune arthritis. Int J Biochem Cell Biol 2015;58:92–6.

192. van Hamburg JP, Asmawidjaja PS, Davelaar N, et al. Th17 but not Th1 cells from early RA patients are potent inducers of MMPs and IL-6, IL-8 upon RASF interaction including autocrine IL-17A production. Arthritis Rheum 2010;63(1):73–83.

193. Colin EM, Asmawidjaja PS, Van Hamburg JP, et al. 1,25-Dihydroxyvitamin D3 modulates Th17 polarization and interleukin-22 expression by memory T cells from patients with early rheumatoid arthritis. Arthritis Rheum 2010;62(1):132–42.

194. Lubberts E, Joosten LAB, Chabaud M, et al. IL-4 gene therapy for collagen arthritis suppresses synovial IL-17 and osteoprotegerin ligand and prevents bone erosion. J Clin Invest 2000;105(12):1697–710.

195. Ehrenstein MR. Compromised function of regulatory T cells in rheumatoid arthritis and reversal by anti-TNF therapy. J Exp Med 2004;200(3):277–85.

196. Nie H, Zheng Y, Li R, et al. Phosphorylation of FOXP3 controls regulatory T cell function and is inhibited by TNF-α in rheumatoid arthritis. Nat Med 2013;19(3): 322–8.

197. Valencia X, Stephens G, Goldbach-Mansky R, et al. TNF downmodulates the function of human CD4+CD25hi T-regulatory cells. Blood 2006;108(1):253–61.

198. Laragione T, Shah A, Gulko PS. The vitamin D receptor regulates rheumatoid arthritis synovial fibroblast invasion and morphology. Mol Med 2012;18: 194–200.

199. Huhtakangas JA, Veijola J, Turunen S, et al. 1,25(OH)2D3 and calcipotriol, its hypocalcemic analog, exert a long-lasting anti-inflammatory and antiproliferative effect in synoviocytes cultured from patients with rheumatoid arthritis and osteoarthritis. J Steroid Biochem Mol Biol 2017. http://dx.doi.org/10.1016/j.jsbmb.2017.01.017.

200. Lam GKW, Petri M. Assessment of systemic lupus erythematosus. Clin Exp Rheumatol 2005;23(5 Suppl 39):S120–32.

201. Mao S, Huang S. Association between vitamin D receptor gene BsmI, FokI, ApaI and TaqI polymorphisms and the risk of systemic lupus erythematosus: a meta-analysis. Rheumatol Int 2014;34(3):381–8.

202. Müller K, Kriegbaum NJ, Baslund B, et al. Vitamin D3 metabolism in patients with rheumatic diseases: low serum levels of 25-hydroxyvitamin D3 in patients with systemic lupus erythematosus. Clin Rheumatol 1995;14(4):397–400.

203. Kamen DL, Cooper GS, Bouali H, et al. Vitamin D deficiency in systemic lupus erythematosus. Autoimmun Rev 2006;5(2):114–7.

204. Peracchi OAB, Terreri MTRA, Munekata RV, et al. Low serum concentrations of 25-hydroxyvitamin D in children and adolescents with systemic lupus erythematosus. Braz J Med Biol Res 2014;47(8):721–6.

205. Foering K, Chang AY, Piette EW, et al. Characterization of clinical photosensitivity in cutaneous lupus erythematosus. J Am Acad Dermatol 2013;69(2): 205–13.

206. Hiraki LT, Feldman CH, Liu J, et al. Prevalence, incidence, and demographics of systemic lupus erythematosus and lupus nephritis from 2000 to 2004 among children in the US Medicaid beneficiary population. Arthritis Rheum 2012; 64(8):2669–76.

207. Carvalho JF, Blank M, Kiss E, et al. Anti-vitamin D, vitamin D in SLE: preliminary results. Ann N Y Acad Sci 2007;1109:550–7.

208. Ben-Zvi I, Aranow C, Mackay M, et al. The impact of vitamin D on dendritic cell function in patients with systemic lupus erythematosus. PLoS One 2010;5(2): e9193.

209. Mok C, Birmingham D, Ho L, et al. Vitamin D deficiency as marker for disease activity and damage in systemic lupus erythematosus: a comparison with anti-dsDNA and anti-C1q. Lupus 2012;21(1):36–42.

210. Ritterhouse LL, Crowe SR, Niewold TB, et al. Vitamin D deficiency is associated with an increased autoimmune response in healthy individuals and in patients with systemic lupus erythematosus. Ann Rheum Dis 2011;70(9):1569–74.

211. Lemire JM, Ince A, Takashima M. 1,25-Dihydroxyvitamin D3 attenuates the expression of experimental murine lupus of MRL/l mice. Autoimmunity 1992; 12:143–8.

212. Abe J, Nakamura K, Takita Y, et al. Prevention of immunological disorders in MRL/l mice by a new synthetic analogue of vitamin D3: 22-oxa-1 alpha,25-dihydroxyvitamin D3. J Nutr Sci Vitaminol (Tokyo) 1990;36(1):21–31.

213. Abou-Raya A, Abou-Raya S, Helmii M. The effect of vitamin D supplementation on inflammatory and hemostatic markers and disease activity in patients with systemic lupus erythematosus: a randomized placebo-controlled trial. J Rheumatol 2013;40(3):265–72.

214. Lima GL, Paupitz J, Aikawa NE, et al. Vitamin D supplementation in adolescents and young adults with juvenile systemic lupus erythematosus for improvement in disease activity and fatigue scores: a randomized, double-blind, placebo-controlled trial. Arthritis Care Res (Hoboken) 2016;68(1):91–8.

215. Aranow C, Kamen DL, Dall 'era M, et al. Randomized, double-blind, placebo-controlled trial of the effect of vitamin D 3 on the interferon signature in patients with systemic lupus erythematosus. Arthritis Rheumatol 2015;67(7):1848–57.

216. Linker-Israeli M, Elstner E, Klinenberg JR, et al. Vitamin D3 and its synthetic analogs inhibit the spontaneous in vitro immunoglobulin production by SLE-derived PBMC. Clin Immunol 2001;99(1):82–93.

217. Yang J, Lu Y-W, Pan H-F, et al. Seasonal distribution of systemic lupus erythematosus activity and its correlation with climate factors. Rheumatol Int 2012;32(8): 2393–9.

218. Marinho A, Carvalho C, Boleixa D, et al. Vitamin D supplementation effects on FoxP3 expression in T cells and FoxP3+/IL-17A ratio and clinical course in systemic lupus erythematosus patients: a study in a Portuguese cohort. Immunol Res 2016;65(1):197–206.

219. Piantoni S, Andreoli L, Scarsi M, et al. Phenotype modifications of T-cells and their shift toward a Th2 response in patients with systemic lupus erythematosus

supplemented with different monthly regimens of vitamin D. Lupus 2015; 24(4–5):490–8.

220. Yan B, Ye S, Chen G, et al. Dysfunctional CD4+,CD25+ regulatory T cells in untreated active systemic lupus erythematosus secondary to interferon-α–producing antigen-presenting cells. Arthritis Rheum 2008;58(3):801–12.

221. Lavi Arab F, Rastin M, Faraji F, et al. Assessment of 1,25-dihydroxyvitamin D3 effects on Treg cells in a mouse model of systemic lupus erythematosus. Immunopharmacol Immunotoxicol 2015;37(1):12–8.

222. Wahono CS, Rusmini H, Soelistyoningsih D, et al. Effects of 1,25(OH)2D3 in immune response regulation of systemic lupus erithematosus (SLE) patient with hypovitamin D. Int J Clin Exp Med 2014;7(1):22–31.

223. Baumgart DC, Carding SR. Inflammatory bowel disease: cause and immunobiology. Lancet 2007;369(9573):1627–40.

224. Xue L-N, Xu K-Q, Zhang W, et al. Associations between vitamin D receptor polymorphisms and susceptibility to ulcerative colitis and Crohn's disease. Inflamm Bowel Dis 2013;19(1):54–60.

225. Wang L, Wang ZT, Hu JJ, et al. Polymorphisms of the vitamin D receptor gene and the risk of inflammatory bowel disease: a meta-analysis. Genet Mol Res 2014;13(2):2598–610.

226. Szilagyi A, Leighton H, Burstein B, et al. Latitude, sunshine, and human lactase phenotype distributions may contribute to geographic patterns of modern disease: the inflammatory bowel disease model. Clin Epidemiol 2014;6:183.

227. Nerich V, Jantchou P, Boutron-Ruault M-C, et al. Low exposure to sunlight is a risk factor for Crohn's disease. Aliment Pharmacol Ther 2011;33(8):940–5.

228. Jantchou P, Clavel-Chapelon F, Racine A, et al. High residential sun exposure is associated with a low risk of incident Crohn's disease in the prospective E3N cohort. Inflamm Bowel Dis 2014;20(1):75–81.

229. Khalili H, Huang ES, Ananthakrishnan AN, et al. Geographical variation and incidence of inflammatory bowel disease among US women. Gut 2012;61(12): 1686–92.

230. Suibhne TN, Cox G, Healy M, et al. Vitamin D deficiency in Crohn's disease: prevalence, risk factors and supplement use in an outpatient setting. J Crohns Colitis 2012;6(2):182–8.

231. Abraham BP, Prasad P, Malaty HM. Vitamin D deficiency and corticosteroid use are risk factors for low bone mineral density in inflammatory bowel disease patients. Dig Dis Sci 2014;59(8):1878–84.

232. Del Pinto R, Pietropaoli D, Chandar AK, et al. Association between inflammatory bowel disease and vitamin D deficiency: a systematic review and meta-analysis. Inflamm Bowel Dis 2015;21(11):2708–17.

233. Torki M, Gholamrezaei A, Mirbagher L, et al. Vitamin D deficiency associated with disease activity in patients with inflammatory bowel diseases. Dig Dis Sci 2015;60(10):3085–91.

234. Ulitsky A, Ananthakrishnan AN, Naik A, et al. Vitamin D deficiency in patients with inflammatory bowel disease: association with disease activity and quality of life. JPEN J Parenter Enteral Nutr 2011;35(3):308–16.

235. Blanck S, Aberra F. Vitamin d deficiency is associated with ulcerative colitis disease activity. Dig Dis Sci 2013;58(6):1698–702.

236. Ham M, Longhi MS, Lahiff C, et al. Vitamin D levels in adults with Crohn's disease are responsive to disease activity and treatment. Inflamm Bowel Dis 2014;20(5):856–60.

237. Garg M, Rosella O, Lubel JS, et al. Association of circulating vitamin D concentrations with intestinal but not systemic inflammation in inflammatory bowel disease. Inflamm Bowel Dis 2013;19(12):2634–43.

238. Cantorna MT, Munsick C, Bemiss C, et al. 1,25-Dihydroxycholecalciferol prevents and ameliorates symptoms of experimental murine inflammatory bowel disease. J Nutr 2000;130(11):2648–52.

239. Zhang H, Wu H, Liu L, et al. 1,25-dihydroxyvitamin D3 regulates the development of chronic colitis by modulating both T helper (Th)1 and Th17 activation. APMIS 2015;123(6):490–501.

240. Laverny G, Penna G, Vetrano S, et al. Efficacy of a potent and safe vitamin D receptor agonist for the treatment of inflammatory bowel disease. Immunol Lett 2010;131(1):49–58.

241. Jørgensen SP, Agnholt J, Glerup H, et al. Clinical trial: vitamin D3 treatment in Crohn's disease - a randomized double-blind placebo-controlled study. Aliment Pharmacol Ther 2010;32(3):377–83.

242. Raftery T, Martineau AR, Greiller CL, et al. Effects of vitamin D supplementation on intestinal permeability, cathelicidin and disease markers in Crohn's disease: results from a randomised double-blind placebo-controlled study. United European Gastroenterol J 2015;3(3):294–302.

243. Wingate KE, Jacobson K, Issenman R, et al. 25-Hydroxyvitamin D concentrations in children with Crohn's disease supplemented with either 2000 or 400 IU daily for 6 months: a randomized controlled study. J Pediatr 2014;164(4): 860–5.

244. Ananthakrishnan AN, Cagan A, Gainer VS, et al. Normalization of plasma 25-hydroxy vitamin d is associated with reduced risk of surgery in Crohn's disease. Inflamm Bowel Dis 2013;19(9):1.

245. Huang Y, Chen Z. Inflammatory bowel disease related innate immunity and adaptive immunity. Am J Transl Res 2016;8(6):2490–7.

246. Wang TT, Dabbas B, Laperriere D, et al. Direct and indirect induction by 1,25-dihydroxyvitamin D3 of the NOD2/CARD15-defensin beta2 innate immune pathway defective in Crohn disease. J Biol Chem 2010;285(4):2227–31.

247. Bartels LE, Jørgensen SP, Bendix M, et al. 25-Hydroxy vitamin D3 modulates dendritic cell phenotype and function in Crohn's disease. Inflammopharmacology 2013;21(2):177–86.

248. Dadaei T, Safapoor MH, Asadzadeh Aghdaei H, et al. Effect of vitamin D3 supplementation on TNF-α serum level and disease activity index in Iranian IBD patients. Gastroenterol Hepatol Bed Bench 2015;8(1):49–55.

249. Ardizzone S, Cassinotti A, Trabattoni D, et al. Immunomodulatory effects of 1,25-dihydroxyvitamin D3 on TH1/TH2 cytokines in inflammatory bowel disease: an in vitro study. Int J Immunopathol Pharmacol 2009;22(1):63–71.

250. Yu S, Bruce D, Froicu M, et al. Failure of T cell homing, reduced CD4/CD8alphaalpha intraepithelial lymphocytes, and inflammation in the gut of vitamin D receptor KO mice. Proc Natl Acad Sci U S A 2008;105(52):20834–9.

251. Cheroutre H, Lambolez F. The thymus chapter in the life of gut-specific intra epithelial lymphocytes. Curr Opin Immunol 2008;20(2):185–91.

252. Khajavi A, Amirhakimi GH. The rachoitic lung: pulmonary findings in 30 infants and children with malnutritional rickets. Clin Pediatr (Phila) 1977;16(1):36–8.

253. Rook GA, Steele J, Fraher L, et al. Vitamin D3, gamma interferon, and control of proliferation of Mycobacterium tuberculosis by human monocytes. Immunology 1986;57(1):159–63.

254. Cannell JJ, Vieth R, Umhau JC, et al. Epidemic influenza and vitamin D. Epidemiol Infect 2006;134(6):1129–40.
255. Ginde AA, Mansbach JM, Camargo CA. Association between serum 25-hydroxyvitamin d level and upper respiratory tract infection in the Third National Health and Nutrition Examination Survey. Arch Intern Med 2009;169(4):384.
256. Jolliffe DA, Griffiths CJ, Martineau AR. Vitamin D in the prevention of acute respiratory infection: systematic review of clinical studies. J Steroid Biochem Mol Biol 2013;136:321–9.
257. Zhang H-Q, Deng A, Guo C-F, et al. Association between FokI polymorphism in vitamin D receptor gene and susceptibility to spinal tuberculosis in Chinese Han population. Arch Med Res 2010;41(1):46–9.
258. Gao L, Tao Y, Zhang L, et al. Vitamin D receptor genetic polymorphisms and tuberculosis: updated systematic review and meta-analysis. Int J Tuberc Lung Dis 2010;14(1):15–23.
259. Lewis SJ, Baker I, Davey Smith G. Meta-analysis of vitamin D receptor polymorphisms and pulmonary tuberculosis risk. Int J Tuberc Lung Dis 2005;9(10): 1174–7.
260. Junaid K, Rehman A, Jolliffe DA, et al. Vitamin D deficiency associates with susceptibility to tuberculosis in Pakistan, but polymorphisms in VDR, DBP and CYP2R1 do not. BMC Pulm Med 2016;16(1):73.
261. Huang L, Liu C, Liao G, et al. Vitamin D receptor gene FokI polymorphism contributes to increasing the risk of tuberculosis. Medicine (Baltimore) 2015;94(51): e2256.
262. McNamara L, Takuva S, Chirwa T, et al. Prevalence of common vitamin D receptor gene polymorphisms in HIV-infected and uninfected South Africans. Int J Mol Epidemiol Genet 2016;7(1):74–80.
263. Wang TJ, Zhang F, Richards JB, et al. Common genetic determinants of vitamin D insufficiency: a genome-wide association study. Lancet 2010;376(9736): 180–8.
264. Wejse C, Olesen R, Rabna P, et al. Serum 25-hydroxyvitamin D in a West African population of tuberculosis patients and unmatched healthy controls. Am J Clin Nutr 2007;86(5):1376–83.
265. Williams B, Williams AJ, Anderson ST. Vitamin D deficiency and insufficiency in children with tuberculosis. Pediatr Infect Dis J 2008;27(10):941–2.
266. Ustianowski A, Shaffer R, Collin S, et al. Prevalence and associations of vitamin D deficiency in foreign-born persons with tuberculosis in London. J Infect 2005; 50(5):432–7.
267. Martineau AR, Honecker FU, Wilkinson RJ, et al. Vitamin D in the treatment of pulmonary tuberculosis. J Steroid Biochem Mol Biol 2007;103(3–5):793–8.
268. Wejse C, Gomes VF, Rabna P, et al. Vitamin D as supplementary treatment for tuberculosis. Am J Respir Crit Care Med 2009;179(9):843–50.
269. Tan BH, Meinken C, Bastian M, et al. Macrophages acquire neutrophil granules for antimicrobial activity against intracellular pathogens. J Immunol 2006;177(3): 1864–71.
270. Rahman S, Rehn A, Rahman J, et al. Pulmonary tuberculosis patients with a vitamin D deficiency demonstrate low local expression of the antimicrobial peptide LL-37 but enhanced FoxP3+ regulatory T cells and IgG-secreting cells. Clin Immunol 2015;156(2):85–97.
271. Olliver M, Spelmink L, Hiew J, et al. Immunomodulatory effects of vitamin D on innate and adaptive immune responses to Streptococcus pneumoniae. J Infect Dis 2013;208(9):1474–81.

272. Romero R, Espinoza J, Gonçalves LF, et al. The role of inflammation and infection in preterm birth. Semin Reprod Med 2007;25(1):21–39.
273. Muehleisen B, Bikle DD, Aguilera C, et al. PTH/PTHrP and vitamin D control antimicrobial peptide expression and susceptibility to bacterial skin infection. Sci Transl Med 2012;4(135):135ra66.
274. Schauber J, Dorschner RA, Coda AB, et al. Injury enhances TLR2 function and antimicrobial peptide expression through a vitamin D-dependent mechanism. J Clin Invest 2007;117(3):803–11.
275. Schauber J, Oda Y, Büchau AS, et al. Histone acetylation in keratinocytes enables control of the expression of cathelicidin and CD14 by 1,25-dihydroxyvitamin D3. J Invest Dermatol 2008;128(4):816–24.
276. Martineau AR, Jolliffe DA, Hooper RL, et al. Vitamin D supplementation to prevent acute respiratory tract infections: systematic review and meta-analysis of individual participant data. BMJ 2017;356:i6583.
277. Khare D, Godbole NM, Pawar SD, et al. Calcitriol [1, 25[OH]2 D3] pre- and posttreatment suppresses inflammatory response to influenza A (H1N1) infection in human lung A549 epithelial cells. Eur J Nutr 2013;52(4):1405–15.
278. Brockman-Schneider RA, Pickles RJ, Gern JE. Effects of vitamin D on airway epithelial cell morphology and rhinovirus replication. PLoS One 2014;9(1):e86755. Rohde GG, ed.
279. Barlow PG, Svoboda P, Mackellar A, et al. Antiviral activity and increased host defense against influenza infection elicited by the human cathelicidin LL-37. PLoS One 2011;6(10):e25333. Kovats S, ed.

Genetic Diseases of Vitamin D Metabolizing Enzymes

Glenville Jones, PhD[a],*, Marie Laure Kottler, MD, PhD[b,c],
Karl Peter Schlingmann, MD[d]

KEYWORDS

• Vitamin D metabolism • Cytochrome P450 • Rickets • Hypercalcemia

KEY POINTS

• This review presents current knowledge of the key activating and inactivating cytochrome P450 (CYP)–containing enzymes involved in vitamin D metabolism in mammals.
• The case for mutations of vitamin D_3-25-hydroxylase/CYP2R1 associated with vitamin D–dependent rickets (VDDR), type 1B, is presented.
• The case for mutations of 25-hydroxyvitamin D_3-1α-hydroxylase/CYP27B1 associated with VDDR, type 1A, is presented.
• The case for mutations of 25-hydroxyvitamin D_3-24-hydroxylase/CYP24A1 associated with idiopathic infantile hypercalcemia is presented.
• Symptoms, diagnosis, treatment, and management of VDDR and idiopathic infantile hypercalcemia are reviewed.

INTRODUCTION

The activation of vitamin D_3 is accomplished by sequential steps of 25-hydroxylation, first in the liver[1] to produce the main circulating form, 25-hydroxyvitamin D_3 [25-(OH)D_3], followed by 1α-hydroxylation in the kidney and extrarenal sites to produce the hormonal form, 1α,25-dihydroxyvitamin D_3 [1,25-(OH)$_2D_3$][2–4] (**Fig. 1**). Although vitamin D_2 undergoes the same hydoxylations as vitamin D_3, this article focuses on the latter because most current knowledge comes from studies of vitamin D_3. Evidence from a variety of mammalian species has revealed that several cytochrome P450 (CYP)

Disclosures: The authors have nothing to disclose.
[a] Department of Biomedical and Molecular Sciences, Queen's University, Room 650, Botterell Hall, Kingston, ON K7L 3N6, Canada; [b] Department of Genetics, University de Basse-Normandie, National Reference Center for Rare Diseases of Calcium and Phosphorus Metabolism, Caen University Hospital, Avenue de la Côte de Nacre, 14033 Caen, France; [c] Team 7450 BIO-TARGEN, Caen-Normandy University, Esplanade de la Paix, 14032 Caen, France; [d] Department of General Pediatrics, University Children's Hospital, Waldeyerstr. 22, D-48149 Muenster, Germany
* Corresponding author.
E-mail address: gj1@queensu.ca

Endocrinol Metab Clin N Am 46 (2017) 1095–1117
http://dx.doi.org/10.1016/j.ecl.2017.07.011
0889-8529/17/© 2017 Elsevier Inc. All rights reserved.

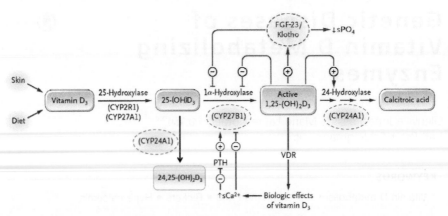

Fig. 1. Calcium and phosphate homeostasis and its close association with the enzymes involved in vitamin D metabolism. (*Adapted from* Schlingmann KP, Kaufmann M, Weber S, et al. Mutations in CYP24A1 and idiopathic infantile hypercalcemia. N Engl J Med 2011;365:412; with permission.)

enzymes—CYP2R1, CYP27A1, CYP3A4, CYP2D25, and perhaps others—are capable of 25-hydroxylation of vitamin D_3 and could be referred to as vitamin D_3-25-hydroxylase but that CYP2R1 is emerging as the physiologically relevant enzyme.[5] The nature of the 25-(OH)D_3-1α-hydroxylase enzyme responsible for 1α-hydroxylation as CYP27B1 is undisputed.[6,7] The third enzyme under focus is the vitamin D inactivating enzyme, 25-(OH)D_3-24-hydroxylase, known as CYP24A1, which is responsible for the side chain hydroxylation of both 25-(OH)D_3 and 1,25-(OH)$_2D_3$.[8]

CYPs are classified into 2 main subtypes based on their subcellular location: microsomal or mitochondrial; vitamin D metabolism features both subtypes.[9] Both microsomal and mitochondrial CYP subtypes are components of electron transport chains; the microsomal CYPs (eg CYP2R1) require a single general purpose protein NADPH-CYP reductase, whereas mitochondrial vitamin D–related CYPs (eg CYP27A1, CYP27B1, and CYP24A1) require the assistance of 2 additional electron-transporting proteins consisting of a general purpose ferredoxin reductase, a general purpose ferredoxin, and a highly specific CYP.[8] Most of the vitamin D–related CYPs catalyze single or multiple hydroxylation reactions on specific carbons of the vitamin D substrate using a transient Fe-O intermediate. The exact site of hydroxylation, termed *regioselectivity*, can be somewhat variable with vitamin D–related CYPs; human CYP24A1 is documented to hydroxylate at C23, C24, or C26.

All vitamin D–related CYP proteins possess approximately 500 amino acids, which makes them 50 kDa to 55 kDa, featuring abundant highly conserved residues that suggest a common secondary structure with multiple highly conserved helices (designated A–L) connected by loops and β-sheet structures.[9] CYPs possess a cysteine residue and 2 other residues near to the C-terminus, which covalently bind and align the heme group, in addition to several other domains for interaction with the electron transferring machinery, such as ferredoxin or NADPH-CYP reductase. The N-terminus inserts into the endoplasmic reticular membrane for microsomal CYPs or the inner mitochondrial membrane for mitochondrial CYPs. The substrate-binding pocket is formed by several secondary structures folded around the distal face of the heme-group so that substrate can be brought to within 3.2 Å of the iron atom for hydroxylation.

Attempts to identify the key substrate-binding residues were originally guided by homology models[10–14] based on 10 to 20 available crystal structures from unrelated soluble prokaryotic CYPs. Recently, the study of the active site of vitamin D–related CYPs has been further advanced by the emergence of x-ray crystallography–derived models of CYP2R1 and CYP24A1, respectively.[15,16] Mutational analyses that pinpoint residues involved in contact with the main functional groups (hydroxyls) or hydrophobic cis-triene of the vitamin D substrate as well as define those amino acid residues that are closest to the hydroxylation-sensitive 1α-position in CYP27B1 or the side-chain C-23 to C-27 carbons in the side-chain hydroxylases (CYP2R1, CYP24A1, and CYP27A1) have also aided knowledge of the structure. These studies require expression of the CYP in question (mutated or wild-type) in a mammalian cell system (eg, V79 Chinese hamster lung fibroblasts) or the use of an in vitro cell-free system where the *Escherichia coli*–expressed CYP is incubated with the relevant mitochondrial or microsomal NADPH generating system.[8,9]

Based on emerging knowledge of the structure of vitamin D–related CYPs, genetic variants found in patients as loss-of-function mutations or polymorphisms can be rationalized, if not predicted. In the following sections, diseases associated with these 3 vitamin D–related CYPs are described: CYP2R1 (vitamin D–dependent rickets [VDDR], type 1B [VDDR-1B]), CYP27B1 (VDDR, type 1A [VDDR-1A]), and CYP24A1 (idiopathic infantile hypercalcemia [IIH]) as well as some of the evidence to support the association of the specific CYP and the pertinent vitamin D hydroxylase.

VITAMIN D_3-25-HYDROXYLASE, CYP2R1: VITAMIN D–DEPENDENT RICKETS, TYPE 1B
Evidence for Association

CYP2R1 is a liver microsomal CYP that is 501 amino acids in size, cloned from mouse and human, and shown by real-time polymerase chain reaction (PCR) to be primarily expressed in liver and testis.[17] Alignment of the CYP2R1 sequences of greater than 200 species reveals a highly conserved structure in comparison to other broad-specificity, xenobiotic-metabolizing CYP2 family members.[18] Initial studies demonstrated that human CYP2R1, unlike all other putative 25-hydroxylases, 25-hydroxylates both vitamin D_2 and vitamin D_3 equally well at physiologically relevant substrate concentrations.[17] Subsequent work[19] using nanomolar substrate concentrations of $[^3H]1\alpha\text{-(OH)}D_2$ has reinforced the finding that transfected mouse and human CYP2R1 enzymes are able to synthesize the predominant in vivo metabolite 1,25-$(OH)_2D_2$, and not 1,24-$(OH)_2D_2$, the minor in vivo product of $1\alpha\text{-(OH)}D_2$, which is the major in vitro product of $1\alpha\text{-(OH)}D_2$ incubated with CYP27A1. Recent work[15] using bacterially expressed human CYP2R1 protein in a solubilized system revealed enzyme kinetic properties consistent with both of the earlier studies.[17,19] Human CYP2R1 showed K_m values of 4.4 μM, 11.3 μM, and 15.8 μM for vitamin D_3, $1\alpha\text{-(OH)}D_2$ and $1\alpha\text{-(OH)}D_3$ respectively, suggesting a high-affinity, low-capacity enzyme given physiologic vitamin D levels in the nanomolar range whereas K_{cat} values of 0.48 mol/min/mol, 0.45 mol/min/mol, and 1.17 mol/min/mol P450 were observed for the same 3 substrates. The regioselectivity of human CYP2R1 was clearly confined to the C-25 position with no peaks corresponding to 24-hydroxylated or 26-hydroxylated products, in sharp contrast to the findings with CYP27A1[15] and lack of activity toward 25-$(OH)D_3$, cholesterol, or 7-dehydrocholesterol.

Strushkevich and colleagues[15] also solved the crystal structure of a functional form of CYP2R1 in complex with vitamin D_3, representing the first crystal structure of a vitamin D–related CYP. The crystal structure generally confirmed the helical nature and binding pocket of CYP2R1 predicted from other CYPs using homology modeling.[10] Co-crystallized vitamin D_3 in the CYP2R1 occupied a position with the side chain pointing toward the heme group, but somewhat paradoxically, it was not optimally placed for hydroxylation, because the C-25 carbon was 6.5 Å from the heme iron.

Another piece of evidence that strengthens the case for CYP2R1 being the vitamin D_3-25-hydroxylase is the finding of a human p.Leu99Pro mutation in a Nigerian family, which results in VDDR-1B[20] (**Fig. 2**A). This disease was postulated 4 decades ago[21] after the elucidation of vitamin D metabolism. The genetic nature of the p.Leu99Pro mutation of CYP2R1 was determined by Cheng and colleagues,[5] a decade after the initial identification of the Nigerian rachitic patient, making patient and family follow-up difficult. Subsequent genetic analysis of exon 2 of CYP2R1 by Cheng and colleagues[5] in 50 Nigerian individuals, however, revealed 1 heterozygote with the p.Leu99Pro mutation, suggesting that there may be a founder gene effect in the Nigerian population, where vitamin D deficiency is prevalent.[22] Although the Leu99 residue is not in a region of the CYP2R1 coding for substrate-binding domain, it is involved in water-mediated hydrogen bonding to the Arg445 amide nitrogen located 3 residues from the heme coordinating Cys448, and thus a p.Leu99Pro mutation probably results in a misfolded protein with little or no enzyme activity. Numerous attempts to bacterially express human CYP2R1 with a p.Leu99Pro mutation, at the same time as the wild-type human CYP2R1, failed, leading Strushkevich and colleagues[15] to conclude that CYP2R1 with p.Leu99Pro is misfolded or shows poor protein stability. In a recent follow-up study,[23] the p.Leu99Pro mutation was transiently expressed in HEK293T cells and shown to be devoid of enzyme activity. Thacher and colleagues[23] also

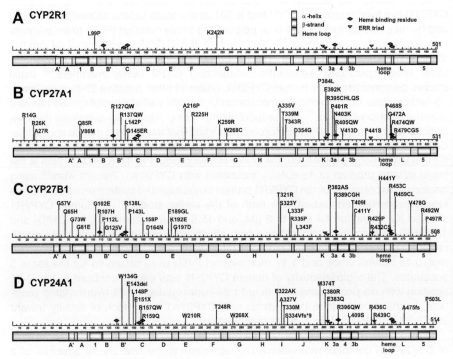

Fig. 2. Location of mutations found in (A) CYP2R1, (B) CYP27A1, (C) CYP27B1, and (D) CYP24A1 proteins. (*Data from* David Prosser, Queen's University, unpublished data, 2017.)

identified a second p.Lys242Asn mutation associated with rickets in a cohort of Nigerian children. Subsequently, Molin and colleagues[24] have identified a total of 6 patients with p.Leu99Pro or another mutation of CYP2R1, namely p.G42_I46del insR in a population of French rachitic patients.

Furthermore, a genome-wide association study of the genetic determinants of serum 25-hydroxyvitamin D (25-[OH]D) concentrations[25] concluded that variants at the chromosomal locus for CYP2R1 (11p15) were the second strongest association of only 4 sites, vitamin D binding protein (VDBP or GC), CYP24A1, and 7-dehydrocholesterol reductase (DHR7) being the others. Variants of the other 25-hydroxylases (eg, CYP27A1) were not associated with serum 25-(OH)D concentrations, arguing that CYP27A1 (**Fig. 2**B) is not involved in 25-hydroxylation of vitamin D at physiologic substrate concentrations.

Although the clinical case for CYP2R1 representing the physiologic 25-hydroxylase has become stronger, the development of a CYP2R1 knockout mouse has provided a slightly different conclusion. Zhu and colleagues[26] 2013 found that ablation of the CYP2R1 gene resulted in a 60% reduction of serum 25-(OH)D$_3$ concentration, but unlike the human situation, the mice showed no signs of rickets. In the same study, Zhu and colleagues[26] reported that the CYP27A1 null mouse had elevated serum 25-(OH)D$_3$ and the CYP2R1/CYP27A1 double-knockout mouse had an even lower serum 25-(OH)D$_3$. The investigators concluded from these mouse studies that CYP2R1 is the major, but not the only, 25-hydroxylase in this species. The lack of rickets in CYP2R1 null mice and the detection of residual 25-(OH)D$_3$ in the serum of these mice and in patients with loss-of-function mutations of CYP2R1 by reliable liquid chromatography tandem–mass spectrometry (LC-MS/MS) methods are independent pieces of evidence that there is some redundancy in the liver vitamin D$_3$-25-hydroxylase family of enzymes that can compensate for the defective CYP2R1.

Symptoms of Vitamin D–Dependent Rickets, Type 1B

VDDR-1B caused by recessive loss-of-function mutations in the CYP2R1 gene encoding 25-hydroxylase is a rare disorder with only a few clinical descriptions published so far (discussed previously). Compared with VDDR-1A (discussed later), however, a milder phenotype can be assumed. The first patients originally reported by Casella and colleagues[20] and genetically analyzed by Cheng and colleagues[5] (CYP2R1-p.Leu99Pro) presented in early childhood (between 2 and 7 years of age) with clinical signs of rickets. The laboratory evaluation of the index patient showed low normal serum calcium levels, low serum phosphate levels, and elevated serum alkaline phosphatase levels. Although serum levels of 1α,25-(OH)$_2$D$_3$ were normal, the patient was found to have low levels of 25-(OH)D$_3$ despite a history of adequate vitamin D intake. A second family of Arabian descent was reported by Al Mutair and colleagues.[27] The 2 affected children presented with progressive bowing of legs and bone pain but without additional signs of rickets at school age. The genetic analysis showed 2 loss-of-function alleles in compound-heterozygous state. More recently, Thacher and colleagues[23] reported the identical p.Leu99Pro variant observed by Cheng and colleagues as well as a novel p.Lys242Gln variant in 2 families with multiple cases of clinical rickets. As discussed previously, the probands from these families as the first patient reported by Casella and colleagues[20] and Cheng and colleagues[5] were all of Nigerian descent. Clinical presentations and laboratory findings in the families reported by Thacher and colleagues[23] are comparable to the initial patient reported by Casella and colleagues.[20] Ages at presentation similarly varied between 2 years and 12 years of age. Two findings reported by Thacher and colleagues[23] deserve special attention. First, the mutation p.Leu99Pro was also detected in homozygous state in the father of 1 family who did not present with skeletal deformities in childhood. Second, in the probands with clinical signs of rickets in the second family, only 1 mutated (p.Leu99Pro) allele was detected arguing either for a gene dosage effect of CYP2R1 with a milder phenotype also observed in patients with only 1 mutated allele or a second mutated allele that was not detected by the mutational analysis. Molin and colleagues[24] recently reported CYP2R1 mutations in 2 French families with VDDR-1B. The index patients of both families presented in infancy and early childhood, respectively, with bowing of lower extremities. Mutational analyses of the CYP2R1 gene detected the previously described p.Leu99Pro mutations in homozygous state in the index patient of family 1 as well as a new variant (p.G42_L46delinsR) in the index patient of family 2. The p.Leu99Pro variant was also detected in homozygous state in 2 siblings as well as a paternal aunt and uncle (suggesting multiple consanguinity). Of these 4 additional homozygous carriers of p.Leu99Pro, 2 (aunt and uncle) had presented in infancy with leg bowing and were fortunately treated with 25-(OH)D$_3$. Of the 2 younger siblings of the index patients, 1 had developed leg bowing but had remained untreated prior to the diagnosis in his elder brother, the younger sister had remained clinically asymptomatic (4 years of age). Biochemical abnormalities found in carriers of homozygous CYP2R1 mutations in both families were in accordance with the previous descriptions. In summary, these clinical findings argue for a milder phenotype in VDDR-1B compared with VDDR-1A, even with the possibility of asymptomatic clinical courses.

Diagnostic Test for Vitamin D–Dependent Rickets, Type 1B

In addition to the radiological findings of rickets in affected children, all VDDR-1B patients present with low serum 25-(OH)D levels. Many different methods are available to measure serum 25-(OH)D, including a variety of antibody-based and LC-MS/MS–based methods.[28] Of these, the LC-MS/MS methods offer greater specificity and sensitivity and still detect a 25-(OH)D value in the 5 to 10 ng/mL range in VDDR-1B. Normal 25-(OH)D values are considered greater than 20 ng/mL, although there is considerable evidence that florid rickets only becomes evident in vitamin D–deficient individuals at 25-(OH)D values less than 12 ng/mL.

Differential Diagnosis of Vitamin D–Dependent Rickets, Type 1B, Versus Other Forms of Rickets

The detection of low serum levels of 25-(OH)D in a child with clinical and radiographic rickets and compatible laboratory findings (low serum calcium, high alkaline phosphatase, secondary hyperparathyroidism) almost automatically guides to the diagnosis of vitamin D deficiency rickets, the most likely differential diagnosis by far. A therapy with vitamin D according to current recommendations is regularly initiated. Although a history of adequate vitamin D intake might raise some doubt, only the lack of response to standardized treatment in a compliant patient leads to a diagnosis of a hereditary defect in vitamin D activation. In contrast to VDDR-1B, patients with VDDR-1A and VDDR-2 exhibit normal serum levels of 25-(OH)D.

Treatment and Management of Vitamin D–Dependent Rickets, Type 1B

In their initial publication, Casella and colleagues[20] report a failure of treatment with vitamin D in appropriate doses to correct biochemical abnormalities and radiographic deformities. In contrast, Al Mutair and colleagues[27] demonstrate a clinical response as well as significant increases in serum 25-(OH)D$_3$ in their 2 patients with 2 CYP2R1 null-alleles under treatment with daily oral vitamin D$_3$ (5000 IU/d and 10,000 IU/d, respectively). Similarly, Thacher and colleagues[23] report a successful challenge with high-dose oral vitamin D (50,000 IU vitamin D_2 as well as vitamin D_3) in their patients: although the observed rise in serum 25-(OH)D was blunted in their probands with mutations in CYP2R1. The investigators report an incremental increase depending on the number of affected alleles (heterozygous vs homozygous CYP2R1-p.Leu99Pro). Also, initially low levels of active 1,25-$(OH)_2D$ increased in response to the administration of vitamin D_2 or D_3. These findings, especially those of Al Mutair and colleagues,[27] suggest the existence of other 25-hydroxylases contributing to the formation of 25-(OH)D when substrate levels are raised by supplementation. This assumption would be in accordance with observations in *Cyp2r1* knockout mice that exhibit markedly reduced but detectable 25-(OH)D levels in homozygous *Cyp2r1* $-/-$ mice and under therapy show a gene-dosage effect on circulating levels of 25-(OH)D. Unfortunately, no long-term medical therapies are reported in these publications. All patients of the described French families received treatment with physiologic doses of 25-$(OH)D_3$ after genetic diagnosis that resulted in a complete resolution of clinical and laboratory abnormalities. These observations together with the pathophysiology of the disease strongly argue for preparations containing 25-$(OH)D_3$ (calcidiol and calcifediol) as the therapeutic option of choice for VDDR-1B.

25-HYDROXYVITAMIN D_3-1α-HYDROXYLASE, CYP27B1: VITAMIN D–DEPENDENT RICKETS, TYPE 1A

Evidence for Association

25-(OH)D–1α-hydroxylase represents a central regulatory axis of the calcium and phosphate homeostatic systems, subject to up-regulation by PTH, low Ca^{2+}, and low PO_4^{3-} levels[29,30] and down-regulation by fibroblast growth factor (FGF)-23[31] (see **Fig. 1**). It was quickly recognized that serum 1α,25-$(OH)_2D_3$ was predominantly made in the kidney[3,32,33] with a parathyroid hormone (PTH)-regulated form located in the proximal convoluted tubule and a calcitonin-regulated form in the proximal straight tubule.[34,35] Numerous investigations also reported an extrarenal 25-(OH) D-1α-hydroxylase activity in several sites, including placenta, bone, keratinocytes, and macrophages.[36–43] In 1997, several groups coincidentally cloned, sequenced, and characterized CYP27B1 from rat, mouse, and human species.[6,7,42,43] Although many of these groups used kidney libraries as the source of the enzyme, other groups reported finding the same CYP27B1mRNA in keratinocyte[43] and human colonic HT-29 cell libraries.[44] Subsequently, it has been confirmed that the CYP27B1 protein is identical in all locations[45] whether renal or extrarenal, although the regulation in these different tissue forms involves different hormones and modulators.

Human CYP27B1 is a 507 amino acid protein with a molecular mass of approximately 55 kDa.[8] CYP27B1 1α-hydroxylates 25-$(OH)D_2$ and 25-$(OH)D_3$ equally efficiently to give the active hormonal form of each vitamin. The genetic condition, VDDR-1A, in which the 1α-hydroxylase enzyme is absent or defective, due to mutation of CYP27B1, was first recognized in the early 1970s by Fraser and colleagues[21] and Scriver and colleagues.[46] They showed that patients had low or absent serum 1,25-$(OH)_2D$ and could be successfully treated using small amounts of synthetic 1,25-$(OH)_2D_3$. VDDR-1A involves a resistant rickets phenotype, characterized by hypocalcemia, hypophosphatemia, secondary hyperparathyroidism, and undermineralized bone. It is essentially cured by physiologic (microgram) amounts of 1,25-$(OH)_2D_3$ or pharmacologic (milligram) amounts of 25-$(OH)D_3$ or vitamin D, which is consistent with a block in 1α-hydroxylation activity.[21] Subsequent work mapped the CYP27B1 gene to 12q13.1-q13.3, which is the same location established for the VDDR-1A disease.[6] Human CYP27B1 mutations occur throughout the gene (**Fig. 2**C) resulting in defective and misfolded proteins with little or no activity.[47–51]

At least 2 groups have created CYP27B1-null mice,[52,53] which exhibit a lack of 1α-hydroxylated metabolites in the blood and tissues, revealing that CYP27B1 is the sole source of 1,25-$(OH)_2$D in the body. The mouse phenotype mirrors human VDDR-1A in terms of resistant rickets. The animals also show a reduction in $CD4^+$ and $CD8^+$ peripheral lymphocytes, and the female mice are infertile[54] unless raised on a rescue diet. Detailed bone histomorphometric analyses of the CYP27B1 and CYP27B1/PTH double-knockout mice established that 1,25-$(OH)_2D_3$ deficiency resulted in epiphyseal dysgenesis and only minor changes in trabecular bone volume.[54] Bikle and colleagues[55] showed that CYP27B1 is also required for optimal epidermal differentiation and permeability barrier homeostasis in the skin of mice. Administration of a normal diet supplemented with either small amounts of 1,25-$(OH)_2D_3$ or use of a high calcium rescue diet largely corrects the mineral metabolism and bone defects seen in the CYP27B1-null mouse.[56–59] Tissue-specific knockout of the mouse Cyp27b1 gene in chondrocytes has been achieved and suggests that local production of 1,25-$(OH)_2D_3$ plays a role in growth plate development[60,61] but not directly—the defect seems due to increased FGF-23.

The availability of specific CYP27B1 mRNA and anti-CYP27B1 protein antibodies has allowed for a more rigorous exploration of the extrarenal expression of the enzyme. Diaz and colleagues[62] used Northern blot analysis and reverse transcriptase–PCR to examine mRNA expression in human synctiotrophoblasts and concluded that there was CYP27B1 expression in human placenta. Using similar techniques, several groups reported low but detectable expression of CYP27B1 in a variety of cultured cell lines and freshly isolated cell explants for example, prostate and colonic cells.[63–65] Immunohistochemistry data from analysis of animal and human tissues have revealed the presence of the CYP27B1 protein in several tissues purported to express 1α-hydroxylase activity, for example, skin, colon, macrophage, prostate, and breast.[63–65] Not all studies have reached the conclusion that CYP27B1 is expressed outside of the kidney in normal, nonpregnant animals. Using a β-galactosidase reporter system, Vanhooke and colleagues[59] found no evidence for expression of CYP27B1 in murine skin or primary keratinocytes, although there was expression in kidney and placenta. It is also possible that the lack of detection of low abundance extrarenal CYP27B1 transcripts is due to some inherent insensitivity of the β-galactosidase reporter system, whereas it is sufficiently sensitive to detect abundant renal CYP27B1 transcripts. There has been some criticism of this work[59] because some mouse tissues, including the kidney, show high endogenous β-galactosidase activity toward the preferred substrate X-Gal, and thus the Vanhooke and colleagues[59] control data might be explained by an artifact.

Despite that the exact function of the extrarenal 1α-hydroxylase remains elusive, there has been intense speculation about the role of this enzyme in health and disease.[66–68] A role for extrarenal CYP27B1 is also consistent with the finding that serum 25-(OH)D levels are associated with various health outcomes from bone health to cardiovascular health. In particular, low serum 25-(OH)D levels are associated with increased mortality for colon, breast, and prostate cancer; increased autoimmune diseases and greater susceptibility to tuberculosis; and increased cardiovascular diseases and hypertension.[66–68] The presence of CYP27B1 in cells of the colon, breast, prostate, monocyte/macrophage, skin, parathyroid gland, and vasculature could explain why serum 25-(OH)D levels are so critical to the normal functioning of these tissues.

Symptoms of Vitamin D–Dependent Rickets, Type 1A

VDDR-1A is the classic and most prevalent form of pseudovitamin D deficiency rickets or hereditary vitamin D–resistant rickets. It is caused by recessive loss-of-function mutations in the CYP27B1 gene encoding 25-(OH)D_3-1α-hydroxylase.[21,47–51] Numerous patients and CYP27B1 mutations have been reported (see **Fig. 2C**). In general, clinical symptoms are comparable to those of vitamin D deficiency rickets, including failure to thrive, muscular hypotonia, and growth retardation. The onset of clinical symptoms is usually during the first year of life. Intrauterine development is undisturbed as maternal normocalcemia and maternal 1,25-(OH)$_2$D$_3$ ensure a sufficient calcium supply. At clinical presentation, affected infants are usually small for age and often lay supine because of muscle weakness and bone pain. They may already exhibit typical clinical signs of rickets, such as a widened anterior fontanel, frontal bossing, and craniotabes (easy depression of the softened parieto-occipital region). A rachitic rosary may be either visible or palpable, enlarged wrists and ankles reflect the widening of the metaphyseal areas. At this early age, however, gross skeletal deformities are still rare. But, if diagnosis and treatment are delayed, severe deformities of the spine and of long bones can occur as well as pathologic fractures. Tooth eruption may be delayed, and erupted teeth show hypoplasia of enamel. In some patients, the initial event is generalized convulsions or tetany. The Chvostek sign (twitching of the upper lip on light finger tapping of the facial nerve) reflects nerve irritability, a consequence of a rapid fall in serum calcium. Furthermore, muscle weakness and potential thorax deformities predispose to pulmonary infections and respiratory insufficiency, which may even be life threatening at least in developing countries or if diagnosis and treatment are delayed.

Radiologic features in patients with VDDR-1A include diffuse osteopenia (mild to severe hypomineralization of the skeleton) and classic rachitic metaphyseal changes: fraying, cupping, widening, and fuzziness of the zone of provisional calcification immediately under the growth plate. These changes are seen better and detected earlier in the most active growth plates, namely, the distal ulna and femur and the proximal and distal tibia. Changes in the diaphyses may not be evident when metaphyseal changes are first detected. They appear later, however, as rarefaction, coarse trabeculation, cortical thinning, and subperiosteal erosions. Looser-Milkman pseudofractures and curvature of the shafts of long bones may be observed, especially in children more than 1 year to 2 years of age.

Diagnostic Test for Vitamin D–Dependent Rickets, Type 1A

In patients with VDDR-1A, vitamin D metabolite assays become critical to the diagnosis. Although the assay for serum 1,25-(OH)$_2$D is rarely ordered as a routine tool, it is a good follow-up test for use when rickets is present along with normal serum 25-(OH)D. Current serum 1,25-(OH)$_2$D assays are based on an antibody generated to 1,25-(OH)$_2$D$_3$ that accurately detects both 1,25-(OH)$_2$D$_2$ and 1,25-(OH)$_2$D$_3$ in the low picogram/milliliter range. Normal values range from 20 pg/mL to 65 pg/mL, whereas VDDR-1A patients have undetectable (<10 pg/mL) values.

Differential Diagnosis of Vitamin D–Dependent Rickets, Type 1A Versus Other Forms of Rickets

A diagnosis of VDDR-1A in patients with calciopenic rickets should be suspected in the presence of normal serum levels of 25-(OH)D_3 if the extended diagnostic work-up yields almost undetectable serum levels for active 1,25-(OH)$_2$D$_3$. Still, establishing an early diagnosis of VDDR-1A is challenging, especially in developing countries where dietary calcium deficiency is common. Furthermore, the laboratory differentiation from hypophosphatemic rickets might still be challenging. On the one hand, increased levels of the phosphaturic hormone FGF-23, as present in most forms of hypophosphatemic rickets, not only provoke renal phosphate wasting but also effectively inhibit CYP27B1 and activate CYP24A1, resulting in low serum levels of 1,25-$(OH)_2D_3$. On the other hand, secondary hyperparathyroidism in VDDR-1A can lead to phosphate deficiency and hypophosphatemia as seen in hypophosphatemic rickets.

Treatment and Management of Vitamin D–Dependent Rickets, Type 1A

The pathophysiology of VDDR-1A involving the defective conversion of 25-$(OH)D_3$ to 1,25-$(OH)_2D_3$ was already postulated by Fraser and colleagues.[21] A few years later, Delvin and colleagues[69] demonstrated the clinical response of affected patients to physiologic doses of calcitriol or 1α-$(OH)D_3$ (whereas high doses of cholecalciferol were shown ineffective). Actual recommendations, therefore, consider long-term therapy with calcitriol as the treatment of choice for VDDR-1A.[70] Usually, initial dosages of 1 μg/d to 2 μg/d are used whereas maintenance doses typically vary between 0.5 μg/d and 1 μg/d. The therapy aims at the correction of clinical, radiologic, and biochemical abnormalities associated with the disease. Some investigators also evaluated the use of the synthetic analog 1α-hydroxyvitamin D_3 (1α[OH]D_3 [alfacalcidiol]). Alfacalcidiol itself is a prodrug with low biological activity; its pharmacologic actions result from its transformation to calcitriol. Because administration of alfacalcidiol is thought to lead to a delayed and moderated rise in serum levels of 1,25-$(OH)_2D_3$, it might provide a wider margin of safety and a lower risk of inadvertent side effects.[71] Both drugs (calcitriol and alfacalcidiol) have a short half-life (hours) that can be of advantage in case of accidental overtreatment. A further important aspect is an adequate calcium supply during the bone healing phase after start of treatment. Calcium supply and dosing of calcitriol are adjusted by monitoring of urinary calcium excretion. Unfortunately, hypercalciuria is a common finding during early treatment with 1,25-$(OH)_2D_3$ and requires frequent renal imaging by ultrasound and assessment of renal function.

25-HYDROXYVITAMIN D_3-24-HYDROXYLASE, CYP24A1: IDIOPATHIC INFANTILE HYPERCALCEMIA
Evidence for Association

The catabolic CYP, CYP24A1, is able to catalyze multiple hydroxylation reactions at carbons C-24 and C-23 of the side chain of both 25-$(OH)D_3$ and its hormonal form, 1,25-$(OH)_2D_3$.[72] It is now believed that CYP24A1, alone, is responsible for the 5-step, 24-oxidation pathway from 1,25-$(OH)_2D_3$ to produce calcitroic acid, a known biliary catabolite[73,74] as well as catalyzing a similar pathway that starts with 23-hydroxylation and culminates in the 1,25-$(OH)_2D_3$-26,23-lactone (see **Fig. 1**).[75,76] Alignment of CYP24A1 from greater than 200 species shows an impressive conservation of residues for at least a good part of the protein.[9] An interesting dichotomy exists at residue 326, where most species possess a CYP24A1 with Ala326 and exhibit 24-hydroxylation to a calcitroic acid product, whereas more primitive organisms have Gly326 and show predominantly 23-hydroxylation to give a 26,23-lactone product.[13] The functional significance of 2 distinct pathways in different species is unknown.[13] In 2010, the crystal structure of rat CYP24A1 was elucidated but with detergent not vitamin D in the active site.[16]

CYP24A1 has been shown to be expressed in many, if not all, target cells containing the vitamin D receptor (VDR), including kidney, bone, and intestine. It is strongly inducible by VDR agonists in such tissues, and this has been confirmed by CYP24A1 mRNA studies.[72,77] This led some investigators to propose that the role of CYP24A1 is primarily to limit or attenuate the action of 1,25-$(OH)_2D_3$ on target cells after an initial round of transcriptional activation in a negative feedback loop.[78] Thus, there is abundant evidence that CYP24A1 exists in normal physiology to catabolize 25-$(OH)D_3$ to prevent its eventual activation to 1,25-$(OH)_2D_3$ and/or to degrade the hormone, 1,25-$(OH)_2D_3$, within its target cells to terminate its biological activity. St-Arnaud and colleagues[79] have recently challenged this solely catabolic role for CYP24A1 by noting the accelerated healing of bone fractures in laboratory animals after the administration of 24-hydroxylated metabolites of vitamin D.

Although CYP24A1 has been clearly established as the key enzyme responsible for vitamin D catabolism, it has become evident that CYP24A1 works in balance with CYP27B1, which is the CYP enzyme responsible for converting 25-$(OH)D_3$ to 1,25-$(OH)_2D_3$ both in the kidney where its role in vitamin D hormone activation was first established and in extrarenal tissues where it seems to play a cell specific role. The emergence of the extrarenal 1α-hydroxylase (CYP27B1) as a mechanism for raising the cellular concentration of 1,25-$(OH)_2D_3$[66,67] has refocused attention on the crucial role of target-cell CYP24A1 as a fine-tuning mechanism to attenuate and eventually reduce the hormone level after gene expression has been modulated. Although the renal CYP24A1 enzyme may function to balance systemic 25-$(OH)D_3$ and 1,25-$(OH)_2D_3$ levels, target cell extrarenal enzyme probably acts in conjunction with CYP27B1 to fine-tune target tissue exposure to the 1,25-$(OH)_2D_3$ hormone.[80]

Vitamin D signaling plays a critical role in regulating bone and mineral homeostasis, and consequently, enzymes, such as CYP24A1, which control vitamin D levels, are regulated by hormones, which are integral to mineral metabolism.[1] In addition to the self-induced regulation of CYP24A1 by 1,25-$(OH)_2D_3$ itself, the enzyme is regulated by such key factors as PTH and FGF-23. 1,25-$(OH)_2D_3$–mediated induction of CYP24A1 expression is significantly attenuated by PTH,[81–83] due to destabilization and increased degradation of CYP24A1 mRNA.[84] As with PTH, FGF-23 also plays a central role in the regulation of mineral homeostasis affecting both expression of genes regulating serum phosphate and those controlling vitamin D metabolism.[85–87] Induction of FGF-23 expression in osteocytes and osteoblasts follows rising serum phosphate and 1,25-$(OH)_2D_3$ levels; subsequently, FGF-23 reduces renal phosphate reabsorption by inhibiting sodium/phosphate (Na/Pi) cotransporter activity[88,89] and indirectly suppresses intestinal phosphate absorption by suppressing renal expression of CYP27B1, thus lowering blood 1,25-$(OH)_2D_3$.[90–93] FGF-23 also controls 1,25-$(OH)_2D_3$ levels by inducing expression of CYP24A1 mRNA in the kidney.[94]

Based on numerous reports in recent years,[95–116] it has become evident that loss-of-function mutations of CYP24A1 (**Fig. 2D**) are one of the principal genetic causes of hypercalcemia. Schlingmann and colleagues[97] reported several families with hypercalcemia and an assortment of homozygous recessive and compound-heterozygous mutations causing defective 25-$(OH)D_3$-24-hydroxylase enzyme activity, elevated serum 1,25-$(OH)_2D_3$, and hypercalcemia, which ultimately result in hypercalciuria, nephrolithiasis, and nephrocalcinosis. This was followed by various publications reporting the same consequences in adults,[98,100] including 1 in a 70-year-old man.[108] Thus, the name, IIH, is a misnomer because the cause of the disease is no longer unknown and is not confined to childhood. In fact, there are at least 3 known diseases under the constellation of IIH:

1. Loss-of-function mutations of CYP24A1 at cytogenetic location 20q13.2 (sometimes known as Lightwood syndrome[117])

2. Williams-Beuren syndrome (WBS) caused by a large deletion on chromosome 7 (cytogenetic location 7q11.23) of 28 genes, including the elastin gene (Online Mendelian Inheritance in Man [OMIM] #194050)
3. Loss-of-function mutations of the Na/Pi cotransporter at cytogenetic location 5q35.3 (also known as SLC34A1)[118]

And there are likely to be more genetic bases for hypercalcemia to be discovered in the future.

There are currently 21 missense and deletion mutations of CYP24A1 described in the literature (see **Fig. 2**D). These mutations must be distinguished from numerous polymorphisms of the CYP24A1 gene. Loss-of-function mutations can be predicted by various computer programs, but comprehensive confirmation of their effects on enzyme activity only come from expression of the defective gene. Schlingmann and colleagues[97] used site-directed mutagenesis of the wild-type human CYP24A1 gene, followed by transient or stable expression of the mutant in V-79 Chinese hamster lung fibroblasts and incubation of the cells with $[1\beta-^3H]1,25-(OH)_2D_3$ to demonstrate loss of enzyme activity. Other investigators[105] have used cultured fibroblasts to show loss of CYP24A1 enzyme function. More recently, Molin and colleagues[115] used LC-MS/MS analysis of the $1,24,25-(OH)_3D_3$ product, instead of use of a radioactive substrate, to demonstrate loss of CYP24A1 enzyme activity.

Dinour and colleagues[113] and Shah and colleagues[114] both reported multiple episodes of hypercalcemia in patients with proved CYP24A1 mutations coinciding with successive pregnancies. It is postulated that the well-documented, increased $1,25-(OH)_2D_3$ production by the placenta during pregnancy[36,37] upsets calcium homeostasis in these individuals and normocalcemia returns after pregnancy is over. Although the heterozygotic newborn has been reported to be normal in such pregnancies, mothers can suffer from the harmful effects of the hypercalcemia, namely renal stones, pancreatitis, and calcification of the placenta.[99,113,114] The gestating female Cyp24a1-knockout mouse fails to carry to term and does not survive pregnancy (St-Arnaud R, PhD, personal communication, 2017).

Symptoms of Idiopathic Infantile Hypercalcemia

IIH was first described in the 1950s[117] in Great Britain during a phase of high supplemental vitamin D (approximately 4000 IU/d) for the prevention of rickets. Affected infants usually present with failure to thrive, weight loss, dehydration, polyuria, constipation, muscular hypotonia, and apathy, typical symptoms of profound hypercalcemia. Even single fatal cases have been described early after initial description of the disease. Concomitant hypercalciuria typically leads to the development of early nephrocalcinosis. Fortunately, clinical symptoms normalize under appropriate therapy. Patients may present, however, with clinical relapses after initial therapeutic measures are discontinued. Patients who receive daily oral low-dose vitamin D prophylaxis against rickets usually present in the second half of the first year of life. In contrast, patients receiving bolus vitamin D prophylaxis that used to be common in some eastern European countries, including the German Democratic Republic and Poland, may become symptomatic after several days to weeks after such an oral bolus of up to 600,000 IU vitamin D.

A majority of patients with biallelic CYP24A1 mutations present with the described clinical picture of classic IIH. A significant percentage of patients with identical (biallelic) CYP24A1 mutations (up to a third[112]), however, remain asymptomatic during infancy and present later in life with recurrent episodes of kidney stones. Laboratory analyses in these patients demonstrate an ongoing activation of vitamin D metabolism (discussed later). Also, patients with the classic initial manifestation in infancy are prone to develop renal sequelae during follow-up. Therefore, long-term surveillance of patients seems mandatory. Moreover, clinical manifestations or exacerbation of the disease during pregnancy and shortly after labor with symptomatic hypercalcemia have been described.[113–115] These observations indicate that adult patients who are able to limit vitamin D activation under physiologic circumstances may develop clinically evident disease if additional risk factors or predisposing conditions emerge, that is, increased vitamin D activation during pregnancy.

In contrast, knowledge of the clinical impact of heterozygous *CYP24A1* mutations is still limited. Data on carriers of heterozygous *CYP24A1* mutations mainly come from studies on family members of index patients with classic biallelic *CYP24A1* mutations. Two of these studies report a significant number of heterozygous relatives with hypercalciuria and nephrolithiasis.[107,115] Laboratory abnormalities include increased values for 1,25-$(OH)_2D_3$ and low levels of intact PTH (iPTH), possibly reflecting insufficient vitamin D degradation. This milder but detectable biochemical phenotype in carriers of a single mutated *CYP24A1* allele might only result in clinically evident disease in the presence of additional contributing factors or circumstances promoting increased vitamin D activation, such as prematurity/early infancy, high doses of exogenous vitamin D, or pregnancy. The initial study cohort already included a patient with a single mutated *CYP24A1* allele who developed symptomatic hypercalcemia after receiving vitamin D bolus prophylaxis, suggesting an increased sensitivity to exogenous vitamin D.[97] Definitely, larger studies exploring the spectrum of biochemical changes and clinical phenotypes in carriers of heterozygous *CYP24A1* mutations are warranted.

Diagnostic Test for Idiopathic Infantile Hypercalcemia

In IIH, it is critical to show that there are 2 genetically mutated *CYP24A1* alleles and that these are loss-of-function mutations not polymorphisms. The value of a reliable rapid screening test for IIH has also been a principal research focus. Kaufmann and colleagues[119] described such an LC-MS/MS method for measuring 24,25-$(OH)_2D_3$ using 100 μL of serum or less, based on derivatization with DMEQ-TAD, a dienophile that couples to all vitamin D metabolites in the blood. 24,25-$(OH)_2D_3$ is the main product of CYP24A1 found in the blood, is indicative of the enzyme activity of the kidney enzyme, and is approximately proportional to the level of the substrate 25-$(OH)D_3$. The absolute concentration of 24,25-$(OH)_2D_3$ is a fairly reliable measure of CYP24A1 enzyme activity in vivo, and the metabolite is low (value <1.0 ng/mL) in most IIH patients with biallelic CYP24A1 mutations, even though most untreated IIH patients have elevated serum 25-$(OH)D_3$ values.[119] A more reliable indicator of IIH, however, due to CYP24A1 mutations, is the ratio of the metabolite to its precursor 25-$(OH)D_3$, namely serum 25-$(OH)D_3$:24,25-$(OH)_2D_3$.[112,115,119,120] The authors have found that this ratio (normal 5–25) rises to greater than 80 and is even more conclusive than serum 24,25-$(OH)_2D_3$ alone because it eliminates the possibility that the patient might have a low serum 24,25-$(OH)_2D_3$ level due to vitamin D deficiency. The authors' experience with this analytic test using the serum 25-$(OH)D_3$:24,25-$(OH)_2D_3$ ratio in more than 100 IIH patients is convincing in that the test does not produce false-negative results.[108,115]

Differential Diagnosis of Idiopathic Infantile Hypocalcemia Versus Other Forms of Hypercalcemia

Despite being rare, symptomatic hypercalcemia is a severe clinical condition that requires a targeted diagnostic work-up and therapy. Next to vitamin D intoxication, the most common etiologies in adulthood comprise primary hyperparathyroidism and malignancy. In infancy and childhood, underlying etiologies are more heterogeneous, including rare hereditary disorders.

The determinations of iPTH and vitamin D metabolites (25-[OH]D$_3$ and 1,25-[OH]$_2$D$_3$) represent central elements of the diagnostic work-up. Largely, 3 categories can be differentiated: PTH-dependent hypercalcemia, vitamin D–dependent-hypercalcemia, and other causes, including vitamin A intoxication, malignancy with production of PTH-related peptide, and hypophosphatasia. These disorders result in low levels of iPTH as well as changes in vitamin D metabolites. High iPTH levels generally point to a primary dysfunction of the parathyroid. The differential diagnoses include primary hyperparathyroidism as well as hereditary defects of the calcium-sensing receptor. Patients with inactivating calcium-sensing receptor mutations display inappropriately high levels of iPTH as well as a concomitant reduction in renal calcium excretion.

The determination of 25-(OH)D$_3$ primarily aims at the exclusion of vitamin D intoxication. Typically, 25-(OH)D$_3$ levels of greater than 200 ng/mL are considered toxic.[121] As patients exhibit an intact regulation of vitamin D activation by CYP27B1 as well as an intact degradation by CYP24A1, they may exhibit normal serum levels of active 1,25-(OH)$_2$D$_3$. In the presence of normal 25-(OH)D$_3$ levels, elevated or inappropriately high levels of 1,25-(OH)$_2$D$_3$ point to a disturbance in vitamin D metabolism. An elevated activity of extrarenal CYP27B1 is present in subcutaneous fat necrosis as well as granulomatous disease, such as sarcoidosis and tuberculosis. Patients with WBS, a contiguous gene syndrome caused by a large deletion of chromosome 7q11.23, also display an increased activity of CYP27B1 that may lead to symptomatic hypercalcemia.

IIH has been shown genetically heterogeneous and may either be caused by mutations in CYP24A1 or in SLC34A1, encoding renal proximal tubular sodium-phosphate cotransporter Na/Pi-IIa. The primary defect in renal phosphate conservation leads to phosphate depletion and a suppression of the phosphaturic hormone FGF-23.[118] Next to its role in phosphate metabolism, FGF-23 limits vitamin D activity by inversely regulating CYP27B1 and CYP24A1. Lack of FGF-23 in patients with renal phosphate wasting, therefore, leads to an increased activity of 1α-hydroxylase, whereas 24-hydroxylase activity is suppressed. The differentiation of these clinical entities is critical for therapy, because patients with Na/Pi-IIa (SLC34A1) defects require phosphate supplementation to normalize the secondary changes in vitamin D and calcium metabolism.

Next to genetic analyses of CYP24A1 and SLC34A1 genes, the determination of 24-hydroxylated vitamin D metabolites (discussed previously) provides a rapid diagnostic method to detect a lack of 24-hydroxylase activity caused by biallelic CYP24A1 mutations. The other known causes of IIH, namely WBS mutations (OMIM #194050) and Na/Pi cotransporter defects,[118] have normal serum 25-(OH)D$_3$:24,25-(OH)$_2$D$_3$ ratios and thus can be distinguished from CYP24A1 defects by a rapid LC-MS/MS assay of the vitamin D metabolites[122] (**Fig. 3**).

Treatment and Management of Idiopathic Infantile Hypercalcemia

In the face of symptomatic hypercalcemia, the acute therapy primarily aims to normalize serum calcium levels and relieve clinical symptoms. Before clarification of the underlying etiology, vitamin D supplementation has to be stopped and, if appropriate, a low-calcium diet should be implemented. Vigorous rehydration with saline solutions always represents a central element of therapy, and doses of up to twice the daily fluid requirement have been described. Pharmacologic treatment comprises therapeutic measures that decrease intestinal calcium absorption, promote renal calcium excretion, inhibit calcium release from bone, and/or inhibit the activation of

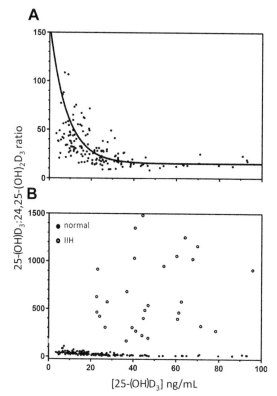

Fig. 3. The ratio of 25-(OH)D$_3$:24,25-(OH)$_2$D$_3$ in idiopathic infantile hypercalcemia patients with mutations in both CYP24A1 alleles in comparison with a group of normal subjects. (*A*) 25-(OH)D$_3$:24,25-(OH)$_2$D$_3$ ratio in a group of individuals with serum 25-OH-D$_3$ in the range 5–100 ng/mL. (*B*) 25-(OH)D$_3$:24,25-(OH)$_2$D$_3$ ratio in a group of patients with idiopathic infantile hypercalcemia (*open circles*) and their normocalcemic parents and siblings (*closed circles*). Note the elevated ratio and serum 25-OH-D$_3$ in IIH patients with a CYP24A1 mutation. (*Adapted from* Kaufmann M, Morse N, Molloy BJ, et al. Improved screening test for idiopathic infantile hypercalcemia confirms residual levels of serum 24,25-(OH)$_2$D$_3$ in affected patients. J Bone Miner Res 2017;32(7):1589–96; with permission.)

vitamin D by CYP27B1.[123] Corticosteroids have been shown to not only lower intestinal calcium absorption but also induce CYP24A1 expression.[72] Unfortunately, a failure to reduce serum calcium levels and hypercalciuria was reported in patients with IIH, arguing for the induction of CYP24A1 as the predominant mode of treatment rather than directing treatment to intestinal calcium absorption.[107] Although furosemide is commonly used to inhibit renal calcium conservation, the data on its therapeutic efficacy are sparse, and it might even worsen volume depletion and augment the risk for renal calcifications and kidney stone formation.

In patients with IIH, the successful use of sodium cellulose phosphate, a nonabsorbable cation exchange resin, has been described.[95,124] Although long-term therapy with sodium cellulose phosphate seems safe and well-tolerated, major concerns involve the risk of calcium depletion, iatrogenic rickets, and an increased intestinal absorption of oxalate that may aggravate the risk of kidney stone formation. Identical considerations and precautions have to be taken into account when implementing a low-calcium diet for long-term therapy (discussed later). In the presence of severe symptomatic hypercalcemia of different etiologies, bisphosphonates, such as pamidronate, have been successfully used to rapidly lower serum calcium levels.[97,102] A class of drugs specifically used in vitamin D–mediated hypercalcemia are azole derivates, such as ketoconazole, that also inhibit mammalian CYP enzymes, including CYP27B1.[96,116,125] Sayers and colleagues[125] were able to show a significant decline in serum levels of 1,25-(OH)$_2$D$_3$ and a stabilization of serum calcium levels after the administration of fluconazole that, compared with ketoconazole, might bear a significantly lower risk of side effects and hepatotoxicity. Finally, a genetic differentiation between CYP24A1 and SLC34A1 defects is critical not only for acute therapy but also during long-term follow-up as phosphate supplementation may be required for patients with SLC34A1 defects.[118]

Little is known about the benefits and risks of omitting vitamin D and implementing a low calcium diet in the long-term therapy for both patient groups. Especially, the risk of vitamin D deficiency with low levels of 25-(OH)D$_3$ despite normal levels of 1,25-(OH)$_2$D$_3$ remains unclear. For patients with CYP24A1 defects, a tendency toward higher serum calcium levels and higher urinary calcium excretion has been observed during the summer months.[112] Although IIH typically manifests after administration of supplemental vitamin D, cutaneous vitamin D synthesis may critically influence the clinical course during follow-up, and patients may require a limitation of sunlight exposure. Definitely, therapy and clinical course of patients with CYP24A1 defects have to be carefully monitored to ensure safety of therapy and to prevent long-term sequelae, including a deterioration of renal function.

REFERENCES

1. Jones G, Strugnell SA, DeLuca HF. Current understanding of the molecular actions of vitamin D. Physiol Rev 1998;78:1193–321.

2. Ponchon G, DeLuca HF. The role of the liver in the metabolism of vitamin D. J Clin Invest 1965;48:1273–9.

3. Fraser DR, Kodicek E. Unique biosynthesis by kidney of a biological active vitamin D metabolite. Nature 1970;228:764–6.

4. Hewison M, Adams J. Extra-renal 1alpha-hydroxylase activity and human disease. Chapter 79. In: Feldman D, Pike JW, Glorieux FH, editors. Vitamin D. 2nd edition. San Diego (CA): Academic Press; 2005. p. 1379–400.

5. Cheng JB, Levine MA, Bell NH, et al. Genetic evidence that the human CYP2R1 enzyme is a key vitamin D 25-hydroxylase. Proc Natl Acad Sci U S A 2004;101: 7711–5.

6. St-Arnaud R, Messerlian S, Moir JM, et al. The 25-hydroxyvitamin D 1alpha-hydroxylase gene maps to the pseudovitamin D-deficiency rickets (PDDR) disease locus. J Bone Miner Res 1997;12:1552–9.

7. Takeyama K, Kitanaka S, Sato T, et al. 25-Hydroxyvitamin D3 1alpha-hydroxylase and vitamin D synthesis. Science 1997;277:1827–30.

8. Jones G, Prosser DE, Kaufmann M. Cytochrome P450-mediated metabolism of vitamin D. J Lipid Res 2014;55:13–31.

9. Nelson DR. The cytochrome p450 homepage. Hum Genomics 2009;4:59–65.

10. Prosser DE, Guo YD, Jia Z, et al. Structural motif-based homology modeling of CYP27A1 and site-directed mutational analyses affecting vitamin D hydroxylation. Biophys J 2006;90:3389–409.

11. Hamamoto H, Kusudo T, Urushino N, et al. Structure-functional analysis of vitamin D 24-hydroxylase (CYP24A1) by site-directed mutagenesis: amino

acid residues responsible for species-based difference of CYP24A1 between humans and rats. Mol Pharmacol 2006;70:120–8.

12. Masuda S, Prosser DE, Guo YD, et al. Generation of a homology model for the human cytochrome P450, CYP24A1, and the testing of putative substrate binding residues by site-directed mutagenesis and enzyme activity studies. Arch Biochem Biophys 2007;460:177–91.

13. Prosser DE, Kaufmann M, O'Leary B, et al. Single A326G mutation converts human CYP24A1 from 25-OH-D3-24-hydroxylase into -23-hydroxylase, generating 1alpha,25-(OH)2D3-26,23-lactone. Proc Natl Acad Sci U S A 2007;104: 12673–8.

14. Annalora AJ, Bobrovnikov-Marjon E, Serda R, et al. Hybrid homology modeling and mutational analysis of cytochrome P450C24A1 (CYP24A1) of the vitamin D pathway: insights into substrate specificity and membrane-bound structure-function. Arch Biochem Biophys 2007;460:262–73.

15. Strushkevich N, Usanov SA, Plotnikov AN, et al. Structural analysis of CYP2R1 in complex with vitamin D3. J Mol Biol 2008;380:95–106.

16. Annalora AJ, Goodin DB, Hong WX, et al. Crystal structue of CYP24A1, a mitochondrial cytochrome P450 involved in vitamin D metabolism. J Mol Biol 2010; 396:441–51.

17. Cheng JB, Motola DL, Mangelsdorf DJ, et al. Deorphanization of cytochrome P450 2R1: a microsomal vitamin D25-hydroxylase. J Biol Chem 2003;278: 38084–93.

18. Nelson DR. Comparison of P450s from human and fungus: 420 Million years of vertebrate P450 evolution. Arch Biochem Biophys 2003;409:18–24.

19. Jones G, Byford V, West S, et al. Hepatic activation & inactivation of clinically-relevant vitamin D analogs and prodrugs. Anticancer Res 2006;26:2589–96.

20. Casella SJ, Reiner BJ, Chen TC, et al. A possible genetic defect in 25-hydroxylation as a cause of rickets. J Pediatr 1994;124:929–32.

21. Fraser D, Kooh SW, Kind HP, et al. Pathogenesis of hereditary vitamin D-dependent rickets. An inborn error of vitamin D metabolism involving defective conversion of 25-hydroxyvitamin D to 1alpha,25-dihydroxyvitamin D. N Engl J Med 1973;289:817–22.

22. Thacher TD, Fischer PR, Pettifor JM, et al. Case control study of factors associated with nutritional rickets in Nigerian children. J Pediar 2000;137:367–73.

23. Thacher TD, Fischer PR, Singh RJ, et al. CYP2R1 mutations impair generation of 25-hydroxyvitamin D and cause an atypical form of vitamin D deficiency. J Clin Endocrinol Metab 2015;100:E1005–13.

24. Molin A, Fillet F, Demers N, et al. Two French families with vitamin D dependency rickets type 1B harbor homozygous expression of CYP2R1 mutations L99P and G42_L46delinsR. Paper presented at: 19th Workshop on Vitamin D. Boston, MA, March 28–31, 2016.

25. Wang TJ, Zhang F, Richards JB, et al. Common genetic determinants of vitamin D insufficiency: a genome-wide association study. Lancet 2010;376:180–8.

26. Zhu JG, Ochalek JT, Kaufmann M, et al. CYP2R1 is a major, but not exclusive, contributor to 25-hydroxyvitamin D production in vivo. Proc Natl Acad Sci U S A 2013;110:15650–5.

27. Al Mutair AN, Nasrat GH, Russell DW. Mutation of the CYP2R1 vitamin D 25-hydroxylase in a Saudi Arabian family with severe vitamin D deficiency. J Clin Endocrinol Metab 2012;97:E2022–5.

28. Jones G. Interpreting vitamin D assay results: proceed with caution. Clin J Am Soc Nephrol 2015;10:331–4.

29. Omdahl JL, Gray RW, Boyle IT, et al. Regulation of metabolism of 25-hydroxy-cholecalciferol by kidney tissue in vitro by dietary calcium. Nat New Biol 1972;237:63–4.
30. Tanaka Y, DeLuca HF. The control of 25-hydroxyvitamin D metabolism by inorganic phosphorus. Arch Biochem Biophys 1973;154:566–74.
31. Liu S, Quarles LD. How fibroblast growth factor 23 works. J Am Soc Nephrol 2007;18:1637–47.
32. Gray RW, Omdahl JL, Ghazarian JG, et al. 25-Hydroxycholecalciferol-1-hydroxylase. Subcellular location and properties. J Biol Chem 1972;247:7528–32.
33. Akiba T, Endou H, Koseki C, et al. Localization of 25-hydroxyvitamin D(3)-1α-hydroxylase activity in mammalian kidney. Biochem Biophys Res Commun 1980; 94:313–8.
34. Kawashima H, Torikai S, Kurokawa K. Calcitonin selectively stimulates 25-hydroxyvitamin D3-1α-hydroxylase in the proximal straight tubule of the rat kidney. Nature 1981;291:327–9.
35. Kawashima H, Kurokawa K. Unique hormonal regulation of vitamin D metabolism in the mammalian kidney. Miner Electrolyte Metab 1983;9:227–35.
36. Weisman Y, Vargas A, Duckett G, et al. Synthesis of 1,25-dihydroxyvitamin D in the nephrectomized pregnant rat. Endocrinology 1978;103:1992–6.
37. Gray TK, Lester GE, Lorenc RS. Evidence for extra-renal 1alpha-hydroxylation of 25-hydroxyvitamin D3 in pregnancy. Science 1979;204:1311–3.
38. Howard GA, Turner RT, Sherrard DJ, et al. Human bone cells in culture metabolize 25-hydroxyvitamin D3 to 1,25-dihydroxyvitamin D3 and 24,25-dihydroxyvitamin D3. J Biol Chem 1981;256:7738–40.
39. Somjen D, Katzburg S, Stern N, et al. 25 hydroxy-vitamin D3-1alpha hydroxylase expression and activity in cultured human osteoblasts and their modulation by parathyroid hormone, estrogenic compounds and dihydrotestosterone. J Steroid Biochem Mol Biol 2007;107:238–44.
40. Gray TK, Maddux FW, Lester GE, et al. Rodent macrophages metabolize 25-hydroxyvitamin D3 in vitro. Biochem Biophys Res Commun 1982;109:723–9.
41. Adams JS, Sharma OP, Gacad MA, et al. Metabolism of 25-hydroxyvitamin D3 by cultured pulmonary alveolar macrophages in sarcoidosis. J Clin Invest 1983;72:1856–60.
42. Monkawa T, Yoshida T, Wakino S, et al. Molecular cloning of cDNA and genomic DNA for human 25-hydroxyvitamin D3 1alpha-hydroxylase. Biochem Biophys Res Commun 1997;239:527–33.
43. Fu GK, Lin D, Zhang MYH, et al. Cloning of human 25-hydroxyvitamin D-1alpha-hydroxylase and mutations causing vitamin D-dependent rickets type 1. Mol Endocrinol 1997;11:1961–70.
44. Jones G, Ramshaw H, Zhang A, et al. Expression and activity of vitamin D-metabolizing cytochrome P450s (CYP1alpha and CYP24) in human non-small cell lung carcinomas. Endocrinology 1999;140:3303–10.
45. Zehnder D, Bland R, Williams MC, et al. Extrarenal expression of 25-hydroxyvitamin D3-1alpha-hydroxylase. J Clin Endocrinol Metab 2001;86:888–94.
46. Scriver CR, Reade TM, DeLuca HF, et al. Serum 1,25-dihidroxyvitamin D levels in normal subjects and in patients with hereditary rickets or bone diseases. N Engl J Med 1978;299:976–9.
47. Miller WL, Portale AA. Vitamin D 1alpha-hydroxylases. Trends Endocrinol Metab 2000;11:315–9.
48. Kitanaka S, Takeyama K, Murayama A, et al. The molecular basis of vitamin D-dependent rickets type 1. Endocr J 2001;48:427–32.

49. Wang X, Zhang MY, Miller WL, et al. Novel gene mutations in patients with 1alpha-hydroxylase deficiency that confer partial enzyme activity in vitro. J Clin Endocrinol Metab 2002;87:2424–30.

50. Kim CJ, Kaplan LE, Perwad F, et al. Vitamin D 1alpha-hydroxylase gene mutations in patients with 1alpha-hydroxylase deficiency. J Clin Endocrinol Metab 2007;92:3177–82.

51. Malloy P, Feldman D. Genetic disorders and defects in vitamin D action. Endocrinol Metab Clin North Am 2010;39(2):333–46.

52. Panda DK, Miao D, Tremblay ML, et al. Targeted ablation of the 25-hydroxyvitamin D 1alpha-hydroxylase enzyme: evidence for skeletal, reproductive and immune dysfunction. Proc Natl Acad Sci U S A 2001;98:7498–503.

53. Dardenne O, Prud'homme J, Arabian A, et al. Targeted inactivation of the 25-hydroxyvitamin D3-1alpha-hydroxylase gene (CYP27B1) creates an animal model of pseudovitamin D-deficiency rickets. Endocrinology 2001;142:3135–41.

54. Xue Y, Karaplis AC, Hendy GN, et al. Genetic models show that parathyroid hormone and 1,25-dihydroxyvitamin D3 play distinct and synergistic roles in postnatal mineral ion homeostasis and skeletal development. Hum Mol Genet 2005;14:1515–28.

55. Bikle DD, Chang S, Crumrine D, et al. 25-hydroxyvitamin D 1alpha-hydroxylase is required for optimal epidemal differentiation and permeability barrier homeoatasis. J Invest Dermatol 2004;122:984–92.

56. Hoenderop JG, Dardenne O, Van Abel M, et al. Modulation of renal Ca2+ transport protein genes by dietary Ca2+ and 1,25-dihydroxyvitamin D3 in 25-hydroxyvitamin D3-1alpha-hydroxylase knockout mice. FASEB J 2002;16:1398–406.

57. Dardenne O, Prodhomme J, Hacking SA, et al. Rescue of the pseudo-vitamin D deficiency rickets phenotype of CYP27B1-deficient mice by treatment with 1,25-dihydroxyvitamin D3: biochemical, histomorphometric and biochemical analyses. J Bone Miner Res 2003;18:637–43.

58. Dardenne O, Prud'homme J, Hacking SA, et al. Correction of the abnormal mineral ion homeostasis with a high-calcium, high-phosphorus, high-lacose diet rescues the PDDR phenotype of mice deficient for the 25-hydroxyvitamin D-1alpha-hydroxylase (CYP27B1). Bone 2003;32:332–40.

59. Vanhooke JL, Prahl JM, Kimmel-Jehan C, et al. CYP27B1 null mice with LacZ reporter gene display no 25-hydroxyvitamin D3-1alpha-hydroxylase promotor activity in the skin. Proc Natl Acad Sci U S A 2006;103:75–80.

60. St-Arnaud R, Dardenne O, Prud'homme J, et al. Conventional and tissue-specific inactivation of the 25-hydroxyvitamin D-1alpha-hydroxylase (CYP27B1). J Cell Biochem 2003;88:245–51.

61. Naja RP, Dardenne O, Arabian A, et al. Chondrocyte-specific modulation of Cyp27b1 expression supports a role for local sythesis of 1,25-dihydroxyvitamin D3 in growth plate development. Endocrinology 2009;150:4024–32.

62. Diaz L, Sanchez I, Avila E, et al. Identification of a 25-hydroxyvitamin D3 1alpha-hydroxylase gene transcription product in cultures of human syncytiotroblast cells. J Clin Enocrinol Metab 2000;85:2543–9.

63. Whitlatch LW, Young MV, Schwartz GG, et al. 25-hydroxyvitamin D-1alpha-hydroxylase activity is diminished in human prostate cancer cells and is enhanced by gene transfer. J Steroid Biochem Mol Biol 2002;81:135–40.

64. Tangpricha V, Flanagan JN, Whitlatch LW, et al. 25-hydroxyvitamin D-1alpha-hydroxylase in normal and malignant colon tissue. Lancet 2001;357:1673–4.

65. Bareis P, Bises G, Bischof MG, et al. 25-hydroxy-vitamin D metabolism in human colon cancer cells dureing tumor progression. Biochem Biophys Res Commun 2001;285:1012–7.

66. Holick MF. Vitamin D deficiency. N Engl J Med 2007;357:266–81.

67. Jones G. Expanding role for vitamin D in chronic kidney disease: importance of blood 25-OH-D levels & extra renal 1alpha-hydroxylase in the classical and non-classical actions of 1alpha,25-dihydroxyvitamin D3. Semin Dial 2007;20:316–24.

68. Adams JS, Hewison M. Update in vitamin D. J Clin Endocrinol Metab 2010;95:471–8.

69. Delvin EE, Glorieux FH, Marie PJ, et al. Vitamin D dependency: replacement therapy with calcitriol? J Pediatr 1981;99:26–34.

70. Glorieux FH. Calcitriol treatment in vitamin D-dependent and vitamin D-resistant rickets. Metabolism 1990;39:10–2.

71. Kubodera N. A new look at the most successful prodrugs for active vitamin D hormone (D hormone): alfacalcidol and doxercalciferol. Molecules 2009;14:3869–80.

72. Jones G, Kaufmann M, Prosser D. 25-hydroxyvitamin D_3-24-hydroxylase (CYP24A1): its important role in the degradation of vitamin D. Arch Biochem Biophys 2012;523:9–18.

73. Makin G, Lohnes D, Byford V, et al. Target cell metabolism of 1,25-dihydroxyvitamin D_3 to calcitroic acid. Evidence for a pathway in kidney and bone involving 24-oxidation. Biochem J 1989;262:173–80.

74. Reddy GS, Tserng K-Y. Calcitroic acid, end product of renal metabolism of 1,25-dihydroxyvitamin D_3 through C-24 oxidation pathway. Biochemistry 1989;28:1763–9.

75. Yamada S, Nakayama K, Takayama H, et al. Isolation, identification, and metabolism of (23S,25R)-25-hydroxyvitamin D3 26,23-lactol. A biosynthetic precursor of (23S,25R)-25-hydroxyvitamin D_3 26,23-lactone. J Biol Chem 1984;259:884–9.

76. Sakaki T, Sawada N, Komai K, et al. Dual metabolic pathway of 25-hydroxyvitamin D_3 catalyzed by human CYP24. Eur J Biochem 2000;267:6158–65.

77. Ohyama Y, Noshiro M, Okuda K. Cloning and expression of cDNA encoding 25-hydroxyvitamin D_3 24-hydroxylase. FEBS Lett 1991;278:195–8.

78. Lohnes D, Jones G. Further metabolism of 1α,25-dihydroxyvitamin D3 in target cells. J Nutr Sci Vitaminol (Tokyo) 1992;Spec No:75–8.

79. St-Arnaud R, Kupscik L, Naja RP, et al. Novel mechanism of action for 24-hydroxylated vitamin D metabolites in fracture repair. 15th Workshop on Vitamin D. Houston, TX, June 16–22, 2012. [abstract: 27].

80. Jones G, Vriezen D, Lohnes D, et al. Side-chain hydroxylation of vitamin D_3 and its physiological implications. Steroids 1987;49:29–53.

81. Zierold C, Reinholz GG, Mings JA, et al. Regulation of the porcine 1,25-dihydroxyvitamin D_3-24-hydroxylase (CYP24) by 1,25-dihydroxyvitamin D_3 and parathyroid hormone in AOK-B50 cells. Arch Biochem Biophys 2000;381:323–7.

82. Shinki T, Jin CH, Nishimura A, et al. Parathyroid hormone inhibits 25-hydroxyvitamin D_3-24-hydroxylase mRNA expression stimulated by 1α,25-dihydroxyvitamin D_3 in rat kidney but not in intestine. J Biol Chem 1992;267:13757–62.

83. Reinhardt TA, Horst RL. Parathyroid hormone down-regulates 1,25-dihydroxy vitamin D receptors (VDR) and VDR messenger ribonucleic acid in vitro and blocks homologous up-regulation of VDR in vivo. Endocrinology 1990;127:942–8.

84. Zierold C, Mings JA, DeLuca HF. Parathyroid hormone regulates 25-hydroxyvitamin D_3-24-hydroxylase mRNA by altering its stability. Proc Natl Acad Sci U S A 2001;98:13572–6.
85. Razzaque MS, Lanske B. The emerging role of the fibroblast growth factor-23-klotho axis in renal regulation of phosphate homeostasis. J Endocrinol 2007; 194:1–10.
86. Fukumoto S. Physiological regulation and disorders of phosphate metabolism–pivotal role of fibroblast growth factor 23. Intern Med 2008;47:337–43.
87. Ramon I, Kleynen P, Body JJ, et al. Fibroblast growth factor 23 and its role in phosphate homeostasis. Eur J Endocrinol 2010;162:1–10.
88. Saito H, Kusano K, Kinosaki M, et al. Human fibroblast growth factor-23 mutants suppress Na+-dependent phosphate co-transport activity and 1α,25-dihydroxyvitamin D_3 production. J Biol Chem 2003;278:2206–11.
89. Shimada T, Hasegawa H, Yamazaki Y, et al. FGF-23 is a potent regulator of vitamin D metabolism and phosphate homeostasis. J Bone Miner Res 2004; 19:429–35.
90. Perwad P, Zhang MY, Tenenhouse HS, et al. Fibroblast growth factor 23 impairs phosphorus and vitamin D metabolism in vivo and suppresses 25-hydroxyvitamin D-1α-hydroxylase expression in vitro. Am J Physiol Renal Physiol 2007;293: F1577–83.
91. Shimada T, Yamazaki Y, Takahashi M, et al. Vitamin D receptor-independent FGF23 actions in regulating phosphate and vitamin D metabolism. Am J Physiol Renal Physiol 2005;289:F1088–95.
92. Bai XY, Miao D, Goltzman D, et al. The autosomal dominant hypophosphatemic rickets R176Q mutation in fibroblast growth factor 23 resists proteolytic cleavage and enhances in vivo biological potency. J Biol Chem 2003;278:9843–9.
93. Larsson T, Marsell R, Schipani E, et al. Transgenic mice expressing fibroblast growth factor 23 under the control of the alpha1(I) collagen promoter exhibit growth retardation, osteomalacia, and disturbed phosphate homeostasis. Endocrinology 2004;145:3087–94.
94. Inoue Y, Segawa H, Kaneko I, et al. Role of the vitamin D receptor in FGF23 action on phosphate metabolism. Biochem J 2005;390:325–31.
95. McTaggart SJ, Craig J, MacMillan J, et al. Familial occurrence of idiopathic infantile hypercalcemia. Pediatr Nephrol 1999;13:668–71.
96. Nguyen M, Boutignon H, Mallet E, et al. Infantile hypercalcemia and hypercalciuria: new insights into a vitamin D-dependent mechanism and response to ketoconazole treatment. J Pediatr 2010;157:296–302.
97. Schlingmann KP, Kaufmann M, Weber S, et al. Mutations in CYP24A1 and idiopathic infantile hypercalcemia. N Engl J Med 2011;365:410–21.
98. Dauber A, Nguyen TT, Sochett E, et al. Genetic defect in CYP24A1, the vitamin D 24-hydroxylase gene, in a patient with severe infantile hypercalcemia. J Clin Endocrinol Metab 2012;97:E268–74.
99. Castanet M, Mallet E, Kottler ML. Lightwood syndrome revisited with a novel mutation in CYP24 and vitamin D supplement recommendations. J Pediatr 2013;163:1208–10.
100. Dinour D, Beckerman P, Ganon L, et al. Loss-of-function mutations of CYP24A1, the vitamin D 24-hydroxylase gene, cause long-standing hypercalciuric nephrolithiasis and nephrocalcinosis. J Urol 2013;190:552–7.
101. Fencl F, Blahova K, Schlingmann KP, et al. Severe hypercalcemic crisis in an infant with idiopathic infantile hypercalcemia caused by mutation in CYP24A1 gene. Eur J Pediatr 2013;172:45–9.

102. Skalova S, Cerna L, Bayer M, et al. Intravenous pamidronate in the treatment of severe idiopathic infantile hypercalcemia. Iran J Kidney Dis 2013;7:160–4.

103. Figueres ML, Linglart A, Bienaime F, et al. Kidney function and influence of sunlight exposure in patients with impaired 24-hydroxylation of vitamin D due to CYP24A1 mutations. Am J Kidney Dis 2015;65:122–6.

104. Streeten EA, Zarbalian K, Damcott CM. CYP24A1 mutations in idiopathic infantile hypercalcemia. N Engl J Med 2011;365:1741–2 [author reply: 1742–3].

105. Nesterova G, Malicdan MC, Yasuda K, et al. 1,25-(OH)2D-24 hydroxylase (CYP24A1) deficiency as a cause of nephrolithiasis. Clin J Am Soc Nephrol 2013;8:649–57.

106. Meusburger E, Mundlein A, Zitt E, et al. Medullary nephrocalcinosis in an adult patient with idiopathic infantile hypercalcaemia and a novel CYP24A1 mutation. Clin Kidney J 2013;6:211–5.

107. Colussi G, Ganon L, Penco S, et al. Chronic hypercalcaemia from inactivating mutations of vitamin D 24-hydroxylase (CYP24A1): implications for mineral metabolism changes in chronic renal failure. Nephrol Dial Transplant 2014;29:636–43.

108. Jacobs TP, Kaufman M, Jones G, et al. A lifetime of hypercalcemia and hypercalciuria, finally explained. J Clin Endocrinol Metab 2014;99:708–12.

109. Wolf P, Muller-Sacherer T, Baumgartner-Parzer S, et al. A case of "late-onset" idiopathic infantile hypercalcemia secondary to mutations in the CYP24A1 gene. Endocr Pract 2014;20:e91–5.

110. Dowen FE, Sayers JA, Hynes AM, et al. CYP24A1 mutation leading to nephrocalcinosis. Kidney Int 2014;85:1475.

111. Jobst-Schwan T, Pannes A, Schlingmann KP, et al. Discordant clinical course of vitamin-D-hydroxylase (CYP24A1) associated hypercalcemia in two adult brothers with nephrocalcinosis. Kidney Blood Press Res 2015;40:443–51.

112. Cools M, Goemaere S, Baetens D, et al. Calcium and bone homeostasis in heterozygous carriers of CYP24A1 mutations: a cross-sectional study. Bone 2015;81:89–96.

113. Dinour D, Davidovits M, Aviner S, et al. Maternal and infantile hypercalcemia caused by vitamin-D-hydroxylase mutations and vitamin D intake. Pediatr Nephrol 2015;30:145–52.

114. Shah AD, Hsiao EC, O'Donnell B, et al. Maternal hypercalcemia due to failure of 1,25-Dihydroxyvitamin-D3 catabolism in a patient with CYP24A1 mutations. J Clin Endocrinol Metab 2015;100:2832–6.

115. Molin A, Baudoin R, Kaufmann M, et al. CYP24A1 mutations in a cohort of hypercalcemic patients: evidence for a recessive trait. J Clin Endocrinol Metab 2015;100:E1343–52.

116. Tebben PJ, Milliner DS, Horst RL, et al. Hypercalcemia, hypercalciuria, and elevated calcitriol concentrations with autosomal dominant transmission due to CYP24A1 mutations: effects of ketoconazole therapy. J Clin Endocrinol Metab 2012;97:E423–7.

117. Lightwood R, Stapleton T. Idiopathic hypercalcaemia in infants. Lancet 1953;265:255–6.

118. Schlingmann KP, Ruminska J, Kaufmann M, et al. Autosomal-recessive mutations in SLC34A1 encoding sodium-phosphate cotransporter 2A cause idiopathic infantile hypercalcemia. J Am Soc Nephrol 2016;27:604–14.

119. Kaufmann M, Gallagher C, Peacock M, et al. Clinical utility of simultaneous quantitation of 25-hydroxyvitamin D & 24,25-dihydroxyvitamin D by LC-MS/MS

involving derivatization with DMEQ-TAD. J Clin Endocrinol Metab 2014;99: 2567–74.

120. Ketha H, Kumar R, Singh RJ. LC-MS/MS for identifying patients with CYP24A1 Mutations. Clin Chem 2016;62:236–42.

121. Jones G. Pharmacokinetics of vitamin D toxicity. Am J Clin Nutr 2008;88: 582S–6S.

122. Kaufmann M, Morse N, Molloy BJ, et al. Improved screening test for idiopathic infantile hypercalcemia confirms residual levels of serum 24,25-$(OH)_2D_3$ in affected patients. J Bone Miner Res 2017;32(7):1589–96.

123. Davies JH, Shaw NJ. Investigation and management of hypercalcaemia in children. Arch Dis Child 2012;97:533–8.

124. Huang J, Coman D, McTaggart SJ, et al. Long-term follow-up of patients with idiopathic infantile hypercalcaemia. Pediatr Nephrol 2006;21:1676–80.

125. Sayers J, Hynes AM, Srivastava S, et al. Successful treatment of hypercalcaemia associated with a CYP24A1 mutation with fluconazole. Clin Kidney J 2015;8:453–5.

Genetic and Racial Differences in the Vitamin D Endocrine System

 CrossMark

Roger Bouillon, MD, PhD, FRCP

KEYWORDS

- Vitamin D • Vitamin D binding protein • CYP2R1 • CYP24A1
- Delta-7-steroid-reductase • 25-Hydroxyvitamin D • Gene polymorphism • Race

KEY POINTS

- The vitamin D status is best assessed by serum 25-hydroxyvitamin D (25OHD).
- Serum 25OHD is highly variable around the world and depends on environmental and genetic factors.
- Twin studies suggest that serum 25OHD is highly genetically driven (explaining overall more than 50% of the variation).
- Genome-wide association study and candidate gene studies conclude that 4 gene polymorphisms (delta-7-steroid-reductase, CYP2R1, CYP24A1, and above all, DBP/GC) explain about 5% of the variations in serum 25OHD.
- Racial differences in DBP/GC only contribute minimally to the wide variations in total or free serum 25OHD concentrations.

Vitamin D is essential for calcium and bone homeostasis and may have many other nonskeletal effects.[1–4] The "nutritional status" of vitamin D is usually assessed by measurements of serum 25-hydroxyvitamin D (25OHD), because this reflects the access to either exogenous (food) or endogenous (skin) synthesis of the parent vitamin D. Indeed, most of the supply of vitamin D is rapidly cleared from serum and is metabolized into 25OHD, with an estimated conversion efficacy of about 25% to 33%, as based on comparison between vitamin D status after oral intake of the parent vitamin D or 25OHD.[5,6] The hormonal status of vitamin D is reflected in serum concentrations of $1,25(OH)_2D$ as the renal conversion of 25OHD into $1,25(OH)_2D$ is tightly feedback-controlled by several hormones.[1–4] The paracrine/autocrine status of vitamin D, being the local conversion of 25OHD into $1,25(OH)_2D$ in several tissues by locally expressed CYP27B1, so far cannot be easily assessed. From several twin studies, one can

The author received speakers fee from Amgen, Abiogen, L'Oréal, Chugai and Teijin and is co-owner of a university patent on vitamin D analogs licenced to Hybrigenix (France).
Clinical and Experimental Endocrinology, KU Leuven, Herestraat 49 ON1 Box 902, Leuven 3000, Belgium
E-mail address: roger.bouillon@kuleuven.be

Endocrinol Metab Clin N Am 46 (2017) 1119–1135
http://dx.doi.org/10.1016/j.ecl.2017.07.014
0889-8529/17/© 2017 Elsevier Inc. All rights reserved.

conclude that the vitamin D status as reflected by serum 25OHD is genetically highly regulated. Indeed, depending on the type of study (**Table 1**), between 25% and even 80% of the variation would be under genetic control. The influence of genes as based on the results of twin studies on serum 1,25(OH)$_2$D is, however, much lower when compared with serum 25OHD (see **Table 1**). Therefore, the obvious question is which genes are involved in the metabolism and action of vitamin D? Indeed, gene polymorphisms may be part of the genetic and racial differences in vitamin D status or action. The potentially large genetic influence on serum 25OHD is rather unexpected because 25OHD is thought to be an excellent indicator of combined (nutritional intake and endogenous synthesis) access to vitamin D. Both types of access to vitamin D are highly dependent on the environmental and lifestyle factors rather than genetic background. Although twin studies are considered the best strategy to overcome environmental and other confounding factors (by comparing nonidentical from identical twins, living in similar situations), possible remaining confounding resulting in overestimation of genetic factors is always a possible concern. In this article, the author summarizes existing data concerning the ethnic, racial, and genetic influences on the vitamin D endocrine system.

ETHNIC AND RACIAL DIFFERENCE IN VITAMIN D STATUS LARGELY DUE TO ENVIRONMENTAL FACTORS

The nutritional intake of vitamin D is dependent on the intake of a few food items with high vitamin D content, such as oily fish. Overall, the intake of vitamin D in most countries around the world is rather low and only contributes to (far) less than 50% (and usually even <20%) of the overall supply. Exceptions are of course populations with high habitual intake of oily fish (or fish oil). Most European populations have a daily oral intake of less than 5 μg[7] and thus well below the minimal requirements of (at least) 10 μg/d for humans of all ages.[8] In populations with a high intake of vitamin D (eg, Iceland), the seasonal variation in serum 25OHD is therefore much lower than the seasonal variation in other countries or regions with a much lower vitamin D intake. There are, indeed, some ethnic differences in choice or access to vitamin D–rich food, but these situations are due to environmental, economic, or cultural factors and not really genetically or racially driven. Differences in food intake are thus unlikely factors involved in the genetic control of serum vitamin D metabolites. Endogenous production of vitamin D, however, may be more sensitive to ethnic, racial, or genetic factors. Access to UV-B irradiation from sunlight is of course dependent on many

Table 1
Genetic determinants of serum 25-hydroxyvitamin D and 1,25(OH)$_2$D

Authors	25OHD, %	1,25(OH)$_2$D, %	Comments
Hunter et al,[76] 2001	43		UK twins
Wjst et al,[77] 2007	80	30	Germany asthma patients
Orton & Ebers,[78] 2011	77		Canadian twins
Engelman et al,[79] 2008	23–41	16–48	US Hispanics and African Americans
Snellman et al,[80] 2009	50		Sweden (summertime)
Shea et al,[81] 2009	25		US Framingham
Karohl et al,[82] 2010	70		Vietnam twin
Mills et al,[83] 2015	86		Australia
Arguelles et al,[84] 2009	36		Chinese adolescents

geographic and related factors (such as latitude, season, and UV-B absorption by clouds, pollution, and physical factors). Obviously, ethnic and racial factors have defined where people live on earth and thus influence their possible access to UV-B light. However, if people migrate to areas beyond their original living area, they will be exposed to the UV-B light of their new environment. A more likely factor contributing to ethnic or racial differences in vitamin D status is skin color because the pigmentation and thickness of the skin have major influences on absorption of UV-B light before it is able to activate the photochemical synthesis of vitamin D from 7-dehydrocholesterol (7-DHC). This implies that dark-skinned Africans need about 5 to 6 times more UV-B light than fair-skinned individuals, whereas people with intermediate skin color or thickness have an intermediate photosynthetic capacity.[9] These skin characteristics are of course largely genetically driven and vary widely along ethnic and racial lines. A second factor defining the endogenous synthesis of vitamin D is the real-life exposure to available UV-B irradiation, depending on lifestyle, outdoor activities, and clothing. Evidently, this is largely dependent on cultural, religious, and other traditional factors, and this is again linked to ethnic or racial determinants.

Regional differences in vitamin D intake around the world may well differ about 10-fold with very low intake (around 1–2 μg/d) in some areas with little or no intake of oily fish or other vitamin D–rich food items up to areas with very high fish consumption such as Scandinavian countries or Japan (mean vitamin D intake of 10 μg/d or more). Regional differences in endogenous vitamin D synthesis are much more difficult to estimate, because there is substantial disagreement in the efficacy of UV-B irradiation in generating vitamin D. Indeed, mainly based on extrapolation of in vitro data on whole body physiology, Holick[10] estimated that a minimal erythema dose of UV-B results in the production of more than 10,000 IU of vitamin D_3. Another study however revealed that a week of sunbathing holiday of Danish young women in the Canary Islands increased serum 25OHD by about 21 nmol/L, and this would be the equivalent of a daily intake of 800 IU.[11] Therefore, it is hard to estimate the vitamin D synthesis based on exposure to sunlight in a real-life situation. People living in Equatorial Africa in fairly "native or Paleolithic circumstances" and thus with near total body potentially exposed to direct sunlight have a mean serum 25OHD of about 115 nmol/L (46 ng/mL).[12] It is important to mention that nobody of both tribes in this study living in a natural environment had serum 25OHD levels less than 50 nmol/L or greater than 171 nmol/L. This seems to indicate that the many mechanisms involved in the protection against vitamin D excess[2] are highly efficient as to avoid vitamin D toxicity due to exposure to sunlight. Indeed, there are very few examples of such UV-B–induced toxicity, and the few cases are not dark-skinned but light-skinned Europeans.[13] This is in line with some non–black-skinned bay watchers exposed to intensive sunlight who had serum 25OHD levels somewhat higher than native Africans in "natural living conditions" (**Table 2**). Black-skinned subjects living in different areas in the world[14] have quite variable 25OHD concentrations with, as expected, lower levels when living further away from the Equator (see **Table 2**). As these black subjects belong to the same "race," it seems unlikely that genes are the reason for this variation in serum 25OHD concentrations. In addition, the within population differences in serum 25OHD are frequently higher than the between population differences even with the same skin color and the same presumed genes. Apart from UV-B irradiation, lifestyle is a major factor defining endogenous vitamin D synthesis, and this includes time spent outside in the sun and clothing habits, and in general, is dependent on the net exposure to UV-B (duration plus time of the day) multiplied by the surface of skin exposed. The complex origin of vitamin D sometimes results in very strange results, whereby people living in very sunny climates have extremely low mean levels

Table 2
Serum 25-hydroxyvitamin D concentrations in unusual circumstances

Circumstance	Population	25OHD, ng/mL[a]
1. High sun exposure	Farmers (Haddock et al,[85] 1982)	56
	Lifeguards (Haddad & Chyu,[86] 1971)	65
	Lifeguards (Better et al,[87] 1980)	60
	Summer outdoor workers (Barger-Lux & Heaney,[88] 2002)	49
2. Native blacks in Africa and Europe[89] (all similar 1,25(OH)2D levels)	Black men living in Kinshasa Congo	26
	Black men living in Belgium	13
	White men living in Belgium	31
3. African populations with intensive sun exposure	Masai and Hadzabe[12,90]	46
	South Africans J'burg children[91]	40
	Gambia healthy children (Thacher et al,[92] 1999)	20
	Healthy children (Prentice et al,[93] 2008)	38
	Healthy adults (Prentice,[94] 2008)	33–36
	Ghana (Durazo-Arvizu et al,[14] 2014)	30
4. Other regions of world	Jamaica (Durazo-Arvizy et al,[14] 2014)	29
	Australian Aboriginals (Vanlint et al,[95] 2011)	23

[a] To convert nmol/L into ng/mL multiply by 0.4.

of 25OHD, such as in the Middle-East and Gulf states.[15] Occasionally, there is even a reversal of the seasonal variation of serum 25OHD with winter values being higher than summer values in some Gulf States by avoiding all sun exposure during the very hot summer months and more sun exposure during "winter" time.[16] When comparing the worldwide distribution of low (<50 nmol/L) to very low (<25 nmol/L) serum 25OHD concentrations (**Table 3**), it is obvious that the native African population living close to the equator has the best vitamin D status, but when living in more moderate climate zones, their mean 25OHD concentrations are lower, indicating that ethnicity or race is not the main driver of the vitamin D status. Similarly, Caucasians living in North America or Australian/New Zealand have a higher mean 25OHD concentration than their ancestors still living in Western or Middle Europe (see **Tables 2** and **3**). The populations of the Middle East and Gulf States and Northern China/Mongolia have the lowest mean vitamin D status, but this is most likely due to lifestyle differences than to genetic mechanisms.

Table 3
World overview of low serum 25-hydroxyvitamin D concentrations

Serum 25OHD Levels	<10–12 ng/mL, %	<20 ng/mL, %
World overview: 168,000 subjects from 44 countries[96]	6.7	37
US: NHANES 2010 data (>12 y)[97]	6.7	26
EU countries (adults): adjusted 25OHD method[98]	13	40
Middle East/N. Africa (Iran & Jordan)[99]	~50	90
African countries (Ghana, Seychelles)[14]	<0.1	7
China: (estimated from meta-analysis in adults)[100]	~37	~72
Mongolia[99]	~50	NA

ETHNIC AND RACIAL DIFFERENCE IN PROTEINS RELATED TO VITAMIN D STATUS OR METABOLISM

Provitamin D (7-DHC), vitamin D, and its metabolites interact with a large series of proteins before they are finally eliminated or inactivated.

Presence of 7-Dehydrocholesterol in Keratinocytes

The presence of 7-DHC in keratinocytes is essential for the photochemical production of vitamin D_3. 7-DHC is the ultimate metabolite before the final de novo synthesis of cholesterol is realized by the enzyme 7-DHC-reductase, or *delta-7-sterol-reductase* (EC 1.3.1.21), using NADPH. The reverse enzyme 7-DHC-dehydrogenase does not exist in mammalian species or birds so that cholesterol itself cannot be converted into vitamin D. Congenital absence of delta-7-sterol-reductase results in the Smith-Lemli-Opitz syndrome, causing many minor and major congenital abnormities because of the absence of cholesterol. The enzyme is regulated by cholesterol itself by end-product inhibition, thereby accelerating the proteasomal degradation of delta-7-sterol-reductase. This may represent an important switch between cholesterol and vitamin D synthesis that needs further exploration.[17] Only massive amounts of vitamin D but not 1,25(OH)$_2$D may modestly decrease delta-7-sterol-reductase activity in some keratinocyte cell lines, so that it is unlikely that the vitamin D endocrine system plays a role in this pathway.[18] Excess 7-DHC should cause overproduction of vitamin D when exposed to UV-B. Such patients are prone to photosensitivity, which appears to be UV-A mediated.[19] Photosensitivity can be severe and can result from even brief exposure to sunlight. Many children cannot tolerate any exposure to sunlight; others can tolerate varying periods of exposure if properly clothed and protected with a UV-A- and UV-B-protection sunscreen. For these reasons, toxicity because of the expected potential overproduction of vitamin D has not been documented.[20] The inverse situation is found in cats (and the feline species) and dogs, who have higher expression of delta-7-sterol-reductase in their keratinocytes, so that there is too little 7-DHC in these cells to be converted into vitamin D on exposure to sunlight. In these animals, vitamin D is truly a vitamin D because they are unable to synthesize vitamin D (dogs[21]; cats[22]). When such animals are treated with a 7-DHC-delta-7-reductase inhibitor, they are, however, able to produce vitamin D during UV-B exposure. Such agents are also able to allow in vitro vitamin D production in either keratinocytes or even several nonkeratinocyte cells.[23,24] Based on these 2 extremes, one could image that variations in 7-DHC content in the skin, based on relative variations in delta-7-sterol-reductase expression or activity, would make people more or less sensitive to the endogenous production of vitamin D. There are limited data suggesting that in old age keratinocytes have a lower content of 7-DHC, but there are no data on genetic or ethnic differences in 7-DHC content of the skin or of delta-7-sterol-reductase activity. The delta-7-sterol-reductase gene is polymorphic (2 SNPs), and GWAS and candidate gene analysis of Caucasian and Chinese populations concluded that serum 25OHD is influenced by this polymorphism.[25-29] This gene effect is, however, small (explaining <2% of the variation in serum 25OHD), and there are no data on relevant ethnic or genetic differences in the predominant delta-7-sterol-reductase gene expression. Overall, delta-7-sterol-reductase has a minor effect on serum 25OHD but does not seem to be the cause of ethnic or racial differences in vitamin D status.

Vitamin D Transport Proteins

Intestinal absorption of vitamin D in normal subjects is high (about 70% based on isotope-labeled studies). The uptake of such a lipophilic molecule was for a long time considered to be mainly passive, but recent data suggest that this uptake is facilitated by specific transport systems also used for cholesterol, such as scavenger receptor class B type 1 (SR-BI) or CD36. Indeed, in vitro or ex vivo studies indicated that cholesterol or α-tocopherol can decrease the uptake of vitamin D in intestinal cells and that overexpression of SR-BI enhances vitamin D absorption.[30] SR-BI is polymorphic, and its gene (SCARB1) variation affects plasma levels of vitamin E, but no such studies are available for vitamin D status.[31] After intestinal uptake, vitamin D is first transported by *chylomicrons*[32] before being delivered to several cells or tissues (such as adipose tissue or liver) or transferred to a specific serum transport protein, DBP.[33] There are no data on ethnic, racial, or genetic differences in such chylomicron transport. In serum, vitamin D and all its metabolites are mostly bound to serum proteins.[34] The *vitamin D binding protein or DBP* and albumin are the main transporters, but DBP has a much higher affinity than albumin for all D metabolites, so that the large majority (>80%) is DBP bound.[34–37] DBP is a member of the DBP/albumin/α-fetoprotein family and is known to be very polymorphic. In fact, it is one of the most polymorphic proteins known[38] because it was originally discovered and named because of that reason as group-specific component or GC (reviewed in ref.[34]). DBP has a single binding site for all D metabolites located in a cleft at the surface of the A domain.[39] The most frequent polymorphism is due to 2 amino acid differences located in the C domain, far away from the binding cleft.[34]

DBP (GC) is the product of 2 autosomal, codominant alleles (GC1 and GC2). Isoelectric focusing allows the further characterization of slow (Gc1S) and fast (Gc1F) subtypes of Gc1, resulting in 6 common phenotypes. More recently, genotyping is the most common way of identifying DBP/GC polymorphisms (**Table 4**). GC2 is due to the presence of lysine instead of threonine (for GC1) at position 436, whereas GC1s and GC1f differ by the presence of glutamic acid instead of aspartic acid as amino acid 432, respectively. The relative frequency of the GC1f allele is high in people living close to the equator (including most African blacks with close to 90% having GC1f), whereas the GC1s frequency is steadily increasing in populations living in more Northern climates (GC1f allele only found in 10% of Northern Europeans). GC2 is rare in Africans but much more frequent in whites.[40] DBP concentrations are usually measured by immunoassays. Powe and colleagues[41] found that African Americans had substantially lower serum DBP concentrations than US Caucasians, and they found this to be due to the relative presence of GC1f allele. Indeed, they observed that homozygous carriers of GC1f had DBP serum concentration less than 50% of that of homozygous GC1s carriers (or GC2 carriers) with intermediate values in heterozygotes. This big racial difference was confirmed in many other studies using the same R&D monoclonal antibody enzyme-linked immunosorbent assay (**Table 5**). This large

Table 4 Common DBP/GC polymorphisms		
Amino Acid	**432 (416)[a]**	**436 (420)[a]**
Gc 1f	Asp	Thr[b]
Gc 1s	Glu	Thr[b]
Gc 2	Asp	Lys
SNP	RS 7041 Asp → Glu	RS 4588 Thr → Lys

[a] Amino acid 432 and 436 is due to renumbering by counting the presequence.
[b] Threonine of Gc1 is O-linked with NAcGalactosamine, Galactose (with or without additional sialic acid).

Table 5
Overview of serum DBP concentration by race and assay methodology

Study	Black	White	Assay
Powe et al,[101] 2011	144 ± 102 (SE)	248 ± 122 (SE)	R&D
Bhan et al,[102] 2012	75	189	R&D
Denburg et al,[103] 2013	100 (50–250) (median IQR)	240 (160–300) (median IQR)	R&D
Powe et al,[41] 2013	168 ± 3 (SE)	337 ± 5 (SE)	R&D
Schwartz et al,[104] 2014	152 ± 107 (SD)	301 ± 210 (SD)	R&D
Aloia et al,[42] 2015	151	264	R&D
Denburg et al,[44] 2016	106	215	R&D
Nielson et al,[46] 2016	277	128	R&D
M'Buyamba-Kabangu et al,[89] 1987	329 ± 54 (Zaire)	329 ± 43 (Belgium)	Polyclonal RID
Winters et al,[105] 2009	491 ± 128 (SD)	529 ± 202 (SD)	Polyclonal (Alpco)
Denburg et al,[44] 2016	380	376	Polyclonal (Alpco)
Nielson et al,[46] 2016	286	291	Polyclonal RID

Abbreviations: IQR, interquartile range; SD, standard deviation; SE, standard error.

difference in DBP concentrations had major consequences for the calculation of free 25OHD and resulted in normal or even slightly higher 25OHD in most African Americans compared with Caucasians despite much lower total 25OHD in African Americans. These data received substantial attention because it seemed to explain at least part of the African American paradox of a low vitamin D status being associated with a decreased risk of fractures in African Americans.[42] Some older studies using polyclonal antibodies for the immunoassay of DBP, however, had not found a racial difference in DBP concentrations.[43] Mass spectroscopy (MS)[44,45] did not confirm a significant difference in DBP between blacks and whites or between GC1f and GC1s carriers. Because well-validated MS/MS assays can be considered as arbiter for defining the relative or even absolute concentrations of analytes, polyclonal antibody immunoassays were thus found to be reliable, whereas the R&D DBP assay is biased by discrimination between DBP polymorphisms by the monoclonal antibodies used.

An overview of DBP assays using a variety of polyclonal antibodies and techniques reveals indeed that there is no consistent racial or ethnic difference in serum DBP (see **Table 5**). The absolute values are, however, very variable depending on the assay (and standard) used, but the relative DBP values are not racially different. Subjects homozygous for GC2, however, have usually a slightly (about 10%) lower serum DBP concentration than GC1 homozygotes, independent on the country of origin or ethnicity[44–48] (**Table 6**). This is in fact the opposite of what was found by the monoclonal R&D DBP assay.[41] The reason for the lower DBP concentration in GC2 carriers is unknown but may be related to differences in catabolism because DBP/GC2 lacks a glycosylation site on amino acid 436.

DBP/GC polymorphism is also well known to be related to serum 25OHD concentrations as found in 4 independent GWAS studies[25–27,49] and several other candidate gene studies (reviewed in ref.[50]), all indicating that this polymorphism has the greatest influence on 25OHD levels of all vitamin D pathway–related polymorphisms.[51,52] The polymorphism coding for GC2 is indeed associated with a 5% to 15% lower serum 25OHD concentration in comparison with subjects with GC1 genotypes.

Table 6
DBP/Gc polymorphism and vitamin D status

Lower Levels of 25OHD in Gc 2-2 Subjects Found in:	Difference (nmol/L)
Danish (2005)[106]	−15
US Hispanics and African Americans (2008)[79]	−x[a]
Dutch (2009)[107]	−10
French (2009)[108]	−8
Belgian COPD patients and controls (2010)[59]	−12
US whites (2010)[109]	−6
Shanghai Chinese (2013)[52]	−6
Finland (2014)[110]	−6
India (2015)[111]	−x[a]

Association between GC genotype and 1,25(OH)$_2$D is less important or less consistent but serum 1,25(OH)$_2$D is better related with serum DBP concentration.
[a] Significantly lower but precise difference not mentioned in article.

Unfortunately, several large GWAS studies did only evaluate the effect of one SNP rs2282679, related to an intron area of the DBP/GC gene, and did not pick up the effects of the 2 major polymorphisms in the DBP/GC gene on 25OHD levels. Indeed, the 2 most common genotypic differences in DBP/GC are found in one of the exons and code for amino acids 432 and 436 (see **Table 4**) (rs 7041 and rs 4588). The mechanism explaining this association with 25OHD levels is unknown. At first sight, it seems attractive to suggest a feedback mechanism for the free 25OHD concentration, whereby the lower serum DBP as found in DBP/GC2-2 homozygotes results in lower serum 25OHD concentrations, in line with similar phenomena for free and total cortisol, testosterone, or thyroid hormones when their specific serum transport protein fluctuates.[35,53] However, there are strong arguments in animals and humans that changes in serum DBP by hormone treatment or infusions do not consistently result in changes in serum 25OHD,[53] and vice versa, deficiency or excess serum 25OHD does not modify the concentration of serum DBP.[34]

As DBP is the main carrier for 25OHD and other vitamin D metabolites, its concentration and affinity are the main drivers of the free concentration of 25OHD and other D metabolites.[35] The free concentration of 25OHD can be directly measured by a recently developed immunoassay (Future Diagnostics, Wijchen, The Netherlands), but the assay still needs further validation beyond normal subjects, and especially in situations with abnormal DBP concentrations.[37,46] Most studies so far have used calculated free 25OHD concentrations based on the law of mass action and assuming either a constant or a genotype-specific affinity for 25OHD. One study[54] found a major difference in affinity with the highest found in GC1f-1f and the lowest in GC2-2 carriers (overall more than 2-fold difference), with intermediate values for GC1s. Three other studies,[54–57] using a better technology, however, did not find a significant genotype-dependent affinity.[34,37] In addition, there is some discrepancy in the absolute value of the Ka between DBP and 25OHD, and this may depend on temperature or pH or buffer conditions used.[56] Several studies found a fairly high correlation coefficient between calculated (using polyclonal antibodies and constant affinity) and directly measured free 25OHD.[45,46] If there is no racial difference in DBP concentration or affinity for 25OHD, then the simple law of mass action predicts that the free 25OHD concentration will closely be in line with the total 25OHD concentration. This was indeed found in blacks because Gambians had both high total and free 25OHD in comparison with African Americans having both low (calculated) free and total 25OHD concentrations,[45,46] whereas their DBP/GC genotypes were very similar as predictable from their common racial background. Directly measured free 25OHD was lower in African Americans in comparison with US whites in the author's studies,[45,46] but others did not find a significant difference.[42]

Serum 1,25(OH)$_2$D concentrations are also under genetic control based on twin studies but to a much lesser extent than serum 25OHD (see **Table 1**). This is unlikely because of genetic, ethnic, or racial differences in DBP (see earlier discussion). There are differences in total 1,25(OH)$_2$D concentrations between blacks and whites (blacks usually having somewhat higher concentrations than whites), but this may be related to differences in habitual calcium intake or may be due to other factors such as yet to be explored polymorphisms in CYP27B1 or CYP24A1. In contrast to 25OHD, free concentrations of 1,25(OH)$_2$D are tightly feedback regulated,[34,35] but there are few large-scale studies to link variations in total or free 1,25(OH)$_2$D to genes, racial or ethnic differences, or late hard end points, such as fractures, falls, cardiovascular and metabolic effects, or mortality. In the MsOS study, 1,25(OH)$_2$D was linked, independently from 25OHD, with inflammation and bone mass.[58] DBP polymorphism, independently from serum 25OHD, is also linked to a wide variety of health problems and especially with chronic obstructive pulmonary disease (COPD),[59,60] but the biological mechanisms are unclear.

VITAMIN METABOLIZING ENZYMES

The 3 major enzymes of the CYP family could each be involved in genetic, ethnic, or racial differences in vitamin D status, metabolism, or action.

CYP2R1 is the major 25-hydroxylase. It is a microsomal enzyme and does not discriminate between vitamin D$_3$ and D$_2$ and has most likely a high-affinity, low-capacity profile all in line with the expected in vivo properties of the hepatic 25-hydroxylase.[61] Biallelic inactivating mutations can cause vitamin D–dependent rickets type 1B (VDDR1B or MIM 600081) characterized by very low (but not null) levels of 25OHD (<10 nmol/L) and normal to high serum 1,25(OH)$_2$D concentrations. The presence of 1,25(OH)$_2$D is remarkable and indicates that at least one other 25-hydroxylase must be present. Several families have now been described, initially from West Africa and Saudi Arabia but more recently also in Caucasians.[61–64]

The disease is autosomal dominant, and the frequency of the mutant allele, based on limited studies, would be around 0.5% in African or African American[61] populations. The gene is polymorphic, and several studies from different areas of the world have confirmed that the minor allele (not the mutated one) frequency is associated with lower serum 25OHD concentrations.[25,26] The effect of this polymorphism has thus been found in all populations studied so far, independent of their region of origin: Caucasians,[65] African Americans,[66] Chinese,[28,52] subjects from the Middle East,[67] natives from Alaska.[68,69] The impact of this polymorphism is thus found in a wide variety of populations around the world and is unlikely to be linked to racial or ethnic differences. Its overall contribution is, however, less than 2% of the overall variation in serum 25OHD.

CYP27B1 is the enzyme responsible for the systemic or local generation of the hormonally active form of vitamin D (1,25(OH)$_2$D). Absence of this gene/protein is responsible for the total loss of the end product. This is in contrast to CYP2R1 and CYP24A1 because biallelic mutations of these genes results in marked but not total loss of end product formation. In several GWAS or other genetic studies, no link between possible polymorphism of this gene and serum 25OHD concentrations has been found in the general population. In one twin study dealing with patients with multiple sclerosis, CYP27B1 polymorphism was associated with serum 25OHD concentrations.[70] Other data are inconclusive.[50] CYP24A1 is the key enzyme responsible for the formation of 24,25(OH)$_2$D or 1,24,25(OH)$_3$D and its further metabolites. This enzyme is considered to be the major catabolizing enzyme, and its loss results in idiopathic hypercalcemia of infancy or an equivalent disease in adults.[71,72] This gene is also polymorphic, and several GWAS studies indicated a modest effect of this polymorphism on serum 25OHD concentrations. Indeed, in most of the studies looking at the effects of polymorphism of DBP/GC, CYP2R1, and delta-7-steroid reductase,[25–27,49] CYP24A1 polymorphism was a weak or inconsistent contributor to the overall variation in serum 25OHD, whereas DBP/GC and CYP2R1 polymorphisms had the greatest effect. The biologic half-life of 25OHD is slightly lower in subjects from Gambia compared with that of UK Caucasians, and the difference may be influenced by DBP genotype or concentration.[73] However, whether these small differences are truly racially driven requires more extensive studies.

Based on many previous studies, low serum 25OHD concentrations are linked to increased mortality risk.[74] One recent study in German subjects confirmed this link and also confirmed the association between serum 25OHD and the SNPs summarized in the present review. However, the SNPS resulting in the low serum 25OHD did not contribute to the mortality risk.[75]

SUMMARY

Several independent twin studies have clearly shown an important genetic influence on the serum concentration of 25OHD, and this effect may explain about 50% of the variation of serum 25OHD. The same studies also suggest a genetic influence on serum 1,25(OH)$_2$D concentrations but to a much lesser extent. No large-scale studies have been done so far for free 25OHD or free 1,25(OH)$_2$D concentrations. Several GWAS studies including a large to very large number of subjects identified at least 3 gene polymorphisms related to serum 25OHD: delta-7-sterol-reductase, CYP2R1, and DBP/GC with a combined effect explaining 5% (at best up to 10%) of the variation in serum 25OHD. This effect is at most similar to the effect of season on serum 25OHD concentrations. The polymorphism of CYP24A1 has more marginal effects, sometimes not or just significant according to several studies. Overall, the large majority of the genetic variation of 25OHD, based on twin studies, is thus not explained so far. The largest effect (greater than the combined effect of the other polymorphisms) is found for polymorphism of DBP/GC, the major serum carrier protein for all vitamin D metabolites. One monoclonal assay for DBP (R&D) found repeatedly markedly low DBP concentrations in African Americans or carriers of GC1f. The use of this monoclonal DBP assay resulted in calculated normal or high free serum 25OHD concentrations in African Americans, when compared with US whites, despite their much lower total 25OHD concentrations. It is now clear that this assay does not properly detect DBP/GC1f (because of its monoclonal antibody epitope profile). Many other studies using polyclonal antibody-based immunoassays revealed (confirmed by MS data) that there is no significant difference in serum DBP between Africans/African Americans and Caucasians. Many studies in different populations using several polyclonal-based immunoassays, however, found that homozygous carriers of DBP/GC2-2 have slightly lower serum DBP and serum 25OHD concentrations (about 5%–15%) than other subjects having other homozygous DBP/GC alleles, with intermediate effects on heterozygous carriers. None of the polymorphisms is known to create a bone or calcium homeostasis–related disease. However, polymorphisms of

DBP/GC may be associated with nonskeletal disorders such as COPD. The polymorphisms related to the vitamin D axis and influencing serum 25OHD are, however, not truly racially or ethnically determined because all polymorphisms are found in all populations studied so far. Only the major driver, DBP/GC polymorphism, is known to have a specific distribution with a clear South-North gradient of GC1f allele, being the most frequent allele in equatorial areas around the world with a steady decrease in the frequency of this allele in favor of GC2s and GC2 in subjects living in a more Northern climate. This trend is observed on a world scale but also within a large country such as France, Saudi Arabia, or Japan. These observations seem to indicate that there has been (or is) a strong evolutionary driver for this shift in allele frequency, and UV-B exposure could be a likely factor. However, no true mechanism explaining these phenomena has been identified. Overall, there are several independent twin studies around the world indicating a strong genetic influence on serum 25OHD concentrations, but the known vitamin D–related gene polymorphism only explains about 5% of the variation in serum 25OHD.

REFERENCES

1. Bouillon R, Carmeliet G, Verlinden L, et al. Vitamin D and human health: lessons from vitamin D receptor null mice. Endocr Rev 2008;29(6):726–76.
2. Bouillon R. Vitamin D: from photosynthesis, metabolism, and action to clinical applications. In: Jameson JL, De Groot LJ, editors. Endocrinology: adult and pediatric. Philadelphia: Saunders/Elsevier; 2016. p. 1018–38.
3. Rosen CJ, Adams JS, Bikle DD, et al. The nonskeletal effects of vitamin D: an Endocrine Society scientific statement. Endocr Rev 2012;33(3):456–92.
4. Bikle DD. Extraskeletal actions of vitamin D. Ann N Y Acad Sci 2016;1376(1):29–52.
5. Cashman KD, Seamans KM, Lucey AJ, et al. Relative effectiveness of oral 25-hydroxyvitamin D3 and vitamin D3 in raising wintertime serum 25-hydroxyvitamin D in older adults. Am J Clin Nutr 2012;95(6):1350–6.
6. Jetter A, Egli A, Dawson-Hughes B, et al. Pharmacokinetics of oral vitamin D(3) and calcifediol. Bone 2014;59:14–9.
7. Spiro A, Buttriss JL. Vitamin D: an overview of vitamin D status and intake in Europe. Nutr Bull 2014;39(4):322–50.
8. Bouillon R. Comparative analysis of nutritional guidelines for vitamin D. Nat Rev Endocrinol 2017;13(8):466–79.
9. Holick MF. Biological effects of sunlight, ultraviolet radiation, visible light, infrared radiation and vitamin D for health. Anticancer Res 2016;36(3):1345–56.
10. Holick MF. Vitamin D deficiency. N Engl J Med 2007;357(3):266–81.
11. Petersen B, Wulf HC, Triguero-Mas M, et al. Sun and ski holidays improve vitamin D status, but are associated with high levels of DNA damage. J Invest Dermatol 2014;134(11):2806–13.
12. Luxwolda MF, Kuipers RS, Kema IP, et al. Vitamin D status indicators in indigenous populations in East Africa. Eur J Nutr 2013;52(3):1115–25.
13. Laurent MR, Gielen E, Pauwels S, et al. Hypervitaminosis D associated with tanning bed use: a case report. Ann Intern Med 2017;166(2):155–6.
14. Durazo-Arvizu RA, Camacho P, Bovet P, et al. 25-Hydroxyvitamin D in African-origin populations at varying latitudes challenges the construct of a physiologic norm. Am J Clin Nutr 2014;100(3):908–14.

15. Bassil D, Rahme M, Hoteit M, et al. Hypovitaminosis D in the Middle East and North Africa: prevalence, risk factors and impact on outcomes. Dermatoendocrinol 2013;5(2):274–98.
16. Al-Daghri NM, Al-Attas OS, Alokail MS, et al. Increased vitamin D supplementation recommended during summer season in the gulf region: a counterintuitive seasonal effect in vitamin D levels in adult, overweight and obese Middle Eastern residents. Clin Endocrinol (Oxf) 2012;76(3):346–50.
17. Prabhu AV, Luu W, Sharpe LJ, et al. Cholesterol-mediated degradation of 7-dehydrocholesterol reductase switches the balance from cholesterol to vitamin D synthesis. J Biol Chem 2016;291(16):8363–73.
18. Zou L, Porter TD. Rapid suppression of 7-dehydrocholesterol reductase activity in keratinocytes by vitamin D. J Steroid Biochem Mol Biol 2015;148:64–71.
19. Anstey A. Photomedicine: lessons from the Smith-Lemli-Opitz syndrome. J Photochem Photobiol B 2001;62(3):123–7.
20. Rossi M, Federico G, Corso G, et al. Vitamin D status in patients affected by Smith-Lemli-Opitz syndrome. J Inherit Metab Dis 2005;28(1):69–80.
21. Hazewinkel HA, Tryfonidou MA. Vitamin D3 metabolism in dogs. Mol Cell Endocrinol 2002;197(1–2):23–33.
22. Morris JG. Ineffective vitamin D synthesis in cats is reversed by an inhibitor of 7-dehydrocholestrol-delta7-reductase. J Nutr 1999;129(4):903–8.
23. Vantieghem K, De Haes P, Bouillon R, et al. Dermal fibroblasts pretreated with a sterol Delta7-reductase inhibitor produce 25-hydroxyvitamin D3 upon UVB irradiation. J Photochem Photobiol B 2006;85(1):72–8.
24. Vantieghem K, Overbergh L, Carmeliet G, et al. UVB-induced 1,25(OH)2D3 production and vitamin D activity in intestinal CaCo-2 cells and in THP-1 macrophages pretreated with a sterol Delta7-reductase inhibitor. J Cell Biochem 2006; 99(1):229–40.
25. Wang TJ, Zhang F, Richards JB, et al. Common genetic determinants of vitamin D insufficiency: a genome-wide association study. Lancet 2010;376(9736): 180–8.
26. Ahn J, Yu K, Stolzenberg-Solomon R, et al. Genome-wide association study of circulating vitamin D levels. Hum Mol Genet 2010;19(13):2739–45.
27. Hiraki LT, Major JM, Chen C, et al. Exploring the genetic architecture of circulating 25-hydroxyvitamin D. Genet Epidemiol 2013;37(1):92–8.
28. Zhang Y, Wang X, Liu Y, et al. The GC, CYP2R1 and DHCR7 genes are associated with vitamin D levels in northeastern Han Chinese children. Swiss Med Wkly 2012;142:w13636.
29. Lu L, Sheng H, Li H, et al. Associations between common variants in GC and DHCR7/NADSYN1 and vitamin D concentration in Chinese Hans. Hum Genet 2012;131(3):505–12.
30. Reboul E, Goncalves A, Comera C, et al. Vitamin D intestinal absorption is not a simple passive diffusion: evidences for involvement of cholesterol transporters. Mol Nutr Food Res 2011;55(5):691–702.
31. Borel P, Moussa M, Reboul E, et al. Human plasma levels of vitamin E and carotenoids are associated with genetic polymorphisms in genes involved in lipid metabolism. J Nutr 2007;137(12):2653–9.
32. Dueland S, Pedersen JI, Helgerud P, et al. Absorption, distribution, and transport of vitamin D3 and 25-hydroxyvitamin D3 in the rat. Am J Physiol 1983; 245(5 Pt 1):E463–7.
33. Dueland S, Bouillon R, Van Baelen H, et al. Binding protein for vitamin D and its metabolites in rat mesenteric lymph. Am J Physiol 1985;249(1 Pt 1):E1–5.

34. Bouillon R, Pauwels S. Vitamin D binding protein. In: Feldman D, Pike JW, Adams J, editors. Vitamin D. London: Elsevier, in press.

35. Bouillon R, Vanassche FA, Vanbaelen H, et al. Influence of the vitamin D-binding protein on the serum concentration of 1,25-dihydroxyvitamin D3-significance of the free 1,25-dihydroxyvitamin D3 concentration. J Clin Invest 1981;67(3): 589–96.

36. Chun RF, Peercy BE, Orwoll ES, et al. Vitamin D and DBP: the free hormone hypothesis revisited. J Steroid Biochem Mol Biol 2014;144 Pt A:132–7.

37. Bikle D, Bouillon R, Thadhani R, et al. Vitamin D metabolites in captivity? Should we measure free or total 25(OH)D to assess vitamin D status? J Steroid Biochem Mol Biol 2017. [Epub ahead of print].

38. Cleve H, Constans J. The mutants of the vitamin D-binding protein - more than 120 variants of the GC/DBP system. Vox Sang 1988;54(4):215–25.

39. Verboven C, Ragijns A, De Maeyer M, et al. A structural basis for the unique binding features of the human vitamin D-binding protein. Nat Struct Biol 2002; 9(2):131–6.

40. Kamboh MI, Ferrell RE. Ethnic variation in vitamin D-binding protein (GC): a review of isoelectric focusing studies in human populations. Hum Genet 1986; 72(4):281–93.

41. Powe CE, Evans MK, Wenger J, et al. Vitamin D-binding protein and vitamin D status of black Americans and white Americans. N Engl J Med 2013;369(21): 1991–2000.

42. Aloia J, Mikhail M, Dhaliwal R, et al. Free 25(OH)D and the vitamin D paradox in African Americans. J Clin Endocrinol Metab 2015;100(9):3356–63.

43. Bouillon R, Jones K, Schoenmakers I. Vitamin D-binding protein and vitamin D in blacks and whites. N Engl J Med 2014;370(9):879.

44. Denburg MR, Hoofnagle AN, Sayed S, et al. Comparison of two ELISA methods and mass spectrometry for measurement of vitamin D-binding protein: implications for the assessment of bioavailable vitamin D concentrations across genotypes. J Bone Miner Res 2016;31(6):1128–36.

45. Nielson CM, Jones KS, Chun RF, et al. Role of assay type in determining free 25-hydroxyvitamin D levels in diverse populations. N Engl J Med 2016; 374(17):1695–6.

46. Nielson CM, Jones KS, Chun RF, et al. Free 25-hydroxyvitamin D: impact of vitamin D binding protein assays on racial-genotypic associations. J Clin Endocrinol Metab 2016;101(5):2226–34.

47. Carpenter TO, Zhang JH, Parra E, et al. Vitamin D binding protein is a key determinant of 25-hydroxyvitamin D levels in infants and toddlers. J Bone Miner Res 2013;28(1):213–21.

48. Lauridsen AL, Vestergaard P, Nexo E. Mean serum concentration of vitamin D-binding protein (Gc globulin) is related to the Gc phenotype in women. Clin Chem 2001;47(4):753–6.

49. Sapkota BR, Hopkins R, Bjonnes A, et al. Genome-wide association study of 25(OH) Vitamin D concentrations in Punjabi Sikhs: results of the Asian Indian diabetic heart study. J Steroid Biochem Mol Biol 2016;158:149–56.

50. Dastani Z, Li R, Richards B. Genetic regulation of vitamin D levels. Calcif Tissue Int 2013;92(2):106–17.

51. Bouillon R. Genetic and environmental determinants of vitamin D status. Lancet 2010;376(9736):148–9.

52. Zhang Z, He JW, Fu WZ, et al. An analysis of the association between the vitamin D pathway and serum 25-hydroxyvitamin D levels in a healthy Chinese population. J Bone Miner Res 2013;28(8):1784–92.

53. Bouillon R, Vandoren G, Van Baelen H, et al. Lack of effect of the vitamin D status on the concentration of the vitamin D-binding protein in rat serum. Endocrinology 1980;107(1):160–3.

54. Arnaud J, Constans J. Affinity differences for vitamin D metabolites associated with the genetic isoforms of the human serum carrier protein (DBP). Hum Genet 1993;92(2):183–8.

55. Kawakami M, Imawari M, Goodman DS. Quantitative studies of the interaction of cholecalciferol ((vitamin D3) and its metabolites with different genetic variants of the serum binding protein for these sterols. Biochem J 1979;179(2):413–23.

56. Bouillon R, van Baelen H, de Moor P. Comparative study of the affinity of the serum vitamin D-binding protein. J Steroid Biochem 1980;13(9):1029–34.

57. Boutin B, Galbraith RM, Arnaud P. Comparative affinity of the major genetic variants of human group-specific component (vitamin D-binding protein) for 25-(OH) vitamin D. J Steroid Biochem 1989;32(1A):59–63.

58. Srikanth P, Chun RF, Hewison M, et al. Associations of total and free 25OHD and 1,25(OH)2D with serum markers of inflammation in older men. Osteoporos Int 2016;27(7):2291–300.

59. Janssens W, Bouillon R, Claes B, et al. Vitamin D deficiency is highly prevalent in COPD and correlates with variants in the vitamin D-binding gene. Thorax 2010; 65(3):215–20.

60. Delanghe JR, Speeckaert R, Speeckaert MM. Behind the scenes of vitamin D binding protein: more than vitamin D binding. Best Pract Res Clin Endocrinol Metab 2015;29(5):773–86.

61. Cheng JB, Levine MA, Bell NH, et al. Genetic evidence that the human CYP2R1 enzyme is a key vitamin D 25-hydroxylase. Proc Natl Acad Sci U S A 2004; 101(20):7711–5.

62. Levine MA, Dang A, ding C, et al. Tropical rickets in Nigeria: mutation of the CYP2R1 gene encoding vitamin D 25-hydroxylase as a cause of vitamin D dependent rickets. Bone 2007;40(6 suppl 1):S60–1.

63. Thacher TD, Fischer PR, Singh RJ, et al. CYP2R1 mutations impair generation of 25-hydroxyvitamin D and cause an atypical form of vitamin D deficiency. J Clin Endocrinol Metab 2015;100(7):E1005–13.

64. Al Mutair AN, Nasrat GH, Russell DW. Mutation of the CYP2R1 vitamin D 25-hydroxylase in a Saudi Arabian family with severe vitamin D deficiency. J Clin Endocrinol Metab 2012;97(10):E2022–5.

65. Nissen J, Rasmussen LB, Ravn-Haren G, et al. Common variants in CYP2R1 and GC genes predict vitamin D concentrations in healthy Danish children and adults. PLoS One 2014;9(2):e89907.

66. Signorello LB, Shi J, Cai Q, et al. Common variation in vitamin D pathway genes predicts circulating 25-hydroxyvitamin D levels among African Americans. PLoS One 2011;6(12):e28623.

67. Elkum N, Alkayal F, Noronha F, et al. Vitamin D insufficiency in Arabs and South Asians positively associates with polymorphisms in GC and CYP2R1 genes. PLoS One 2014;9(11):e113102.

68. Fohner AE, Wang Z, Yracheta J, et al. Genetics, diet, and season are associated with serum 25-hydroxycholecalciferol concentration in a Yup'ik study population from southwestern Alaska. J Nutr 2016;146(2):318–25.

69. Xu X, Mao J, Zhang M, et al. Vitamin D deficiency in Uygurs and Kazaks is associated with polymorphisms in CYP2R1 and DHCR7/NADSYN1 genes. Medical science monitor. Int Med J Exp Clin Res 2015;21:1960–8.

70. Orton SM, Morris AP, Herrera BM, et al. Evidence for genetic regulation of vitamin D status in twins with multiple sclerosis. Am J Clin Nutr 2008;88(2): 441–7.

71. Schlingmann KP, Kaufmann M, Weber S, et al. Mutations in CYP24A1 and idiopathic infantile hypercalcemia. N Engl J Med 2011;365(5):410–21.

72. Cools M, Goemaere S, Baetens D, et al. Calcium and bone homeostasis in heterozygous carriers of CYP24A1 mutations: a cross-sectional study. Bone 2015; 81:89–96.

73. Jones KS, Assar S, Harnpanich D, et al. 25(OH)D2 half-life is shorter than 25(OH)D3 half-life and is influenced by DBP concentration and genotype. J Clin Endocrinol Metab 2014;99(9):3373–81.

74. Bouillon R, Van Schoor NM, Gielen E, et al. Optimal vitamin D status: a critical analysis on the basis of evidence-based medicine. J Clin Endocrinol Metab 2013;98(8):E1283–304.

75. Ordonez-Mena JM, Maalmi H, Schottker B, et al. Genetic variants in the vitamin D pathway, 25(OH)D levels, and mortality in a large population-based cohort study. J Clin Endocrinol Metab 2017;102(2):470–7.

76. Hunter D, De Lange M, Snieder H, et al. Genetic contribution to bone metabolism, calcium excretion, and vitamin D and parathyroid hormone regulation. J Bone Miner Res 2001;16(2):371–8.

77. Wjst M, Altmuller J, Braig C, et al. A genome-wide linkage scan for 25-OH-D(3) and 1,25-(OH)2-D3 serum levels in asthma families. J Steroid Biochem Mol Biol 2007;103(3–5):799–802.

78. Orton SM, Ebers GC. Heritability of serum vitamin D concentrations: twin studies. Am J Clin Nutr 2011;93(3):667–8 [author reply: 668].

79. Engelman CD, Fingerlin TE, Langefeld CD, et al. Genetic and environmental determinants of 25-hydroxyvitamin D and 1,25-dihydroxyvitamin D levels in Hispanic and African Americans. J Clin Endocrinol Metab 2008;93(9):3381–8.

80. Snellman G, Melhus H, Gedeborg R, et al. Seasonal genetic influence on serum 25-hydroxyvitamin D levels: a twin study. PLoS One 2009;4(11):e7747.

81. Shea MK, Benjamin EJ, Dupuis J, et al. Genetic and non-genetic correlates of vitamins K and D. Eur J Clin Nutr 2009;63(4):458–64.

82. Karohl C, Su S, Kumari M, et al. Heritability and seasonal variability of vitamin D concentrations in male twins. Am J Clin Nutr 2010;92(6):1393–8.

83. Mills NT, Wright MJ, Henders AK, et al. Heritability of transforming growth factor-beta1 and tumor necrosis factor-receptor type 1 expression and vitamin D levels in healthy adolescent twins. Twin Res Hum Genet 2015;18(1):28–35.

84. Arguelles LM, Langman CB, Ariza AJ, et al. Heritability and environmental factors affecting vitamin D status in rural Chinese adolescent twins. J Clin Endocrinol Metab 2009;94(9):3273–81.

85. Haddock L, Corcino J, Vazquez MD. 25(OH)D serum levels in the normal Puerto Rican population and in subjects with tropical sprue and paratyroid disease. P R Health Sci J 1982;1:85–91.

86. Haddad JG, Chyu KJ. Competitive protein-binding radioassay for 25-hydroxy-cholecalciferol. J Clin Endocrinol Metab 1971;33(6):992–5.

87. Better OS, Shabtai M, Kedar S, et al. Increased incidence of nephrolithiasis (N) in lifeguards (LG) in Israel. Adv Exp Med Biol 1980;128:467–72.

88. Barger-Lux MJ, Heaney RP. Effects of above average summer sun exposure on serum 25-hydroxyvitamin D and calcium absorption. J Clin Endocrinol Metab 2002;87(11):4952–6.

89. M'Buyamba-Kabangu JR, Fagard R, Lijnen P, et al. Calcium, vitamin D-endocrine system, and parathyroid hormone in black and white males. Calcif Tissue Int 1987;41(2):70–4.

90. Luxwolda MF, Kuipers RS, Kema IP, et al. Traditionally living populations in East Africa have a mean serum 25-hydroxyvitamin D concentration of 115 nmol/l. Br J Nutr 2012;108(9):1557–61.

91. Pettifor JM, Prentice A. The role of vitamin D in paediatric bone health. Best Pract Res Clin Endocrinol Metab 2011;25(4):573–84.

92. Thacher TD, Fischer PR, Pettifor JM, et al. A comparison of calcium, vitamin D, or both for nutritional rickets in Nigerian children. N Engl J Med 1999;341(8): 563–8.

93. Prentice A, Ceesay M, Nigdikar S, et al. FGF23 is elevated in Gambian children with rickets. Bone 2008;42(4):788–97.

94. Prentice A. Vitamin D deficiency: a global perspective. Nutr Rev 2008;66(10 Suppl 2):S153–64.

95. Vanlint SJ, Morris HA, Newbury JW, et al. Vitamin D insufficiency in Aboriginal Australians. Med J Aust 2011;194(3):131–4.

96. Hilger J, Friedel A, Herr R, et al. A systematic review of vitamin D status in populations worldwide. Br J Nutr 2014;111(1):23–45.

97. Schleicher RL, Sternberg MR, Lacher DA, et al. The vitamin D status of the US population from 1988 to 2010 using standardized serum concentrations of 25-hydroxyvitamin D shows recent modest increases. Am J Clin Nutr 2016; 104(2):454–61.

98. Cashman KD, Dowling KG, Skrabakova Z, et al. Vitamin D deficiency in Europe: pandemic? Am J Clin Nutr 2016;103(4):1033–44.

99. Arabi A, El Rassi R, El-Hajj Fuleihan G. Hypovitaminosis D in developing countries-prevalence, risk factors and outcomes. Nat Rev Endocrinol 2010; 6(10):550–61.

100. Zhang W, Stoecklin E, Eggersdorfer M. A glimpse of vitamin D status in Mainland China. Nutrition 2013;29(7–8):953–7.

101. Powe CE, Ricciardi C, Berg AH, et al. Vitamin D-binding protein modifies the vitamin D-bone mineral density relationship. J Bone Miner Res 2011;26(7): 1609–16.

102. Bhan I, Powe CE, Berg AH, et al. Bioavailable vitamin D is more tightly linked to mineral metabolism than total vitamin D in incident hemodialysis patients. Kidney Int 2012;82(1):84–9.

103. Denburg MR, Kalkwarf HJ, de Boer IH, et al. Vitamin D bioavailability and catabolism in pediatric chronic kidney disease. Pediatr Nephrol 2013;28(9):1843–53.

104. Schwartz JB, Lai J, Lizaola B, et al. A comparison of measured and calculated free 25(OH) vitamin D levels in clinical populations. J Clin Endocrinol Metab 2014;99(5):1631–7.

105. Winters SJ, Chennubhatla R, Wang C, et al. Influence of obesity on vitamin D-binding protein and 25-hydroxy vitamin D levels in African American and white women. Metabolism 2009;58(4):438–42.

106. Lauridsen AL, Vestergaard P, Hermann AP, et al. Plasma concentrations of 25-hydroxy-vitamin D and 1,25-dihydroxy-vitamin D are related to the phenotype of Gc (vitamin D-binding protein): a cross-sectional study on 595 early postmenopausal women. Calcif Tissue Int 2005;77(1):15–22.

107. Fang Y, van Meurs JBJ, Arp P, et al. Vitamin D binding protein genotype and osteoporosis. Calcif Tissue Int 2009;85(2):85–93.
108. Sinotte M, Diorio C, Berube S, et al. Genetic polymorphisms of the vitamin D binding protein and plasma concentrations of 25-hydroxyvitamin D in premenopausal women. Am J Clin Nutr 2009;89(2):634–40.
109. Bu FX, Armas L, Lappe J, et al. Comprehensive association analysis of nine candidate genes with serum 25-hydroxy vitamin D levels among healthy Caucasian subjects. Hum Genet 2010;128(5):549–56.
110. Pekkinen M, Saarnio E, Viljakainen HT, et al. Vitamin D binding protein genotype is associated with serum 25-hydroxyvitamin D and PTH concentrations, as well as bone health in children and adolescents in Finland. PLoS One 2014;9(1): e87292.
111. Lafi ZM, Irshaid YM, El-Khateeb M, et al. Association of rs7041 and rs4588 polymorphisms of the vitamin D binding protein and the rs10741657 polymorphism of CYP2R1 with vitamin D Status among Jordanian patients. Genet Test Mol Biomarkers 2015;19(11):629–36.

UNITED STATES POSTAL SERVICE® Statement of Ownership, Management, and Circulation (All Periodicals Publications Except Requester Publications)

1. Publication Title	2. Publication Number		3. Filing Date
ENDOCRINOLOGY AND METABOLISM CLINICS OF NORTH AMERICA	000 – 275		9/18/2017

4. Issue Frequency	5. Number of Issues Published Annually	6. Annual Subscription Price
MAR, JUN, SEP, DEC	4	$337.00

7. Complete Mailing Address of Known Office of Publication (Not printer) (Street, city, county, state, and ZIP+4®)

ELSEVIER INC.
230 Park Avenue, Suite 800
New York, NY 10169

Contact Person
STEPHEN R. BUSHING

Telephone (Include area code)
215-239-3688

8. Complete Mailing Address of Headquarters or General Business Office of Publisher (Not printer)

ELSEVIER INC.
230 Park Avenue, Suite 800
New York, NY 10169

9. Full Names and Complete Mailing Addresses of Publisher, Editor, and Managing Editor (Do not leave blank)

Publisher (Name and complete mailing address)

ADRIANNE BRIGIDO, ELSEVIER INC.
1600 JOHN F KENNEDY BLVD. SUITE 1800
PHILADELPHIA, PA 19103-2899

Editor (Name and complete mailing address)

STACY EASTMAN, ELSEVIER INC.
1600 JOHN F KENNEDY BLVD. SUITE 1800
PHILADELPHIA, PA 19103-2899

Managing Editor (Name and complete mailing address)

PATRICK MANLEY, ELSEVIER INC.
1600 JOHN F KENNEDY BLVD. SUITE 1800
PHILADELPHIA, PA 19103-2899

10. Owner (Do not leave blank. If the publication is owned by a corporation, give the name and address of the corporation immediately followed by the names and addresses of all stockholders owning or holding 1 percent or more of the total amount of stock. If not owned by a corporation, give the names and addresses of the individual owners. If owned by a partnership or other unincorporated firm, give its name and address as well as those of each individual owner. If the publication is published by a nonprofit organization, give its name and address.)

Full Name	Complete Mailing Address
WHOLLY OWNED SUBSIDIARY OF REED/ELSEVIER, US HOLDINGS	1600 JOHN F KENNEDY BLVD. SUITE 1800 PHILADELPHIA, PA 19103-2899

11. Known Bondholders, Mortgagees, and Other Security Holders Owning or Holding 1 Percent or More of Total Amount of Bonds, Mortgages, or Other Securities. If none, check box ► ☐ None

Full Name	Complete Mailing Address
N/A	

12. Tax Status (For completion by nonprofit organizations authorized to mail at nonprofit rates) (Check one)
The purpose, function, and nonprofit status of this organization and the exempt status for federal income tax purposes:
☒ Has Not Changed During Preceding 12 Months
☐ Has Changed During Preceding 12 Months (Publisher must submit explanation of change with this statement)

13. Publication Title

ENDOCRINOLOGY AND METABOLISM CLINICS OF NORTH AMERICA

14. Issue Date for Circulation Data Below

JUNE 2017

15. Extent and Nature of Circulation			Average No. Copies Each Issue During Preceding 12 Months	No. Copies of Single Issue Published Nearest to Filing Date
a. Total Number of Copies (Net press run)			447	341
b. Paid Circulation (By Mail and Outside the Mail)	(1)	Mailed Outside-County Paid Subscriptions Stated on PS Form 3541 (Include paid distribution above nominal rate, advertiser's proof copies, and exchange copies)	198	165
	(2)	Mailed In-County Paid Subscriptions Stated on PS Form 3541 (Include paid distribution above nominal rate, advertiser's proof copies, and exchange copies)	0	0
	(3)	Paid Distribution Outside the Mails Including Sales Through Dealers and Carriers, Street Vendors, Counter Sales, and Other Paid Distribution Outside USPS®	118	95
	(4)	Paid Distribution by Other Classes of Mail Through the USPS (e.g. First-Class Mail®)	0	0
c. Total Paid Distribution (Sum of 15b (1), (2), (3), and (4))			316	260
d. Free or Nominal Rate Distribution (By Mail and Outside the Mail)	(1)	Free or Nominal Rate Outside-County Copies included on PS Form 3541	50	81
	(2)	Free or Nominal Rate In-County Copies included on PS Form 3541	0	0
	(3)	Free or Nominal Rate Copies Mailed at Other Classes Through the USPS (e.g. First-Class Mail)	0	0
	(4)	Free or Nominal Rate Distribution Outside the Mail (Carriers or other means)	0	0
e. Total Free or Nominal Rate Distribution (Sum of 15d (1), (2), (3) and (4))			50	81
f. Total Distribution (Sum of 15c and 15e)			366	341
g. Copies not Distributed (See Instructions to Publishers #4 (page #3))			81	0
h. Total (Sum of 15f and g)			447	341
i. Percent Paid (15c divided by 15f times 100)			86.34%	76.25%

* If you are claiming electronic copies, go to line 16 on page 3. If you are not claiming electronic copies, skip to line 17 on page 3.

16. Electronic Copy Circulation		Average No. Copies Each Issue During Preceding 12 Months	No. Copies of Single Issue Published Nearest to Filing Date
a. Paid Electronic Copies	►	0	0
b. Total Paid Print Copies (Line 15c) + Paid Electronic Copies (Line 16a)	►	316	260
c. Total Print Distribution (Line 15f) + Paid Electronic Copies (Line 16a)	►	366	341
d. Percent Paid (Both Print & Electronic Copies) (16b divided by 16c × 100)	►	86.34%	76.25%

☒ I certify that 50% of all my distributed copies (electronic and print) are paid above a nominal price.

17. Publication of Statement of Ownership
☒ If the publication is a general publication, publication of this statement is required. Will be printed in the DECEMBER 2017 issue of this publication.   ☐ Publication not required.

18. Signature and Title of Editor, Publisher, Business Manager, or Owner

STEPHEN R. BUSHING - INVENTORY DISTRIBUTION CONTROL MANAGER

Date 9/18/2017

I certify that all information furnished on this form is true and complete. I understand that anyone who furnishes false or misleading information on this form or who omits material or information requested on the form may be subject to criminal sanctions (including fines and imprisonment) and/or civil sanctions (including civil penalties).

PS Form 3526, July 2014 (Page 1 of 4 (see instructions page 4))   PSN: 7530-01-000-9931   PRIVACY NOTICE: See our privacy policy on www.usps.com.

PS Form 3526, July 2014 (Page 3 of 4)   PRIVACY NOTICE: See our privacy policy on www.usps.com

Moving?

Make sure your subscription moves with you!

To notify us of your new address, find your **Clinics Account Number** (located on your mailing label above your name), and contact customer service at:

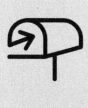

Email: journalscustomerservice-usa@elsevier.com

800-654-2452 (subscribers in the U.S. & Canada)
314-447-8871 (subscribers outside of the U.S. & Canada)

Fax number: 314-447-8029

Elsevier Health Sciences Division
Subscription Customer Service
3251 Riverport Lane
Maryland Heights, MO 63043

*To ensure uninterrupted delivery of your subscription, please notify us at least 4 weeks in advance of move.

Printed and bound by CPI Group (UK) Ltd, Croydon, CR0 4YY

08/05/2025

01864703-0005